FROM LIVING DEAD TO LIVING WONDERFULLY

Michael Poteshman

Michael had it all: wife, kids, friends, house, cars... but as he sat despondent in a far corner of his home, too miserable to enjoy any of it, life seemed irrelevant. By the age of 49, his health problems were out of control. His doctors' advice amounted to eating low-fat or fat-free foods, exercising, and taking prescription drugs. Although he followed this advice, Michael's health continued to decline, and his anxiety became more persistent.

If this sounds familiar, there are millions like you and him. Guess what? **It is NOT entirely your fault; there are extenuating circumstances causing your body to misbehave, even though you've been trying to be healthy. It is not entirely your fault that you're gaining weight and having food cravings, and it is not entirely true that some of these problems are age related.** Michael had serious health problems in the past, and now, at the age of 53, he looks and feels better than in his thirties. He has no food cravings, no brain fog, and he's not taking any medication. He now weighs less than he did in high school.

From Living Dead to Living Wonderfully is the story of one man's journey from a Living Dead existence of declining health, being overweight, having high blood pressure, high cholesterol, acid reflux, excruciating headaches, and anxiety, to transforming his life and the lives of many around him into picture of health, and ultimately Living Wonderfully!

This book chronicles the common health crisis that affects significant numbers of people today, and demonstrates easy, step-by-step techniques to reverse years of health decline. The "Living Wonderfully" system has been applied repeatedly and successfully. <u>**All is done without medications or prohibitive dieting**</u>.

Are you ready for the journey to Living Wonderfully?

REAL RESULTS FROM REAL PEOPLE WHOSE LIFE WAS TRANSFORMED AFTER EXPERIENCING THE LIVING WONDERFULLY LIFESTYLE

Name: Anatoly, M.
Age: 40
Ailments: High blood pressure, kidney stones, trouble sleeping, snoring, obesity
*Living Wonderfully Outcomes:

- Blood pressure normalized within two weeks
- PH Level stays at the prescribed level; no longer experiences pain or symptoms associated with kidney stones. PH level normalized within four weeks
- Snoring stopped gradually over the course of two months
- Went from waist size 42 to 28
- Total weight loss 95 lbs. (43 kg.) within 120 days
- No longer taking any medications

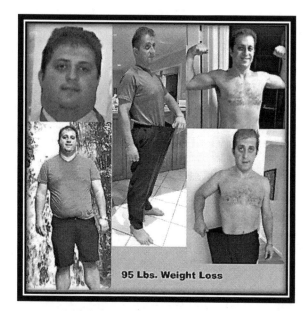

95 Lbs. Weight Loss

Name: Karina, P.
Age: 48
Ailments: Obesity, insomnia, anxiety, persistent coughing at night, chronic postnasal drip
*Living Wonderfully Outcomes:

- Insomnia went away within two weeks; sleep pattern fully restored
- Anxiety went away within one month
- Night coughs stopped within one month
- Postnasal drip stopped within two weeks
- Total weight loss 60 lbs. (27 kg.) within five months

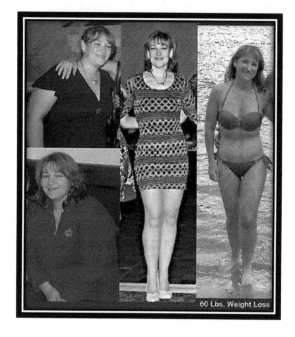

60 Lbs. Weight Loss

Name: Slava, S.
Age: 50
Ailments: High blood pressure, high cholesterol, heart disease, allergies, obesity, acid reflux, stomach ulcers, insomnia, anxiety, migraine headaches, and chronic headaches

*Living Wonderfully Outcomes:

- Blood pressure normalized within eight to ten weeks
- Acid reflux symptoms went away within three weeks
- Stomach ulcers healed within one month
- Cholesterol numbers normalized within two month
- Allergy symptoms went away within two weeks
- Sleep pattern restored within two months
- Anxiety symptoms subsided within two months, and completely went away within three month
- Migraine headaches went away within one week
- Chronic headaches went away within one week
- Weight loss: 30 lbs. within two months; the rest in additional four months. Total weight loss of 40 lbs. (18 kg.) within six months
- No longer taking any medications

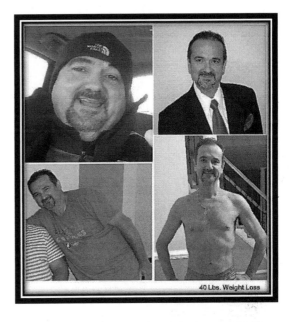

40 Lbs. Weight Loss

Name: Michael, P.
Age: 53
Ailments: High blood pressure, high cholesterol, allergies, heart disease, obesity, acid reflux, pre diabetes, insomnia, anxiety

*Living Wonderfully Outcomes:

- Blood pressure fully normalized within one month
- Acid reflux symptoms went away within three days
- Cholesterol normalized in less than a month
- Allergy symptoms went away within two weeks
- Sleep pattern restored within two weeks
- Blood sugar normalized within two weeks
- Anxiety symptoms subsided within one week, and completely went away within one month
- Total weight loss 60+ lbs. (27 kg.) within 120 days
- No longer taking any medications

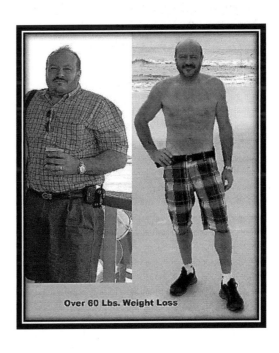

Over 60 Lbs. Weight Loss

Name: Alex, C.

Age: 47

Ailments: Acid reflux, trouble sleeping, obesity, gout

***Living Wonderfully Outcomes:**

- Acid reflux symptoms went away within three weeks
- Gout symptoms have not reoccurred
- Sleep pattern restored within one month
- Weight loss: 40 lbs. in 90 days, and 15 lbs. in additional 30 days. Total weight loss of 55 lbs. (25 kg.) within 120 days
- No longer taking any medications

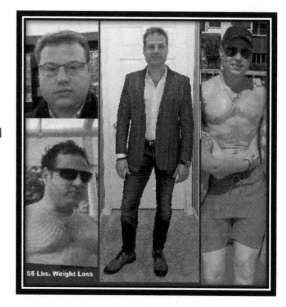

Name: John, A.

Age: 24

Ailments: Frequent physical and mental fatigue, acne, excess weight

***Living Wonderfully Outcomes:**

- Physical fatigue went away within two days
- Mental fatigue diminished within one week
- Acne cleared within two weeks
- Improved cognition (clear thinking) and mental fitness
- Vast increase in strength, specifically geared toward explosiveness in MMA (Mixed Martial Arts)
- Retention of energy - working day job and then training in MMA at night with energy to spare
- Easy to keep weight off
- Total weight loss 20 lbs. (9 kg.) within 60 days

…And many more stories of Living Wonderfully successes!

*Results may vary from person to person, as all of us are unique

ISBN-13: 978-1-7320728-0-0 (Living Wonderfully, LLC)
ISBN-10: 1-7320728-0-9

For more information:
http://livingwonderfully.org

Edited by: Carolyn Hunger
Illustrations by: Kevin Aguillon and Michael Poteshman
Contributions by: Karina Poteshman, Allan Poteshman, George Poteshman, Leonard Kazanov, MD, FAAEM, and Anatoly Mendelson

Disclaimer

Although the information in this book was obtained through credible sources and/or documented studies, the author is not a medical doctor. As such, the author and/or publisher cannot assume any medical responsibility for any information as it relates to any and all material in this book. Before attempting to perform any of the procedures, ingest any vitamins and/or supplements, eat any foods, perform any exercise(s), or perform any activities whether diet related or otherwise that are described in this book, readers are advised to consult with a competent medical professional. While the author and/or publisher made every effort to include credible internet links or sources for studies and articles, the author and/or publisher do not assume any responsibility or liability for errors, omissions, change or full or partial removal of content, or change of web addresses for any third-party websites, medical and/or research papers, studies, and/or publications, as the author has no control over such changes and/or content.

Here' what people say about this book:

"This was definitely an eye opener! Michael Poteshman did a fabulous job on this book! He blew me away with all the information he included on the topic of toxic foods, something that I had no idea that my entire family was ingesting almost daily. Dairy, among the rest of the chapters were equally as eye opening. The interesting phenomenon took place when my husband began to have sound sleep, and started waking up refreshed only two days after he read the chapters on sleep and Insulin. This is a necessary read for anyone wanting to learn more about cutting out toxic foods and overall health and wellness. I highly recommend it!"
Rena Madatova , RN

"This is a phenomenal work. The author in a careful and systematic way lays out the argument as to why, what, and how we eat impacts us so greatly. More often than not, in a negative way.
The Chapters are organized in such a way that a personal story that starts with despair and desperation draws the reader in deeply. It was difficult for me to put this book down.
The multitude of nutritional concepts are then presented in such a way as to be completely understandable.
Are some of the points presented highly controversial? Yes. Do they still make perfect sense? Yes. Do you still need to consult your physician for ongoing health needs? Absolutely.
But reading this book will fundamentally transform your life as it has mine. I personally lost nearly 50 pounds. My blood pressure significantly improved. I became more energetic. And most importantly, and to those that care to listen, I share my story of success.
If for nothing else after you read this book and even should you choose to ignore all that is presented, it will make you wiser as to what you put in your body.
I highly recommended it."
Leonard Kazanov, MD, FAAEM

"Wow! What a kick in the groin, so to speak! Michael Poteshman opens readers' eyes as they have never been opened! This is a definite boost for anyone who wants to preserve or improve their health for the rest of their lives, detoxify the natural way, and easily lose weight without prohibitive diets or special diet pills. This book is excellent for those who want to streamline their exercise routine with proper nutrition and without the use of toxic chemicals! It is hard to believe that this information is not more widespread. Thank you for bringing this "Living Wonderfully" concept full circle!"
Stephen Smith, CPT, SNS, U.S. Army Veteran

"By nature, I'm a cynic, and was quite distrustful when I heard through a friend about Michael's Living Wonderfully program. I was also aware that Michael helped many people with his lifestyle routine. No matter, my distrust stemmed from being on many different diet programs, diet regiments, and other diet related tactics in the past; none of which worked long term. Furthermore, I was taking blood pressure and kidney stones medications. Unfortunately, despite my past dieting adventures the dosages of these medications have not been reduced, as I continued to suffer from the same ailments despite such adventures of erratic weight loss and almost immediate weight gain.

All of the dieting insanity came to a complete stop when I was introduced to an extremely logical Living Wonderfully lifestyle. I was one of the privileged few who read Michael Poteshman's book in manuscript. The entire crux of his book is to improve or restore health, and all the other benefits including weight loss will follow.

To make a long story short, I'm off all prescription and over the counter medications. As a result of the improved health, I lost 95 Lbs., something that I could not have dreamed of in the past. I went from size 42 pants to size 28. Sounds astounding? Not really, because it makes perfect sense. Your body has no other alternative but to get healthy and get rid of unnecessary weight and other ailments, and not the other way around, as methodically described in the book. As Michael put it, I also live this dream of health, every single day, and loving every minute of it through improved energy, stamina, and zest for life!

I strongly recommend this book to anyone who wants to improve their health and as a wonderful side effect, lose couple, or many of unneeded pounds, as I have."

Anatoly Mendelson, EPBU CTO at ActionNet, Inc.

"A truly well researched book without any gimmicks or salesmanship! This writing has not only been helpful to me, but I've been using it consistently as a reference with my clients. Michael Poteshman was very direct in presenting evidence in a very forthright manner. He deciphered medical jargon and other terminology in order to make this an easy read. Furthermore, the concepts that he presents yield easily achievable, and most importantly, solid results in weight loss and wellness. I highly recommend it."

Fernando Huber, General Manager, Gold's Gym, CPT

"As a competitive MMA (Mixed Martial Arts) fighter I could not believe that my well established eating pattern was not only ruining my performance in the ring, but also my mental fitness. That completely changed when I joined the Living Wonderfully lifestyle! Wow, what a change! After following Michael's program, my energy went through the roof, especially working a day job and then training in MMA at night, with energy to spare.

On the second day after starting the program I woke up energized, as if I had three cups of coffee, but I didn't have any. Not only that, but my thought process became clearer. Besides losing 20 lbs., the most incredible improvements were in cardio fitness, as well as vast increase in strength, specifically geared towards explosiveness.

Thank you Michael for introducing me to this incredible Living Wonderfully system which is now a HUGE part of my life!"

John Amos, Retired U.S. Army, Competitive Mixed Martial Arts fighter

I dedicate this writing to my wife, my "Rock", who has stuck with me through thick and thin, when anyone else would have given up. It is her efforts and her push towards getting me out of the "Living Dead" existence that changed not only my life, but the life of my entire family, friends, and many others who have read and will read this writing.

I love you!

TABLE OF CONTENTS

ACKNOWLEDGEMENTS

I was frustrated when I began to compose this acknowledgement page, as it was overwhelming to name every person who has influenced me and provided moral support and encouragement while writing this book. I will concentrate on the people who directly helped to bring this book to life.

First and foremost, I would like to thank my wife, Karina, who has been my inspiration at every step, and the main reason for the existence of this book. I thank my son, Allan, for reading multiple iterations over the past three years. He declared that he can now recite the entire manuscript from memory. I am also grateful to my son, George, for reviewing my work from the perspective of a pre-med student, and for his significant contribution to Alcohol chapter.

I thank Dr. Leonard Kazanov, MD, FAAEM, for reading my work, even while on vacation with his family. His contributions from a medical perspective are greatly appreciated.

The manuscript was edited by Carolyn Hunger. I am grateful for her excellent and thorough work reviewing grammar, word usage, and flow, especially considering the volume of material reviewed.

I am thankful for the contributions of a very talented artist, Kevin Aguillon. His drawings represented both the context and the appropriate tone of each section or chapter.

My deep appreciation goes out to Anatoly Mendelson, the biggest success story of the Living Wonderfully lifestyle so far, for his specific recommendations on several chapters.

I'm grateful to Adelina Mititelu for giving this book a thorough read through, and providing a perspective that hits upon the needs of young women and millennials.

Lastly, a very special note of thanks to all the hard working librarians throughout counties in Maryland, as well as Washington, DC. Their assistance was invaluable in ordering books, retrieving, and in many cases, locating and pulling the scientific articles and studies that were used extensively to bring this book forward.

PREFACE – UNDERSTANDING THE MEANING BEHIND THIS BOOK

The end of life is inevitable! As living beings, we're susceptible to a common denominator: mortality. No matter what our ambitions, our dreams, our accomplishments and our successes, whether derived from wealth or fame, we will eventually be equalized by the inevitable final outcome of death. So, what is left? Money? Power? Unless we possess immense influences, one hundred years from now, no one will remember what type of car we drove, or the type of house we lived in. What we have left after we're gone are our deeds and memories that will live on in people that we affected during our lifetime. Those who have been affected in a positive way by our deeds will inevitably remember, continue to pass on our advice, and continue to guide others to a better and easier path in life.

I fervently believe that this is my calling, as without the help of doctors who were just treating symptoms and not the root cause of the problem, or diet gurus who sell only a temporary fix, I overcame serious health adversities. That I am alive and able to write this today is in and of itself a miracle!

I strongly believe that if I didn't conquer these adversities in time, I would now be dead and this book would never have taken place. Thus, if I can save or prolong lives of many in a similar condition, or on their way to similar health predicaments to those that I experienced, my life will take on a more significant meaning.

This book came to be as a result of my struggles with health, and the ensuing suffering of my family, specifically my wife. She endured sadness and constant worry as a consequence of my inability to cope with life's daily toils. She always suspected that doctors were trying to sustain my condition by covering up symptoms rather than addressing the root cause of the problem. As will be illustrated later in the book, she was unequivocally correct in her suspicions.

By the age of 49 my health problems were out of control; I was literally dying. Doctors' visits only offered more drugs or higher doses of the already prescribed medical cocktail for my astronomically high blood pressure, elevated cholesterol, acid reflux, excruciating headaches, and anxiety. When I was 38, my cardiologist told me, "We'll do our best to keep you alive for as long as we can." How's that for a death sentence? My doctors' "cure" amounted to eating low-fat or fat-free foods, doing exercise, and taking prescription drugs. Although I followed my doctors' advice, my health continued to decline and my anxiety became more persistent. Looking at the past 15 years, I was the "profit center" not only for different doctors, but for the pharmaceutical industry. I was on several toxic medications that manifested themselves into other symptoms where additional liver-toxic medications were prescribed to treat the side effects of the initially prescribed drugs.

If this sounds familiar, there are millions like you and me. Therefore, the first order of the day is to understand how you got to the shape that you're currently in. Guess what? **It's NOT entirely** your fault; there are extenuating circumstances causing your body to misbehave, even though you've been healthy for as long as you can remember. **It is not entirely your fault that you're having food cravings**, and **it is not entirely true that some of these problems are age related.** I had serious health problems in the past, and at the age of 53, I look and feel better than in my thirties. I have no food cravings, no brain fog, and I'm **not** taking any medication!

Please don't think of me as an anti-medicine nut. There are many circumstances where modern medicine is crucial, especially in cases of trauma. But when it came to my condition, <u>medicine was part of the problem</u>.

Doctors' advice and a slew of prescription medications did not make me feel better, but only exacerbated my already declining condition. My health only began to turn around when I learned everything I possibly could about flavor enhancers and chemicals in food and beverages that were poisoning my body.

Consequently, after 15 years of suffering, **I'm completely off <u>all medications</u>; both prescription and over the counter**, and Living Wonderfully as the title of this book affirms! Some may say it is impossible, and some may even say that it is miraculous, and this is only an isolated incident. I say that it is not just easy, but this lifestyle is extremely simple to maintain.

Together we will attempt to ease, or in some cases overcome the illnesses and health problems that you may be experiencing, as I have conquered mine. Even if you are not on prescription medications, and just want to drop some pounds, this is the book for you. The information encompassed in this writing may serve as a preventative to a lot of diseases.

The whole point of this book is not to "Live Dead" or have a marginally acceptable existence, but to live a full and fulfilling life. In other words, "Living Wonderfully" isn't a food-only proposition, but your state of mind will play a major role in your transformation. Together, we will be tuning up your emotional state, as you will experience how every piece of the "Living Wonderfully" puzzle fits together. As this puzzle is uncovered, the unexpected turnaround of years of health decline is imminent!

The chapter overview, which follows, will give you a glimpse into the rest of the story of how I went from Living Dead to Living Wonderfully. You can do it too.

CHAPTER OVERVIEW

I will address critical evidence in a provocative chapter titled "MEDICINE IS MY FRIEND – MEDICINE IS MY FOE", as well as "IN PRIVATE NIGHTMARE", and "LIGHT AT THE END OF THE TUNNEL" chapters where we will examine medical treatment of chronic diseases from a sobering perspective. As to the question "IS REVERSAL OF HEART DISEASE POSSIBLE?", this chapter will demonstrate that despite my doctors' advice, heart disease can actually be stopped dead in its tracks, and in most cases, completely reversed.

In the controversial "DAIRY" chapter I describe why I would never touch dairy products or feed them to my kids… And yes, I will answer the probiotic question as it relates to yogurt in one of the most important chapters of the book, "THE TWO BRAINS PHENOMENON OR GUT HEALTH."

In the "HYDROGENATED OIL" chapter, you will learn that run of the mill peanut butter contains an ingredient that causes a slew of health problems, including cancer.

How would you like to eat artificially colored fresh fish? How about colorful foods that are a suspect in making your kids hyperactive? It's coming up in the "SYNTHETIC FOOD DYES" chapter.

In the "ENHANCED MEAT" chapter, you will learn about chemicals that are being added to your raw meat and how to avoid them.

The "ARSENIC" chapter will illustrate a poison that's added to pork, poultry, and is also present in drinking water.

We will be uncovering the "STEROID HORMONES FOR CATTLE AND SHEEP", as well as "ANTIBIOTICS" across almost all animal species that we consume.

The "WHEAT" chapter may stir controversy as it reveals the toxicity and addiction that originate from this seemingly benign grain, in addition to other undesirable "wonders."

Once you've read the "NITRATES AND NITRITES" chapter, you will be horrified to learn how this ingredient that's found in lunch meats, hot dogs, fish, and even beer, contributes to heart disease, diabetes, different types of cancer, Alzheimer's disease, and mortality.

In the "SUGAR" chapter, you will learn that eating a certain ingredient speeds up the aging process of your skin in addition to fertilizing cancer cells. I will also describe why drinking fruit juices is not exactly good for you. In fact, according to a study, orange juice and honey are not the perfect remedy for cold as we were led to believe.

There are other questionable foods and beverages that you will read about in the "FOODS TO AVOID" section. A sizable portion of the book is devoted to "UNCOVERING THE WORLD OF EXCITOTOXINS." This chapter will outline the why and how of consuming foods with MSG or Monosodium Glutamate that can be found in a lot of the processed and restaurant foods may lead to weight gain, elevated blood pressure, brain lesions, among many other frightening consequences. **We will establish that dieting may be futile for as long as you continue to consume MSG.** Furthermore, **drinking sodas with artificial sweeteners may actually contribute to weight gain**, and not what the industry has been telling us for years.

After you've read the "PROPYLENE GLYCOL" chapter, you may not look the same way at your ice cream or birthday cakes ever again.

I will also answer a question that I get all the time, "Which alcohol type is better and contains less calories?" It's coming up in the "ALCOHOL" chapter.

I rattle a lot of cages with the "SOYBEAN PRODUCTS: THE GOOD, THE BAD, AND THE UGLY" chapter where I show how unfermented soy wreaks havoc on our bodies in addition to containing substances that interfere with the absorption of different nutrients. You will also learn about soy products that are actually beneficial. In addition, I describe the dangers behind the GMO or genetically modified fruits and vegetables, and why I would never eat them myself or feed them to my family.

Besides foods that were ruining my health, equally as crucial factors were keeping me from enjoying the health I once had.

In "THE TWO BRAINS PHENOMENON OR GUT HEALTH" chapter, you will witness how your gut affects your brain, and what it has to do with your mood, sex drive and performance, learning abilities, cardiovascular system, muscles, and even social behavior. I will also show how to improve gut health without medications.

We will uncover that normalizing your sleep pattern is much easier than you may have thought in the "SLEEP, WEIGHT GAIN OR WEIGHT LOSS" chapter.

What about fats and cholesterol? Are they good or bad for you? Even though my doctor was keeping me on a low-fat, cholesterol-free diet, the answer in "LOW-FAT-FAT-FREE MYTH" chapter may surprise you.

The "DIETS-SHMIETS: DO THEY REALLY WORK? ANY OF THEM?" chapter will show why conventional diets may exacerbate your weight gain in the long run.

In the "DETOX-WHY AND HOW?" section I will share the easy and enjoyable ways to not only detoxify your body naturally, but your mind as well. The "FOOD DETOX AND RESULTING WEIGHT LOSS" chapter will outline how to detox and drop some pounds by eating foods that will be a part of your daily "Living Wonderfully" routine.

Because this book encompasses almost every aspect of health-wellness, the "YOUR STATE OF MIND" chapter will demonstrate how to observe and get rid of unrelenting thoughts and perform a very easy mind cleansing exercise.

The "VITAMINS AND MINERALS-FACT OR FICTION" chapter will demonstrate the best way to deliver Vitamins and minerals into your body despite what conventional wisdom has been telling us for decades.

"INSULIN-THE MOST POWERFUL COMMON DENOMINATOR" chapter shows how Insulin may affect your health in a negative or positive way, and what to do in order to normalize the production of this key hormone that's at the center of our existence.

Hunger levels will be introduced in the "EATING TO LIVE" chapter where we will attempt to modify and fine-tune our incorrectly learned eating habits.

Finally, in the "GOLDEN RULES TO EATING WONDERFULLY" section we will look at the aspect of cooked food that may shock you. We will uncover what our everyday cooked foods have to do with overburdening the immune system. You will also witness the **unconditional and delicious way of eating that will provide benefits for the rest of your life that you never thought possible to achieve**. Everything that's described in this section is available at your local supermarket and/or farmer's market without the need for wasting money on dietary products or prepared foods.

The "PORTION SIZE, PORTION CONTROL, DESSERTS, COFFEE, AND SNACKING" chapter will uncover that having a full stomach is not taboo. My wife weighs 125 Lbs. (57 kg.) and eats as much food as I do, as our food portions are huge. We will also discuss why drinking coffee may not do any favors for your waistline.

"EATING WONDERFULLY ON THE GO" may simplify your life, as I describe what to look for when bringing your own lunch to work or occasionally ordering at a restaurant. Difficult food scenarios will also be discussed, as from time to time we may have no other alternative but to comply with unavoidable menus or an overbearing boss.

The "SHOPPING LIST" chapter will summarize what to look for when purchasing vegetables and safer animal products.

The last chapter of the book consists of "LIVING WONDERFULLY RECIPES" that are not only delicious and easy to prepare, but jam-packed with nutrients.

WHY TAKE MY ADVICE?

So, who died and made me the authority on nutrition, wellness, and happiness? No one died. In fact, several people who first read this book in manuscript actually improved or restored their health. So, why should you take my word for what's written in this book?

First, my background and training is not only based on computer science, project management, IT implementation, and business analysis, but I am also wellness certified (CWC or Certified Wellness Coach). My experience as a president and vice president in large and small corporations has taught me to focus on hard data and rational numbers, not trends and pop-culture. I base decisions on empirical evidence after thorough investigation and comparison. Thus, I do not have any preconceived notions from any institutions that promote industry standards and typical medical practices, because no one from the medical community has been able to get to the root of my progressively worsening health problems.

I recovered from decades of suffering only after I conducted my own in-depth independent research into the "wonders" of the modern Western diet and treatment methods to cure my progressively deteriorating condition of hypertension, elevated blood sugar, high cholesterol, acid reflux, and anxiety. **What I have is hard and indisputable evidence and, most importantly, mind-blowing results!**

My "Living Wonderfully" system has been applied repeatedly and successfully. One of my many success stories involves a physician whose life was fundamentally transformed, as he was able to significantly improve his blood pressure, and lost nearly 50 lbs. (23 kg.). His powerful testimony at the beginning of the book pays homage to his transformation.

HOW TO READ THIS BOOK

This entire writing was driven by a single event that my wife uncovered, snowballing into extensive research that changed my life as well as the life of my family, friends, and even total strangers with whom I shared the manuscript.

Although some people insisted that I title this book as an "Encyclopedia for Living Wonderfully", I believe the word "Encyclopedia" would somewhat overstate the content. Instead, it is a compilation of real life noteworthy subjects that will simplify your journey to Living Wonderfully. After you've read this book, you will be in possession of crucial tools to assist in influencing the course of the inevitable – mortality, by uncovering the dangers that have been hidden from all of us up until now. As such, this book is organized chronologically into six sections with their respective chapters:

1. THE JOURNEY INTO HEALTH DESTRUCTION
   CHAPTER 1
2. MONOSODIUM GLUTAMATE AND OTHER TOXIC WONDERS
   CHAPTER 2 - 3
3. WHAT NOT TO EAT? FOODS TO AVOID
   CHAPTERS 4 – 16
4. UNCOVERING MYTHS AND WIDELY DISTRIBUTED UNTRUTHS ABOUT FAT, DIETS, MEDICINE, VITAMINS, GUT HEALTH, REVERSAL OF HEART DISEASE, SLEEP, INSULIN, AND HOW TO EAT TO LIVE
   CHAPTERS 17 – 25
5. DETOX – WHY AND HOW?
   CHAPTERS 26 – 29

6. GOLDEN RULES TO EATING WONDERFULLY FOR LIFE
   CHAPTERS 30 – 36

Because this book conveys extensive detail into revitalization of health, I don't recommend speed-reading or skipping chapters. While written in easy to understand language, every chapter is designed to serve a specific purpose that dovetails into the overall outcome – improved health. In order to achieve success for "Living Wonderfully", concentrate on each section and its respective chapters until you have achieved complete comprehension and absorption of the material. It's that important! I recommend reading no more than two chapters per day. Some of the lengthier sections and chapters may take longer:

- Section 2. - MONOSODIUM GLUTAMATE AND OTHER TOXIC "WONDERS"
- Chapter 4. "SUGAR"
- Chapter 23. "SLEEP, WEIGHT GAIN OR WEIGHT LOSS"
- Chapter 24. "INSULIN – THE MOST POWERFUL COMMON DENOMINATOR"
- Section 5. "DETOX – WHY AND HOW?"
- Section 6. "GOLDEN RULES TO EATING WONDERFULLY FOR LIFE"

I recommend book-marking sections that require additional attention, especially something that often affects you in a negative way. Thus, going back and re-reading certain bookmarked chapters may prove beneficial, as you may find a nugget of information that has eluded you during the initial reading.

If you're not completely clear on a subject, take a look at the endnotes, i.e. reference number(s) above the text. Those numbers correspond to the records in the "References" section. Please don't be afraid of glancing through the References section as it was designed to be as straightforward as possible. Although I used scientific studies to convey the information, in many cases, you will find web links that can point to additional material or even help with expanding your knowledge. **This is the primary reason that whenever possible, I used sources that are available to everyone – the Internet**, not just sources that are only available in certain libraries or are found in certain obscure publications. That way, after you've read this book, the transition to becoming your own architect of Living Wonderfully will be seamless, as you will know what to look for if you require additional knowledge on the subject of health.

Without further ado, let's begin the journey to solving the exciting puzzle to Living Wonderfully one chapter at a time. I believe that you will be thrilled with the results.

Section 1. The Journey into Health-Destruction

Chapter 1 **In Private Nightmare**

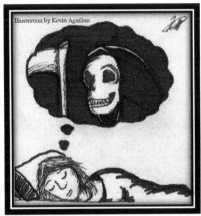

Looking back at my life, I was a Living Dead creature at the age of 48, whose life was suspended with no possibility of ever returning to normal. …And what is normal anyway? My sense of enthusiasm and craving for life became prematurely subdued as the relationships that I forged for decades with my friends and colleagues were marginalized, and at times, felt like a nuisance. I didn't care about what would happen each day, as long as I was left to my private hell, alone with my miserable thoughts of existence. Deep in my mind I understood that what I was feeling, doing, and eating was wrong, but I did not have the strength, energy, or desire to get out of this miserable place.

Recalling my life in the past few years, I welcomed this feeling of sorrow as it gave me a place to escape and actually provided a degree of absurd and illogical comfort. "Tranquility" was my favorite word as I was wallowing in my private hellish pool of misery that I regarded as my permanent and wonderfully melancholic residence. I simply stopped caring.

There are many dismal examples that I can cite where my state of mind was not only ruining my life, but the life of my entire family. One example that sticks in my mind is our family cruise vacation. I spent the entire trip lying in bed in total darkness. My wife was only successful in getting me out of the room to eat. As I didn't want to smile at anyone or even exchange pleasantries with the service staff or fellow passengers, I ate in for almost the entire cruise. I just wanted to be left alone.

My kids, on the other hand, persuaded me to go on one of the island tours. That was one of the most disturbing episodes that I have experienced, and one that I had inadvertently imparted upon my family.

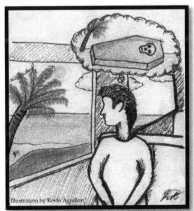

Having just had breakfast on the ship that consisted of the usual eggs, bacon, sausage, croissant, skim milk, and mixed fruit with "diet" whipped cream, I was feeling especially down. …There it was, the beautiful island of Ocho Rios, Jamaica, and here I was, looking through the window of the tour bus and despising every moment. My clouded mind had decided that the sun was too bright and the water was too tranquil, it didn't even look like the ocean; it looked like a ridiculous turquoise bathtub. According to my sarcastically gloomy assessment, this place looked more like a burial ground, which I determined would serve well if I were to just drop dead here, right this minute.

Both my kids and my wife saw that I was upset and tried to get me out of this state of mind, but I asked them not to bother me. I rationalized my unhappiness by explaining that I didn't see the logical point behind this unnecessary sightseeing exercise in the first place.

When the bus arrived at its destination, I asked my family to continue the tour without me. While they were on tour, I sat on a bench in the shade for almost two hours. I was pondering, "When my time comes, should I be buried in the sand on the beach, or just be thrown in the middle of the ocean?" In fact, both scenarios seemed quite acceptable. When my wife and kids returned, all I wanted was to go back on the ship to resume my usual lying in bed, in the darkness of the state room. So, I promptly returned to my misery, and our so-called vacation continued.

Sitting in the same room for hours, staring into space, watching television programs, and not even being able to remember what the shows were about had been my way of life for over half a decade. The salvation to this existence was predominantly fast food restaurants, and my favorite, Chinese food and Vietnamese Pho soup establishments. Afterwards, I was back in the same room, staring into space. There was not a happy thought that entered my mind even though a person in a normal state of well-being should have been delighted to be in my shoes, minus the depressing state of existence.

SICK AND SICKER

Since the age of 34, I had been on a slew of medications to control my high blood pressure, cholesterol, and acid reflux. Over the years, the doses had been substantially increasing as I was getting sicker. Several years prior to this writing, I was rushed to the hospital in an ambulance with tightness in my chest, where cardiac catheterization was performed on my heart. Cardiac catheterization is a procedure where a flexible tube is inserted through the groin, neck, or arm, and is pushed through the respective artery into the heart. It's done in order to assess whether there is an accumulation of plaque or if there is blockage in the arteries.

Several days later I had a follow-up appointment with the cardiologist who had initially ordered the catheterization procedure. He looked at the results and unequivocally told me that I would have to be on blood pressure and cholesterol medications for the rest of my life because of the blockages in my arteries. He also mentioned that because of my family history of heart attacks and strokes, I would be more likely to suffer the same fate as my mother and both of my grandmothers if I didn't adhere to the regular medical routine. My paternal grandmother died of a heart attack, and my maternal grandmother died of a stroke. My doctor advised me to stay away from fatty foods as I had progressive heart disease. Low-fat and fat-free were the foods that were recommended.

IN DESPAIR

Although I was feeling incredibly down after the doctor's grim evaluation of my overall condition and progressing health problems, my wife talked me into joining the gym "for the sake of the family." She also made certain that I stayed on a low-salt, low-fat, or fat-free diet as the doctors had instructed. I was on a strict, low-calorie regimen, going to the gym regularly, and very, very slowly losing some weight, but the blood pressure and the rest of the problems were not going away. In fact, my blood pressure had skyrocketed to new heights, and the headaches became even more profound and frequent.

After six months of going to the gym and eating "low-fat-tasteless-plastic-garbage", as I called it, I was telling my wife about how useless this entire exercise was. Although the fitness training marginally helped with the weight problem, it wasn't effective in lessening my overall condition. I continued to experience feelings of desperation and anxiety, hypertension, increased headaches, and very bad acid reflux. My sleep was completely disjointed, with an inability to sleep for more than one to two hours at a time. The routine of constantly drinking water and taking antacid medications in the middle of the night, or simply getting out of bed because it was intolerable to remain still with my eyes open, became my way of life. In addition, while out of bed at 3 or 4 o'clock in the morning, the attempt to read a book that only made partial sense became sadly acceptable. Thus, the increase of the brain fog and feeling down was the miserable reality that I had to accept.

If that weren't enough, my legs were driving me absolutely crazy during the night. It was the sensation where I had to constantly keep my legs in motion. Later on, while doing research, I found out that I had "Restless Leg Syndrome" as will be discussed in the subsequent sections. In essence, I continued to be a "Living Dead humanoid" that exercised and followed doctor's advice, but without any possibility of a normal existence.

The good news is that decades of suffering came to a screeching halt on one very significant day. In fact, it was a true turning point in my life at the age of 49. First, however, it had to get much, much worse before it could get better.

A SOMBER PRELUDE TO AN EYE OPENING

During one autumn Saturday, my wife and I went to the gym in the morning, and then shopping immediately thereafter. On the way to the mall, we stopped by my favorite Pho restaurant. Pho is a Vietnamese soup that consists of beef or chicken broth, rice noodles, meats of different varieties, and some vegetables on the side, such as bean sprouts and hot green chilies. I always believed in the soothing and satisfying effects of this huge bowl of soup, and how nourishing and wonderful it felt while I was consuming it. Now that I had finished an exhausting workout, I was visualizing how this wonderfully tasting soup would really hit the spot. My wife, not being a big fan of this particular dish, decided to have some tea instead, just to keep me company. This time, the soup was a little different. It was more delicious than usual and tasted very rich. It was clearly out of this world good. I ordered a large bowl, but it didn't feel like I had enough even though the portion that I consumed could have probably fed two people. The feeling that I can describe was something along the lines of bizarre. My stomach felt like it was extremely full, but my mouth felt tingly and actually craved more Pho. I understood that I had enough, but I ordered another small bowl of just broth because I didn't want the extra calories from rice noodles. As I was consuming broth, I experienced a peculiar sensation. My stomach felt even fuller, almost to the point of bursting and my taste buds were running amok. It felt like I needed more soup.

Luckily, cooler heads prevailed. After drinking the remaining broth, my wife and I left the restaurant while I was telling her that it was her loss for missing out on a most incredible and delicious meal. I was also telling her that I had this crazy sensation of "my mouth being hungry", as I was attributing this tingling sensation to this soup being "that good." This strange sensation was driving me crazy. I thought to myself, perhaps I needed to have a glass of diet soda to cleanse my palate. We stopped by a convenience store and picked up a 32 oz. cup of diet soda which was extremely satisfying. Unfortunately, I wasn't aware at the time that diet soda sweetened with Aspartame would contribute to wreaking havoc on my already exhausted system. After having diet soda, the tingling sensation on my tongue somewhat subsided, but gave me the usual headache and brain fog. As the day progressed, the headache partially went away.

While driving back home from the mall, I began to see shiny flat lights that resembled silver mirrors scattered around my vision range in a random pattern. I knew what was in store for me because this wasn't the first time. I immediately pulled over and asked my wife to drive because I could hardly see where I was going. As usual, this vision impairment was followed by an excruciating headache; only this time it was unbearable. The rest of the trip home was a blur.

Although I was never a big fan of headache medicine, I took two pills, but the headache did not subside. I tripled the dosage, and the headache became somewhat tolerable. Consequently, I experienced the most incredible brain fog where I couldn't put together cohesive sentences.

Once again I went to bed in a zombie-like miserable state, and as usual woke up shortly thereafter. Only this time, instead of my customary one to two hours, I slept for only 15 minutes, but it seemed like I slept through the entire night. The headache was absolutely awful, and it felt like something was pushing on my chest. The anxiety that I experienced was nearly impossible to tolerate. The persistent feeling that something terrible was going to happen in conjunction with my declining physical condition felt like the "beginning of the end." My overall state of being can only be described as complete enveloping of desperation, misery, hopelessness, and anguish. I left the bedroom, and for the rest of the night and the following morning stayed in the next room on the couch, staring into space. I couldn't even watch television because changing images were driving me insane due to shifts in colors. In addition, the persistent bright flashes of light that emanated from the screen were intolerable. It was not the first time, and I believed that it certainly wasn't the last.

At six o'clock in the morning of the following day, my wife woke up to find me in an almost catatonic state, staring at the wall. When I saw her come in, I began to cry uncontrollably. Considering that I have always been a strong person, I experienced similar emotions when I lost members of my family or a friend. This time, tears were streaming from my eyes, and I confided to my wife that I was tired and completely drained of being ill with this condition that was obviously irreversible. The doctors, unfortunately, had absolutely no idea what was happening to me, even the workouts at the gym and our nightly walks were not helping.

The sad reality was that I couldn't even go to the hospital in order to ease this pain. A similar event took place following a meal at my favorite Chinese restaurant several years prior to this one. My wife called an ambulance, and I was rushed to the hospital at 2:00 A.M. The doctors thought that this type of a headache and escalating blood pressure was due to a brain aneurism (bulging or bursting artery in the brain), so I had to undergo a spinal tap. A spinal tap is performed to determine whether or not there is blood, bacteria, or other substances present in the spinal fluid. In my case, the doctor was looking for the presence of blood. The standard procedure is the insertion of a needle between vertebrae where the spinal fluid is extracted. After numerous attempts, the doctor extracted the spinal fluid, and to my relief, no blood was present.

In order to ease my condition, I was given morphine, "to calm you down" as the nurse had put it. A few hours later, I was sent home with the advice that I needed to increase the dosage of my blood pressure medication. We'll discuss the wonders of prescription medications later, as I'm dedicating a considerable amount of time to this subject in order to open the reader's mind to this "trend."

Back to the story, but now with the promise of the light at the end of the tunnel. Before I digressed, we left off where my wife came into the room where I was crying uncontrollably. She did not need to ask me what was wrong. She already knew that I had yet another anxiety attack. This time I suffered from slurred speech, the usual awful headache, and blurry vision with shiny lights. Furthermore, I had shortness of breath to the point that I thought that my lung capacity was so diminished that I could only hold a little bit of air. I also had a runny nose, and for some reason, kept sneezing.

My wife suggested taking me to the hospital. I told her that there is no way that I would even consider going to the hospital again because the hospital staff had absolutely no idea what I had, let alone how to treat my condition. The only thing that was certain is that medical professionals at the hospital would undoubtedly dispense a dose of morphine "to calm me down."

The very mention of the hospital got me extremely irritated. I was very short with my wife, and quite agitated. Later on, through research, I learned that my reaction was something that is referred to as "MSG Rage", where out of the blue the emotions begin to flare.

I was rude and uncooperative, yet my loving wife of 25 years decided that instead of going to work, she would stay home in order to look after me, or as I later learned, she was afraid of the worst.

Chapter 2 LIGHT AT THE END OF THE TUNNEL - UNCOVERING THE WORLD OF EXCITOTOXINS

Illustration by Kevin Aguillo

As I was tormenting myself in this private nightmare, sitting in the same room for 12 hours, my wife was on her computer trying to get to the bottom of this alarming situation. Within 15 minutes of searching different websites, she began to ask me questions about my symptoms. Every question that she asked mirrored my symptoms specifically and accurately, down to my sneezing. She walked into the room and declared that she knew exactly what was happening to me for all these years. She was smiling through her tears. She stated unequivocally, "I'm more than positive that you can be fixed, and your suffering may be coming to an end sooner than you think!" I responded by telling her that there are no quick fixes to the health crisis that I experienced in the past decade. Her answer was simple, "We have overcome many obstacles together. Consider this another tough one; have faith!"

She literally took me by the hand and led me out of my "room of suffering" and set me down in front of the computer. Since my vision was partially impaired, she sat next to me and began reading out loud from the list of symptoms that paralleled mine precisely. Although she used a number of websites to assess my symptoms, the chart of "Commonly Reported Symptoms of MSG Toxicity"[1] on the next page will undoubtedly give you a glimpse into what she uncovered: the wonders of the excitotoxin known as Monosodium Glutamate or MSG.

Commonly Reported Symptoms of MSG Toxicity

Based on books by Neurosurgeon, Dr. Russell Blaylock (Excitotoxins: The Taste that Kills) and Toxicologist, Dr. George Schwartz (In Bad Taste: The MSG Symptom Complex)

Numbness or paralysis	Mouth lesions, sores
Swelling of hands, feet, face	Diarrhea
Mitral valve prolapse	Nausea
Arrhythmias or paroxysmal atrial fibrillation (which can lead to stroke)	Vomiting
Rise or drop in blood pressure (a fluctuation)	Stomach cramps and gas
Tachycardia (rapid heartbeat)	Irritable bowel, colitis, and/or constipation
Angina (pain in and around heart and ribs)	Swelling of/or painful rectum
Heart palpitations (change in heart beat, or irregularities, such as atrial fibrillation)	Spastic colon
Shuddering, shaking, chills	Extreme thirst
Tendinitis and joint pain, TMJ	Water retention and bloating (stomach swells)
Arthritic-like pain Muscle aches - legs, back, shoulders, neck	Abdominal discomfort
Flu-like symptoms	Asthma symptoms
Stiffness - jaw, muscles	Shortness of breath
Heaviness of arms, legs	Chest pain
Mental dullness	Tightness of chest
Depression	Runny nose and sneezing
Dizziness, light headedness	Postnasal drip
Disorientation, mental confusion, bi-polar	Bronchitis-like symptoms
Anxiety or panic attacks	Hoarseness, sore throat
Hyperactivity, especially in children (A.D.H.D.)	Chronic cough - sometimes a tickle cough
Attention Deficit Disorder (A.D.D.)	Gagging reflex
Behavioral problems - delinquency, rage, and hostility	Skin rash - hives, itching, rosacea-like reaction
Feelings of inebriation	Mouth lesions, small waxy bits in throat, tonsils
Slurred speech	Tingling numbness on face, ears, arms, legs, or feet
Balance problems	Flushing, tingling, burning sensation in face or chest
Aching teeth	Extreme dryness of mouth, "cotton mouth", or irritated tongue
Seizures, tremors	Dark circles or bags under eyes, face swelling
Loss of memory	Urological problems, nocturia, uncontrollable bladder or swelling of prostate
Lethargy	Difficulty focusing
Sleeping disorders - insomnia or drowsiness (chronic fatigue)	Pressure behind eyes
Migraine headaches - facial or temporal Eye symptoms - tired or burning eyes to blurry vision, optic neuritis	Seeing shiny lights
Neurological diseases: ALS, Parkinson's, M.S.	Burning sinuses, broken sinus capillaries
Prostate, infertility, thyroid problems	Gastro esophgeal reflux
Ear problems - tinnitus or Meniere's Disease	Cartilage, connective tissue damage
Gout-like condition (usually knees)	Gall bladder or gall bladder like problems
Kidney pain - Loin Pain	Hematuria Syndrome
Restless Leg Syndrome	Awareness During Sleep Paralysis (ADSP)
Mastocytosis	

Retrieved from:
Anglesey, D.L. (2011). Symptoms of MSG Toxisity Chart. Home - MSGMYTH. Retrieved from http://msgmyth.com/msg_symptoms.html
Anglesey, D. L. (2011). Battling the MSG myth: a survival guide and cookbook (Revised ed.). Kennewick, Wash.: Front Porch Productions.

Because my mind was dulled with pain, anxiety, and over-the-counter headache medicine, I couldn't fully appreciate the magnitude of what she just read. I stared at her blankly, and said that the information she discovered is inconsequential, since MSG is a flavor enhancer that is used in many foods to wake up flavors. I pointed out, "If it were so bad and dangerous, it would be banned." She smiled at me and said, "I'm not done yet; there is more."

She clicked another tab on the computer screen and indeed, there was more; a lot more! It was the feedback about my favorite Pho restaurant where only the day before I enjoyed the most wonderfully delicious meal. After she read some of the reviews, even my cloudy mind was able to put two and two together. I still couldn't believe that ingesting MSG could wreak such havoc on my system. The reasoning behind my disbelief of solid facts was simple. I never had any limitation of what I ate in the past and where I ate it, especially something as benign as soup. But after she read the reviews, it began to sink in.

Below are a few quotes from some of the past restaurant customers. These quotes were taken from the Yelp website.

"…One day while eating my Pho a delivery person wheeled in a huge sack of MSG on a hand truck! It was like a big sack of rice but was MSG. I saw that and it clicked, so that's the problem. The problem is that they use too much MSG!!!! An outrageous amount of MSG!…" [2],[a]

The customer feedback above was not the only MSG reference. Here are some snippets from other reviews in order not to burden readers with having to read different responses in their entirety:

- "…I recognize their use of MSG and there is A LOT! You know that tingle you get in your mouth with that slightly sweet flavor followed by anxiety when your finished eating? Congratulations, you now know how to recognize MSG…"[3]
- "…Be prepared to drink a lot of water after a meal here! Loads of MSG…"[4]
- "Soup tastes like MSG." "I suspect there might be too much MSG! (I actually was paying extra close attention to my mental state afterward to see if there were any major mood changes or altered states.) "[5]
- "I thought it was yummy until an hour later when I got very thirsty - there must be some MSG in the pho!"[6]
- "MSG. I was wondering why we felt the need to drink so much water when we were eating their pho. I later learned from other Yelp reviews that the reason we were always so thirsty is because they *load* it up with MSG; they go crazy with it."[7]
- "…saucy MSG-filled (my dad says crack-filled) goodness?" [8]
- "…they poured a ton of MSG into this dish because I keep on downing water the whole day."[9]

I have to be as fair as I possibly can, as there was also excellent feedback. I can attest to that, as the soup was truly delicious; but now we know why.

After my wife finished reading the information that pertained to this substance, she said that our entire family had to abstain from restaurant food until we experienced positive changes in health. That meant that we also had to abstain from all processed foods. I told her that I don't believe in these fairy tales because millions of people eat "this stuff" and nothing happens to them (yes, I was in denial). To which she replied, "What have you got to lose? If it doesn't work, we can always go back to our old way of eating "junk." Just give it one month out of your life, please? If not for yourself, just do it for your family!"

---

[a] Before publishing this book, I searched for the link to the negative review of the MSG being wheeled on the hand truck, but it was removed. The rest of the links were active at the time.

Although I was not in a cooperative state of mind, I reluctantly succumbed to the notion that there was enough logic in what my wife was telling me. As the information she found was backed by tangible evidence, and many pages of credible research, I was willing to go along with her wishes. And so it began, slowly, although I continued to be in denial, until I began to see irrefutable and fantastic results.

IN DENIAL

Although this section is only partially related to MSG, it has almost everything to do with getting out of the "Living Dead" existence. Hence, this short section not only applies to this chapter, but to the entire book.

> "…denial is a defense mechanism in which a person, faced with a painful fact, rejects the reality of that fact. They will insist that the fact is not true despite what may be overwhelming and irrefutable evidence."
> (Juan, 2006)[10]

Even though I told my wife that I would give up foods that were loaded with MSG, I was in complete denial. How could any food that tastes that good be so bad for you? My unsophisticated excuse has always been the same. Food companies are using government approved MSG to make food taste better. I believed that people who publish the anti-additive articles had nothing better to do but cause alarm without any basis. I felt that these are busybodies who want to create panic.

As you can tell, I was very definitive in my denial. In the past, if anyone started a discussion about food chemicals, preservatives, or artificial sweeteners, I dismissed them outright. I guess I wasn't sick enough to really grasp what these chemicals were capable of doing to a human body. I believed that if any substance was government approved, it meant that it was safe. Unfortunately, in order to get through my thick analytical skull, I had to reach a point in my life where there were no other choices. All of the alternatives have been already exhausted. The low-fat foods, regular visits to my doctors, slew of medications, and even exercise did not work, hence my repudiation of clear facts.

Long before my wife pointed out the direct correlation between my symptoms and my diet, I actually was somewhat familiar with the detrimental effects of MSG and other food additives and flavor enhancers. Only five years prior to this writing, a colleague who was into health and wellness shared several articles and even studies on excitotoxins. When I got an article in an email, I read it and completely dismissed it, as millions of Americans do. But because I promised my wife and my kids that I would abstain from processed and restaurant foods, as well as diet beverages with Aspartame, I began to search for this "old" communication. To my surprise, it was in my email Sent folder where I shared it with my wife almost five years earlier. It should have been an eye-opening and educational read, but at the time seemed completely insignificant.

In hindsight, how much heartache, nerves, devastation, and sleepless nights could have been saved if we only accepted even a small portion of information that my colleague was trying to share with us? But we were in denial, especially yours truly.

The reason that I'm telling you all this is that I completely understand that I'm not the only one who's been in denial. There are many more of us who are set in old, familiar, and even contented ways. It is a mechanism that gives us a degree of comfort. Until we kick the denial habit, we will be <u>unable</u> to overcome our health adversities. I'm certain that you are familiar with the concept that old habits, whether good or bad, are very hard to break. We all have them, and we all hold onto them like old comfortable shoes, for as long as we can. Before I started "Living Wonderfully", I was in complete denial because I love food, especially processed food, because of its taste. I was making excuse after excuse, including <u>lying to myself</u> as my health was deteriorating.

"When a person is in denial, they engage in distractive or escapist strategies to reduce stress and help them cope."
(Juan, 2006)[11]

I'm no longer in denial! I'm "Living Wonderfully!" I will let the pictures below speak for themselves:

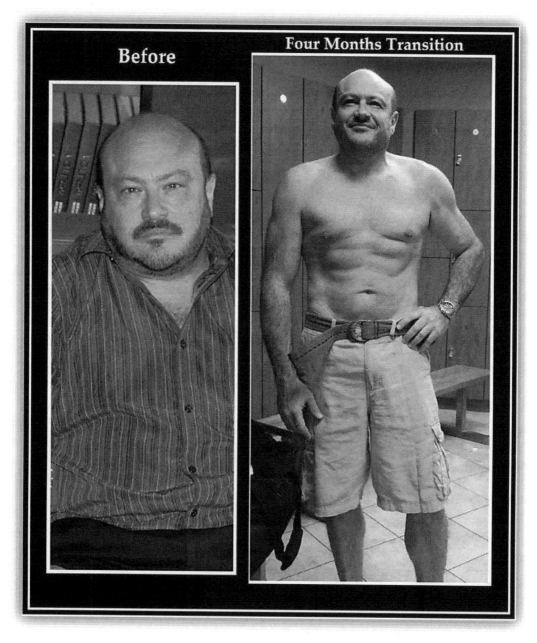

Believe it or not the sad guy in the photo on the previous page on the left, was celebrating his 24th wedding anniversary at a restaurant. At the time I thought that this particular celebration was my last, but as you can tell by the picture on the right, there will be many, many more!

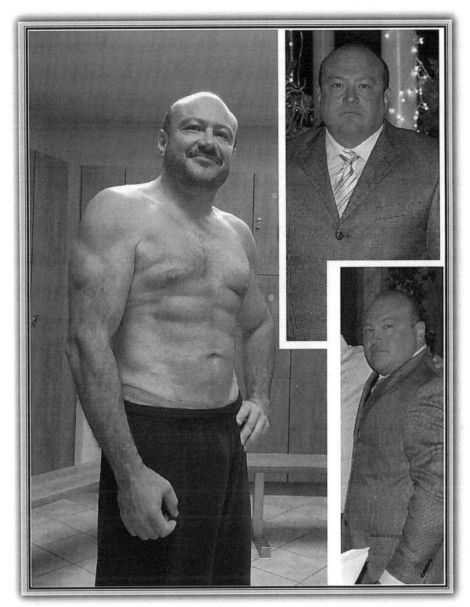

When I show the above comparison to people, I always get feedback such as, "The guy on the right looks old." The photos on the right were taken during my 20th wedding anniversary; I was 44 years of age as compared to 50 years of age on the left. That same photo was featured in the Gold's Gym's Fittest Fathers contest where I was nominated and won their 50th Anniversary competition. That's right, I went from being almost dead for two decades to becoming one of the 50 fittest fathers. I'm done with being unhappy and in denial!

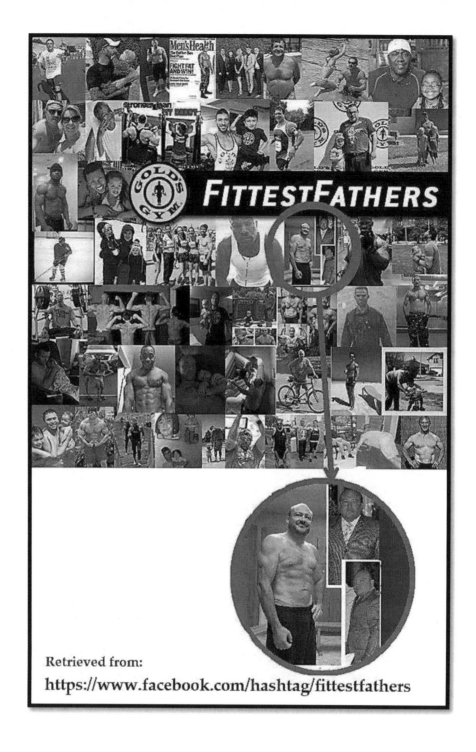

Finally, my wife was so proud of my accomplishments that she asked me for a selfie for her cell phone. Well, here it is – I am 53, three years after I began my journey. My weight stayed off, my mood renewed, because every day is a happier day. As you can see on the photograph on the next page, I'm Living Wonderfully and enjoying every minute of it!

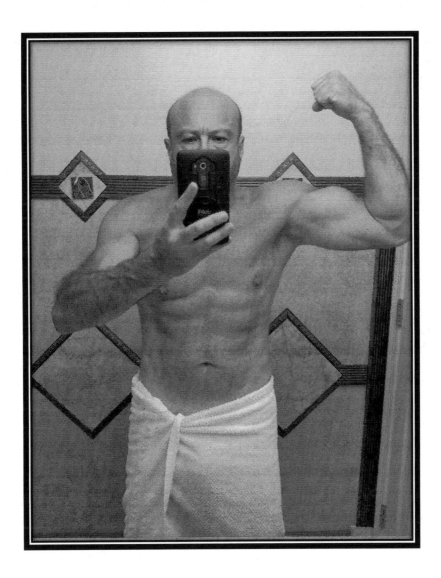

I'm aware that some of the things that I will be talking about in this book may sound peculiar to some people. I know firsthand, as it sounded strange to me as I was gathering vital material to improve my life. I also thought that foods and some of the procedures that allowed the body to purge decades of toxins were completely weird. These were new concepts and philosophies that I never heard of or experienced, or would have subscribed to at any time. That was only one year prior to this writing.

The bottom line is that it all works, not only well, but in the **life-saving** way! **I'm a believer because I live it every single day, and the results are nothing short of miraculous! As such, the word denial is no longer in my vocabulary.**

Keeping all of this in mind, **I ask of you to set aside any preconceived notions about foods and beverages (diet sodas especially), doctors, pharmaceuticals, food additives, preservatives, hearsay or learned activities related to wellness for the remainder of this book.** I believe that you will be very pleased with the outcome. Together we will uncover the mystery of "Living Wonderfully" one piece at a time. But before we delve into uncovering this awesomely wonderful mystery, we need to get some definitions out of the way.

IMPORTANT DEFINITIONS

I didn't introduce the definition of the word "excitotoxin" at the beginning of this chapter, as I didn't want to turn this book into a scientific lecture from the get go. Now that you have been with me for a little while, it is very important to outline this definition.

"Excitotoxin: a substance added to foods and beverages that literally stimulates neurons to death, causing brain damage of varying degrees. Can be found in such ingredients as Monosodium Glutamate (MSG), Aspartame (NutraSweet®), cysteine, hydrolyzed protein, and aspartic acid."
(Blaylock, 1998)[12]

If you decide to drink diet soda that contains Aspartame, which I drank in obscene amounts in the past, or put your favorite ranch dressing on your salad, more likely than not, you are ingesting excitotoxins. Here's what happens to your brain. Your food tastes terrific because the excitotoxin substance fools your brain into thinking that a particular "almost food" is actually worthy of ingesting. In other words, MSG greatly improves the taste of food[13] that otherwise may taste mediocre. You generate almost an "aaahhh" sensation of satisfaction. As a result, your brain cells become exceedingly excited to the point that they are overburdened with excitement before their demise only a few hours after the ingestion of these excitotoxins.[14] Board Certified Neurosurgeon, Dr. Russell Blaylock, who has conducted research on excitotoxins, said it best:

"When neurons are exposed to these substances, they become very excited and fire their impulses very rapidly until they reach a state of 'extreme exhaustion'. Several hours later these neurons suddenly die as if the cells were excited to death."
(Blaylock, 2012)[15]

Perhaps you have already noticed that I've been using the term "almost food." I use this term because I cannot consciously call certain products that are manufactured for human consumption, "food." "Almost food" is my facetious characterization of foods that may be detrimental to health or should not be consumed; period!

Now that you have insight into what excitotoxins represent, please keep this definition in the back of your mind. In the next few sections you will learn various side effects that may rear their ugly heads as a result of consuming some of the most delicious "almost foods" that are spiked with so-called flavor enhancers or excitotoxins. For starters, let's look at why a majority of people are gaining weight even though they're on a permanent diet as I used to be.

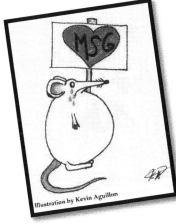

Illustration by Kevin Aguillon

Have you ever seen a fat mouse or a rat? I certainly haven't, as mice and rats are typically not overweight in nature unless they are fed MSG. Check for yourself. Insert the words "Images of MSG mice" into your search engine, and you will get an incredible number of photos of fat mice that were fed MSG. Unfortunately, I don't have the rights to those images, so they're not part of this book.

Indeed, when the laboratory mice or rats are fed MSG, even in <u>low doses</u>, they gain weight very rapidly. Here's what one of the studies concluded:

"We can conclude that MSG administration in rats even at very low doses is efficient to induce weight gain, altered thyroid function and histology"
(Khalaf & Arafat, 2015)[16]

Histology = Study of the microscopic material

It is a well-known fact throughout the scientific community, hence the term "Monosodium Glutamate (MSG)-obese rats."[17] Unfortunately, this excitotoxin is added to the predominant number of processed foods. That's correct, not only in Asian, fast food, and other well-known and not so well-known restaurants, but these "almost foods" are in abundance on <u>every supermarket shelf</u>.

"Monosodium glutamate was proved as obesogenic food additive"
(Savcheniuk, Virchenko, Falalyeyeva, Beregova, Babenko, . . . 2014)[18]

Obesogenic = tending to cause obesity

So what do you think? If the laboratory mice or rats are being fed Monosodium Glutamate in order to fatten them up for experimental purposes, how would MSG affect us, the unsuspecting consumer? That's right, just like with mice and rats, exposure to MSG will eventually make you gain weight, and here's how:

"Leptin is a hormone released by fat cells that is known to indicate fullness, or satiety, in the brain."
(UT Southwestern Medical Center, 2011) [19]

Think of the Leptin hormone as a "messenger." As the human messenger travels from office to office in order to deliver timely packages or information, so does Leptin. The primary function of all hormones is to travel from one part of the body to another or from one set of cells to the next. The hormone Leptin serves as a messenger from your fat cells to the brain where, under ideal conditions, it delivers a message about your energy reserves. When you are hungry, lesser amounts of Leptin are produced, and the brain transmits to your systems to eat more, but as you get fuller, the Leptin production increases. [20] Once that happens, the brain transmits to all systems, "I'm full; Stop eating!" But does your brain get this message?

"If the body is exposed to too much Leptin, however, it will become resistant to the hormone."
(UT Southwestern Medical Center, 2011)[21]

Dr. Ka He, a Chair and Professor of Epidemiology and Biostatistics at Indiana University Bloomington, led the association of MSG consumption and weight gain study while at the University of North Carolina. Dr. He pointed out that there are substantial implications for public health when consuming MSG: [22]

"'MSG consumption may cause Leptin resistance,' Dr. He said, so that the body cannot properly process the energy it receives from food. That, Dr. He added, could explain why people who ate more MSG gained weight regardless of how many calories they consumed."(Marcus, 2011)[23]

I believe that I have to highlight the last couple of words of the previous sentence; **"...people who ate more MSG gained weight <u>regardless of how many calories they consumed</u>."**

Keep in mind that hormone Leptin is not only involved in regulating of metabolism or how we process calories, but in part, **it influences our mood, and even affects how we handle our stress levels**, among others.[24] As Byron J. Richards, Board Certified Clinical Nutritionist has noted:

"Leptin is the king of hormones, the commander and chief of virtually everything that takes place in your body."
(Richards, 2009)[25]

I will not bore you with additional details about numerous functions of this hormone. I just wanted you to see that **the same hormone that controls your satiety has a lot to do <u>with your emotional state</u>**. If your brain is resistant to the effects of Leptin, what other problems may rear their ugly heads?

So, while you were finishing a meal, your fat cells, through the messenger Leptin, sent a message to your brain that you had enough food, and your nutrition levels are exactly where they should be. Everything is hunky-dory, or so we think. The problem is that we just had a meal containing excitotoxin MSG, and perhaps chased it with a diet drink containing excitotoxin Aspartame, which we will be discussing in the next chapter.

For some unknown reason, although we're full, we seem to want to eat more. This is the precise symptom that I described at the beginning of this chapter. Even if cooler heads prevail, and we stop eating, we want to go for a sugary dessert or a snack, or some sort of carbohydrate substance in order to make us feel better or help us get rid of the nagging craving sensation.

While "the messenger Leptin" is coursing through your system and increasingly bombarding your brain with the message that you have eaten enough, your brain becomes desensitized to the receipt of this vital information. Dr. Russell Blaylock, Board Certified Neurosurgeon, pointed out, "It has been shown that you can produce [sic] Leptin insensitivity very easily with MSG." (Blaylock, R. Interview by Adams, M., 2006) [26] He also noted that in a study on animals that were exposed to MSG, they preferred foods high in carbohydrate and sugar content as opposed to foods that were high in protein. [27] Furthermore, besides having an uncontrollable appetite, their metabolisms were unmanageable due to the desensitization to Leptin.[28]

In May 2011, Reuters published an article under the heading, "MSG linked to weight gain."[29] The subheading was sobering: "The flavor enhancer Monosodium Glutamate (MSG), most often associated with

Chinese food and after-dinner headaches, may also be enhancing waistlines, a new study finds." (Marcus, 2011)[30] I don't think that I need drill down further of how MSG is enhancing waistlines.

Consequently, the downward spiral begins. As you continue to put on weight, and become overweight, your production of Leptin continues to climb.

"99.9 % of the overweight population make way too much Leptin from their extra pounds of fat. All this extra Leptin actually clogs Leptin function, sort of like a traffic jam, and induces a problem called Leptin resistance – which means that even though there is far too much Leptin it isn't getting into your brain correctly…"
(Richards, 2009) [31]

That's right, **it's not entirely your fault that even though you're exercising and dieting, you're having a difficult time getting rid of excess weight!**

PRO-MSG PROPAGANDA

Many proponents of the excitotoxin MSG are flooding the Internet with posts, trying to justify that Monosodium Glutamate is not responsible for the weight gain of millions. One of the most fascinating arguments is that Chinese people consume Monosodium Glutamate regularly and "nothing happens to them." This argument is being repeated despite studies that have been published on the excitotoxicity of this substance. In fact, when I began to dig for information in order to verify what was making me sick and overweight, I found that the Internet was flooded with pro-MSG articles.

No matter how much one repeats that same fallacious argument, it remains fallacious. The food industry would lose billions of dollars in revenue if more people were aware of the dangers of ingesting this excitotoxin.

As I only operate on facts and rigid results of research, and not anecdotal substantiation, here is hard evidence from a study I located in the *Obesity Research Journal,* as well as, in the US National Library of Medicine - National Institutes of Health (NIH).

Bear with me for the next couple of paragraphs, as it will get a bit technical, but once you get through it, I believe that your opinion about consumption of excitotoxins will completely change. It is only one piece of the puzzle to "Living Wonderfully", as there is much more.

I present to you a sample of **"<u>human</u>"** study entitled *"Association of Monosodium Glutamate intake with overweight in Chinese adults: the INTERMAP Study."*[32] Here's what the study was all about:

"Animal studies indicate that Monosodium Glutamate (MSG) can induce hypothalamic lesions and Leptin resistance, possibly influencing energy balance, leading to overweight. This study examines the association between MSG intake and overweight in the human species."
(He, K., Zhao, L., Stamler, J., Daviglus, M., Dyer, A., Horn, L. V., et al., 2008)[33]

This was not a small sample study, as it involved 752 Chinese adults ranging between the ages of 40 to 59, 48% of which were women. The participants that were picked at random were sampled from three rural villages from the north and south of China. The majority of participants home-cooked their meals and didn't use processed food. Because it was a controlled study, people were adding measured amounts of MSG to their foods; 0.33 grams per day.

If we put all of the scientific data aside, and only concentrate on two summation sentences from the study, the results are indisputable:

1. "Prevalence of overweight was significantly higher in **MSG users than nonusers**", and
2. "**...**MSG intake may be associated with increased risk of overweight independent of physical activity and total energy intake in humans." (He, K., Zhao, L., Stamler, J., Daviglus, M., Dyer, A., Horn, L. V., et al., 2008) [34]

I'm certain that you noticed the wording "independent of physical activity and total energy intake in humans." [35]

What that means is that <u>it makes no difference whether you exercise or eat small amounts of food</u>, you're at risk of gaining weight when ingesting MSG.

That was one of the big reasons that even though I was exercising, eating small portions of fat-free and low-fat "almost foods", I was resistant to weight loss. Sadly, the predominant majority of the low-fat "garbage" that I consumed was loaded with ingredients that contained MSG.

Another piece of information that's worth mentioning is **MSG affecting Thyroid gland in a negative way, which is "indicative of hypothyroidism" or underactive thyroid to be exact.** [36] [37] Because underactive thyroid does not produce enough hormones, the **metabolism slows down**, which may not only cause **weight gain**, but chronic inflammation of the thyroid gland itself. [38] [39] There are many other symptoms of hypothyroidism which include stiff muscles, dry skin, sleep apnea, slowing of the motor activity; even abnormally heavy bleeding during menstruation, and many more. [40] We will be expanding on the subject of Thyroid in the "**ALCOHOL**" among other chapters later in the book.

There is a lot more scientific information of MSG being the reason behind weight gain. I believe that we have enough evidence to dismiss any efforts by MSG proponents to muddy the waters.

And there you have it! Fat rats and mice, overweight people including those of Chinese decent, hypothalamic lesions in the brain, resistance to Leptin, uncontrollable cravings, stubborn weight retention despite dieting, underactive thyroid, all among the undesirable "MSG Wonders" as will be described next.

ADDITIONAL UNDESIRABLE CONSEQUENCES

There is a vast number of undesirable side effects when one eats "almost foods" and drinks "almost beverages" that are spiked with excitotoxins. Even though you are already aware of MSG and weight gain, there are many more detrimental side effects of Monosodium Glutamate. We will not go into all of them, but will only concentrate on a few major ones which I experienced.

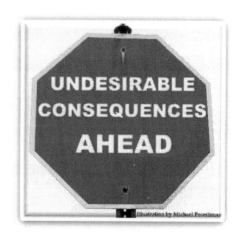

HIGH BLOOD PRESSURE

At the beginning of the book I talked about my problem with high blood pressure even though I was going to the gym, taking blood pressure medication, and eating tasteless fat-free "garbage" that the doctors instructed me to eat. Nothing was helping; not even regular trips to the gym. When I eventually began to get off MSG and other chemicals, all of a sudden my decades of high blood pressure began to normalize.

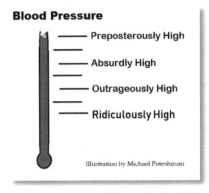

Consider another study on MSG entitled "Monosodium Glutamate is related to a higher increase in blood pressure over 5 years: findings from the Jiangsu Nutrition Study of Chinese adults."[41]

The human study evaluated 1,227 men and women between 2002 and 2007 and concluded that Monosodium Glutamate was linked to a substantial increase in blood pressure:

> "MSG intake was associated with a significant increase in SBP and DBP."
> (Wittert, G., Gill, T., Taylor, A., Pan, X., Dai, Y., Yuan, B., et al., 2011)[42]

SBP = Systolic Blood Pressure or a top number which represents the amount of pressure in your arteries when your heart contracts

DBP = Diastolic Blood Pressure or a bottom number which refers to the amount of pressure between heart beats

The conclusion of the study really hit the nail on the head as it was established that even people who were taking blood pressure medication were susceptible to the increase in blood pressure because of the independent effects of MSG.

> "MSG intake may have independent BP-increasing effects, especially among women and those taking hypertension medications at baseline and follow-up." (Wittert, G., Gill, T., Taylor, A., Pan, X., Dai, Y., Yuan, B., et al., 2011)[43]

That was truly an eye opening moment! I finally understood that **while I was going to the gym and taking elephant doses of hypertension medication, I continued to see my blood pressure rise astronomically**, especially the diastolic. I was unknowingly aggravating my declining condition because I continued to ingest these "almost foods" that contained MSG. Fat-free or low-fat made no difference! Guess what? I'm now off these drugs, as I'm surely off anything that may contain MSG.

Although this research has been available to medical professionals since 2008, my doctors didn't take me off MSG when my blood pressure was jumping through the roof. Instead they were slowly killing me with stronger prescriptions that caused additional side effects. Once again, I have to give my doctors of not so distant past, the benefit of the doubt, as their medical school classes may not have included lectures on the side effects of MSG. We will be discussing prescription medications in a later chapter.

As I mentioned at the beginning of the book, my legs were driving me absolutely crazy during the night. I couldn't fall asleep and stay asleep. It was the sensation where I had to constantly move my legs in order to get relief from this crawly-pins-and-needles feeling. I later discovered that my condition was called Restless Leg Syndrome or RLS.

As I was doing my research on MSG, I came upon a study that was directed by an associate professor of neurology, Richard P. Allen, Ph.D. at the Johns Hopkins University School of Medicine. The study linked high levels of glutamate in the brain with Restless Leg Syndrome. [44] [45]

The researchers used an MRI "...to image the brain and found glutamate — a neurotransmitter involved in arousal — in abnormally high levels in people with RLS. [46] The more glutamate the researchers found in the brains of those with RLS, the worse their sleep" (Johns Hopkins News and Publications, 2013). [47]

As for me, my RLS stopped dead in its tracks a short time after I discontinued eating foods that contained MSG and other MSG-containing chemicals! **Remember, the G in MS<u>G</u> is glutamate!**

SWELLING OF THE UVULA

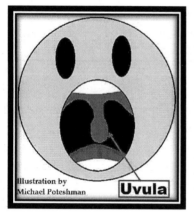

Illustration by
Michael Poteshman   **Uvula**

The uvula is a piece of flesh that hangs in the back of the throat. It happens to be an organ that produces saliva and helps with speech among other functions.[48]

On several occasions after eating buffet style at my ex-favorite Asian restaurant that shall remain nameless, my father and I experienced severe swelling of the uvula. After one of those restaurant outings my father was treated at the hospital and kept overnight. He experienced severe difficulty breathing and swallowing due to acute edema (swelling) of the uvula and the surrounding area. At the time, we were guessing that we were both allergic to seafood, although I had similar reaction when I ate certain processed and restaurant foods. Our thinking was utterly flawed, as when any type of seafood ranging from shrimp to scallops, and even crabs, calamari, fish and other seafood delicacies were prepared at home, we never experienced any type of swelling or inflammation.

A case report entitled "Chinese Restaurant Syndrome" outlined a comparable condition that my father and I experienced several times in the past. Without going into details, here's an excerpt from the report:

"Angioedema of the uvula after ingestion of MSG can be fatal unless patients and physicians are aware of unusual reaction to MSG. Many deaths can be avoided with timely diagnosis and treatment."
(Bawaskar, H. & Bawaskar, P., 2017) [49]

The conclusion was as sobering as the discussion above:

"Severe reaction to MSG, a common active ingredient in Chinese cooking may result in fatal outcome if not treated in time. Delayed occurrence of serious symptoms are to be expected."
(Bawaskar, H. & Bawaskar, P., 2017)[50]

The swelling of my uvula became extinct, just like the Dodo bird, ever since I stopped eating processed foods or any type of foods that may contain MSG and other additives, artificial colors, preservatives, or flavorings.

MSG MOOD SWINGS AND RAGE

Illustration by Michael Poteshman

Approximately nine years prior to writing this book, I was in charge of a sizable program for the federal government. One of my staff members was a technically experienced gentleman who was hired to handle IT customer support. Let's call him Fred for the sake of not revealing his real name. Fred had mood swings that were dreaded by the entire team. Recalling those events of the past, his episodes were especially pronounced after lunch. That's when Fred became jittery and almost hostile to the customers and the members of his team. After several complaints, my government client brought these outbursts to my attention. When I contacted Fred and inquired about the issues at hand, he became enraged and raised his voice. He told me that "these people didn't know what they were doing", and that he had to "hold their hands" in order to teach them the "stupid" things that "they should have known in the first place." I asked him to lower his voice, but that made him even more enraged and irrational. I courteously asked him to leave the premises until further notice.

When I came to the office the next morning, my assistant informed me that Fred was already at work. She also told me that his wife left a message begging me to call her as soon as I got into the office. Although I had reservations about talking to the spouse of a disgruntled employee, I returned her call. Before I was able to say a word, she began to tearfully apologize for her husband's behavior. She explained that this was not his first time that he snapped at people, as he did the same thing at the previous job. She further explained that these episodes only happened when he ate certain foods, or after he ate out at a restaurant. She went on to say that they could not afford for him to lose another job because of their financial situation. She promised me that if I gave him another chance, she would make certain to pack his lunches. She also pointed out that Fred would not deviate from his routine of <u>not eating out</u> as "he knows what happens to his head when he eats the wrong kind of food." I believed her story not only because of her genuine presentation of facts, but due to my past observation of Fred's behavior. Fred wasn't irrational all the time. In fact, when he was level-headed, he exhibited an appropriate level of professionalism.

Because I'm a firm believer in giving people second chances, I went back to my government contact and explained the situation. The client agreed with my assessment to give Fred another chance. As a result, I instituted a 60-day probationary period, to which Fred agreed.

The entire month passed, and Fred was doing extremely well. His customer service skills seemed to be in order. One week into the second month of his probationary period, my government contact stormed into my office, extremely upset. He said that Fred insulted and screamed at two employees when they asked him a simple question. In fact one of the ladies went home crying, and said that she would not return to work until steps are taken to insulate her from Fred's abuse. I believe that you can deduce the fate that Fred had suffered as the result of his irrational aggression.

But was it really Fred's fault? You be the judge. As you've read in the foreword of this book, I was suffering from a similar condition not so long ago. I had no idea that only seven years after Fred's "episode", out of the blue, I would become more enraged and gratuitously emotional. Utterly insignificant events were setting me off without provocation. Talking about road rage…

In his book, "In bad taste - The MSG symptom complex", George R. Schwartz, MD., lists an extensive number of diseases and conditions that are caused or exacerbated by the use of MSG. In addition to mood swings, one of the symptoms is MSG-Rage reactions.[51] The book references an MSG-sensitive killer in the 1984 "McDonald's Massacre" in San Ysidro, California. This massacre resulted in 20 people losing their lives, and 20 injured before the police sharpshooter took out this killer.[52]

After the analysis by the *International Journal of Biosocial Research*, Dr. Robert Hall of Chaminade University of Honolulu concluded that evidence supported "psychotic reaction" to MSG.[53] The part of the brain thought to be responsible for this rage reaction is the amygdala, which is also stimulated by Monosodium Glutamate.[54]

Furthermore, the responses of **mood, rage, and stress, are controlled by the hypothalamus/pituitary gland**.[55] [56] [57] [58] Without going into long scientific details, I'll quote a conclusion of yet another study:

According to a 1995 study, "…results indicate that MSG is harmful to the function of the hypothalamus-pituitary-target system of neonatal rats." (Gong, S., Xia, F., Wei, J., Li, X., Sun, T., Lu, Z., et al., 1995)[59]

There are other examples of MSG-induced conditions such as **depression in all age groups**,[60] allergies[61] [62] **that I used to suffer from year round**, oxidative damage,[63] brain lesions,[64] **liver inflammation and dysplasia** (pre-cancerous condition where cells undergo abnormal changes),[65] dizziness, headaches, pressure and a burning sensation in the chest or face or shoulders,[66] [67] destruction of arcuate nucleus **neurons in the brain**,[68] among other undesirable "wonders" that we already discussed. Children are also affected in a profound way. A good example is Attention Deficit Hyperactivity Disorder (ADHD).[69] [70]

We will not go into additional health adversities that this substance may cause because I believe that you get the point. Instead we will concentrate on how to identify foods that are spiked with MSG.

EAT THIS AT YOUR OWN RISK!

Let's speak hypothetically. Suppose you come across your favorite cup of ramen noodles, can of soup, potato chips, sausages, or even tea bags and coffee with a warning label that would look something like this:

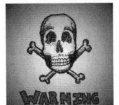

"WARNING: The consumption of this product may trigger your body to store excess fat,[71][72] cause oxidative damage,[73] headaches, mood swings, rage, depression in all age groups,[74]sleeplessness, nausea, raise your blood pressure, cause brain lesions and destruction to parts of the brain, increase in appetite, and trigger cravings and thirst!!!"[75][76][77][78]

Illustration by Kevin Aguillon

Would you purchase such a product? Most likely, you'd say a big "NO!" But because I've been in those shoes, and have consumed my share of these "almost foods", unbeknownst to you, you say "yes" to these so-called food products practically on a daily basis. Let's take a trip to your local grocery store and explore.

I was in a supermarket with my digital camera in hand, inconspicuously walking through the aisles and turning the "almost food" items towards my camera and snapping pictures for this book. All of a sudden, I was approached by the store manager and a security officer.

The manager asked me, "Why are you taking pictures?" I explained that I was doing research for a book that told the story of how I went from "Living Dead to Living Wonderfully." I also mentioned that pictures were for the type of products that I eliminated from my diet. After I finished explaining, the manager asked his security guard to return to his post, and offered me his help. Because I never refuse free help, we went through the aisles, as <u>he</u> was singling out products for my picture taking.

Here's the outcome of our picture taking. Unfortunately, I didn't include all of the images because there were simply too many. As much as possible, I fully or partially removed the manufacturer's name from the labels because I don't want to single out any company. It is up to us, the educated consumer, to decide what is good and what is bad for our health.

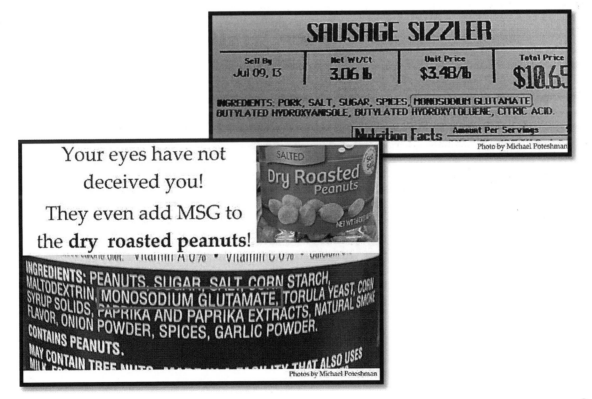

SAUSAGE SIZZLER

Sell By	Net Wt/Ct	Unit Price	Total Price
Jul 09, 13	3.06 lb	$3.48/lb	$10.65

INGREDIENTS: PORK, SALT, SUGAR, SPICES, MONOSODIUM GLUTAMATE BUTYLATED HYDROXYANISOLE, BUTYLATED HYDROXYTOLUENE, CITRIC ACID.

Nutrition Facts — Amount Per Servings

Photo by Michael Poteshman

Your eyes have not deceived you!

They even add MSG to the **dry roasted peanuts!**

SALTED
Dry Roasted Peanuts
NET WT 16OZ

INGREDIENTS: PEANUTS, SUGAR, SALT, CORN STARCH, MALTODEXTRIN, MONOSODIUM GLUTAMATE, TORULA YEAST, CORN SYRUP SOLIDS, PAPRIKA AND PAPRIKA EXTRACTS, NATURAL SMOKE FLAVOR, ONION POWDER, SPICES, GARLIC POWDER. CONTAINS PEANUTS.
MAY CONTAIN TREE NUTS... THAT ALSO USES MILK...

Photos by Michael Poteshman

2-23

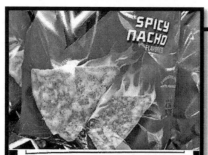

SPICY NACHO FLAVORED

Ingredients: Corn, Vegetable Oil (Sunflower, Corn, and/or Canola Oil), Maltodextrin (Made From Corn), Salt, Whey, Monosodium Glutamate Buttermilk, Romano Cheese (Cow's Milk, Cheese Cultures, Salt, Enzymes), Cheddar Cheese (Milk, Cheese Cultures, Salt, Enzymes), Corn Starch, Onion Powder, Garlic Powder, Dextrose, Natural and Artificial Flavor, Spices, Lactose, Sodium Caseinate, Artificial Color (Including Yellow 6 Lake, Red 40 Lake, Yellow 6, Red 40, Yellow 5, Blue 1), Citric Acid, Sugar, Lactic Acid, Skim Milk, Disodium Inosinate, and Disodium Guanylate. **CONTAINS MILK INGREDIENTS.**
Photos by Michael Poteshman

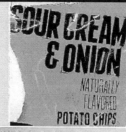

SOUR CREAM & ONION NATURALLY FLAVORED POTATO CHIPS

INGREDIENTS: POTATOES, VEGETABLE OIL (CONTAINS ONE OR MORE OF: CORN, SUNFLOWER, OR CANOLA OIL), WHEY POWDER, SOUR CREAM POWDER (CREAM, NONFAT DRY MILK, CULTURES), ONION POWDER, MALTODEXTRIN, DEXTROSE, SALT, MONOSODIUM GLUTAMATE, SKIM MILK POWDER, NATURAL FLAVORING, SPICE.
Photo by Michael Poteshman

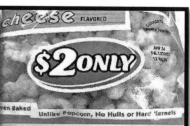

cheese FLAVORED

$2 ONLY

Oven Baked   Unlike Popcorn, No Hulls or Hard Kernels

Ingredients: Enriched Corn Meal (Corn Meal, Ferrous Sulfate, Niacin, Thiamin Mononitrate, Riboflavin, Folic Acid), Vegetable Oil (Corn, Canola, and/or Sunflower Oil), Cheese Seasoning (Whey, Cheddar Cheese [Milk, Cheese Cultures, Salt, Enzymes], Canola Oil, Maltodextrin [Made from Corn], Natural and Artificial Flavors, Salt, Whey Protein Concentrate, Monosodium Glutamate, Lactic Acid, Citric Acid, Artificial Color [Yellow 6]), and Salt. **CONTAINS MILK INGREDIENTS.**
Photos by Michael Poteshman

Cream of Mushroom SOUP

INGREDIENTS: WATER, MUSHROOMS, VEGETABLE OIL (CORN, COTTONSEED, CANOLA, AND/OR SOYBEAN), MODIFIED FOOD STARCH, WHEAT FLOUR, CONTAINS LESS THAN 2% OF: SALT, CREAM (MILK), DEHYDRATED WHEY, SOY PROTEIN CONCENTRATE, MONOSODIUM GLUTAMATE, YEAST EXTRACT, FLAVORING, DEHYDRATED GARLIC.
Photos by Michael Poteshman

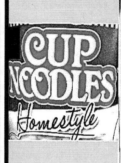

CUP NOODLES Homestyle

INGREDIENTS: ENRICHED FLOUR (WHEAT FLOUR, NIACIN, REDUCED IRON, THIAMINE MONONITRATE, RIBOFLAVIN, FOLIC ACID), VEGETABLE OIL (PALM OIL, HYDROGENATED PALM OIL), SALT, CONTAINS LESS THAN 2% OF: BETA CAROTENE COLOR, CARAMEL COLOR, CITRIC ACID, CONCENTRATED LIME JUICE, DISODIUM GUANYLATE, DISODIUM INOSINATE, DISODIUM SUCCINATE, EGG WHITE, GARLIC POWDER, HYDROLYZED CORN PROTEIN, HYDROLYZED SOY PROTEIN, LACTOSE, MALTODEXTRIN, MODIFIED CORN STARCH, MONOSODIUM GLUTAMATE, NATURAL AND ARTIFICIAL FLAVOR, ONION POWDER, POTASSIUM CARBONATE, POWDERED CHICKEN, SHRIMP EXTRACT POWDER, SHRIMP POWDER, SODIUM ALGINATE, SODIUM CARBONATE, SODIUM PHOSPHATE, SODIUM TRIPOLYPHOSPHATE, SOY LECITHIN, SOYBEAN, SPICE AND COLOR, TBHQ (PRESERVATIVE), WHEAT, YELLOW 5.
CONTAINS WHEAT, SOYBEAN, EGG, MILK AND SHRIMP.

THE ORIGINAL Ranch.

Photos by Michael Poteshman

Calcium 0%   Iron 0%

INGREDIENTS: VEGETABLE OIL (SOYBEAN AND/OR CANOLA), WATER, EGG YOLK, SUGAR, SALT, CULTURED NONFAT BUTTERMILK, NATURAL FLAVORS (MILK, SOY), LESS THAN 1% OF: SPICES, DRIED GARLIC, DRIED ONION, VINEGAR, PHOSPHORIC ACID, XANTHAN GUM, MODIFIED FOOD STARCH, MONOSODIUM GLUTAMATE, ARTIFICIAL FLAVORS, DISODIUM PHOSPHATE, SORBIC ACID AND CALCIUM DISODIUM EDTA AS PRESERVATIVES, DISODIUM INOSINATE, DISODIUM GUANYLATE. **CONTAINS: EGG, MILK, SOY.** **GLUTEN-FREE.**

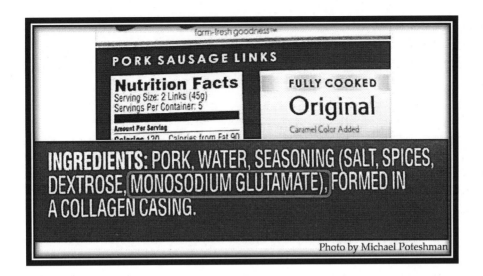

PORK SAUSAGE LINKS

Nutrition Facts
Serving Size: 2 Links (45g)
Servings Per Container: 5

Amount Per Serving
Calories 120   Calories from Fat 90

FULLY COOKED
Original
Caramel Color Added

INGREDIENTS: PORK, WATER, SEASONING (SALT, SPICES, DEXTROSE, MONOSODIUM GLUTAMATE), FORMED IN A COLLAGEN CASING.

Photo by Michael Poteshman

These few examples represent what my family and I used to eat almost on a daily basis. No wonder I was stuck in a rut.

The following two items are straight MSG powder in a shaker container. A lot of restaurants, and even some of our family acquaintances, sprinkle this stuff directly on all of their food. Believe it or not, they even put this stuff on their desserts.

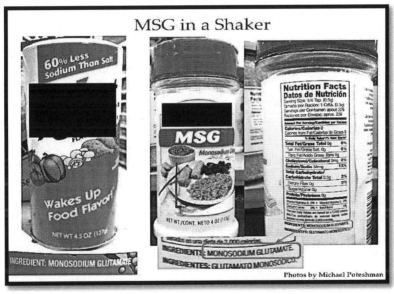

MSG in a Shaker

Photos by Michael Poteshman

You may be puzzled about my sentence: I have absolutely no problems with labels that clearly state "Monosodium Glutamate" in plain English, as the food manufacturers are giving us a choice whether or not we elect to purchase their product or to avoid it. As far as I'm concerned, these labels are practically synonymous with warnings on cigarette packs. The words Monosodium Glutamate should have the same meaning as the hypothetical warning label that I presented at the beginning of this section. The problem is not with the manufacturers who actually spell out the words "Monosodium Glutamate" in their list of ingredients. The problem is in the hidden names. By the end of the next section you will be able to distinguish between the type of stuff masquerading under the MSG covers of something seemingly benign.

"The F.D.A. permits M.S.G. made by certain manufacturing techniques to be called natural flavors or seasonings on food labels."
-The New York Times- [79]

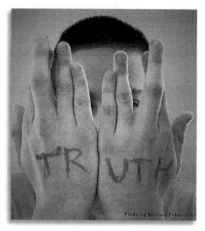

"Natural Flavor" sounds really healthy, doesn't it? As the unsuspecting and gullible consumers that my wife and I once were, we bought the "almost food" containing this ingredient without a second thought. It's because everything that's natural is obviously healthy. Isn't it? I don't think so!

Also, who likes bland food? I certainly don't, so when I see that one of the food ingredients is "seasoning" or "spice" without telling me what the seasoning and/or spices are, I keep as far away from these "almost food" choices as I possibly can.

The U.S. Food and Drug Administration (FDA) has a very long definition for natural flavor or flavoring. I will quote a very small excerpt from the FDA. You will find the rest of the definition in the **Appendix IV** and **Appendices A - F** at the end of this book:

"The term natural flavor or natural flavoring means the essential oil, oleoresin, essence or extractive, protein hydrolysate, distillate, or any product of roasting, heating or enzymolysis, which contains the flavoring constituents derived from a spice…"
(FDA, 2014)[80]

What a mouthful! It is important to keep in mind that not all "spices" or "natural flavors" contain MSG, as they may contain other ingredients that are listed in the **Appendices A - F** at the end of this book. Some so-called spices are benign, and some are plainly scary even without the added MSG. But the manufacturers tell us that they use these terms to keep their proprietary secret recipes close to their vest. It may be true in some cases, but what about other really scary hidden names? Natural flavors can come from almost any natural product or material, even though you may logically believe that a certain natural substance is not at all edible.

For example, how would you like to eat secretions from a beaver's anus masquerading as natural flavors? These natural flavors are more specifically identified as raspberry, strawberry, or even vanilla.[81] [82] Indeed, the brown slimy substance known as "castoreum" that's discharged from the beaver's anus as well as the sack that secretes this stuff, gets extracted by a hot alcohol solution[83] and brought to you as natural flavor. A beaver's castoreum sack and its secretions are obviously natural, but do we really want to consume this stuff? Although FDA regards castoreum as "GRAS" or Generally Recognized as Safe, [84] why not just name this stuff by its real name? Well, they can't and they won't because if the honest ingredient list existed where secretions from the beaver's "butt" were spelled out, none of us would ever purchase such product. Instead, when I called a certain ice cream manufacturer as well as a particular Vitamin water producer, I was told by both that the flavor is proprietary and they can't reveal their trade secrets. But you already know what their trade secrets are. Just as an FYI, castoreum is not only utilized in foods, but it is used extensively in perfumes.[85]

Back to MSG and its deceptive names. According to Reuters, *"MSG is one of the world's most widely used food additive. Although it tends to be more popular in Asian countries, Americans manage to get their share in processed foods, from chips to canned soups, even when it's not labeled as such"* (Marcus, 2011).[86] The last couple of words are worth repeating, "…**even when it's not labeled as such.**"

Let's look at a couple of other examples of hidden ingredients. How about different names for Hydrolyzed Vegetable Protein? Sounds benign, doesn't it?

Indeed, hydrolyzed protein may sound healthy, except that this ingredient may contain as much as 40% or even 50% of Monosodium Glutamate, depending on the manufacturer.[87]

The FDA regulation states that manufacturers must use specific food source names from which a particular "hydrolyzed vegetable protein" and "hydrolyzed protein" were derived.[88] That, unfortunately, does not lessen the amount of MSG that is contained in a specific hydrolyzed protein. Here are some examples of how foods that contain these proteins must be labeled:

"Hydrolyzed wheat gluten", "hydrolyzed soy protein", and "autolyzed yeast extract" are examples of acceptable names. "Hydrolyzed Casein" is also an example of an acceptable name…"
(FDA, 2014)[89]

Here are more ingredients that contain MSG, but are not labeled as such:
Autolyzed Yeast or Yeast Extract which may contain between 10% and 20% MSG, and sometimes even higher; Cassenate with its approximate MSG content of 12%; Disodium Guanylate, Ribonucleotides, Disodium Inosinate which are considered MSG enhancers.[90] When mixed with MSG, Ribonucleotides cause "powerful MSG effects with increased neurological actions" (Schwartz, 1999).[91] So there's no ambiguity, below is the chart that will make it easier for you to do your food shopping:

Certain Sources of MSG	Possible Sources and additives that frequently contain MSG
Monosodium Glutamate	Soy sauce
Sodium Caseinate	Carrageenan or vegetable gum, Seasonings or spices
Protein isolate[92]	Bouillon, broth or stock (may be listed as chicken stock or chicken broth)
Autolyzed yeast	Chicken, beef, pork, smoke flavorings

Certain Sources of MSG	Possible Sources and additives that frequently contain MSG
Vegetable hydrolyzed protein	Barley malt
Plant hydrolyzed protein	Malt extract, malt flavoring
Yeast extract	Whey protein
Plant protein extract	Soy protein
Hydrolyzed oat flour	Textured protein
Hydrolyzed Casein[93]	Soy protein isolate or concentrate
Calcium Caseinate	Whey protein isolate or concentrate
Certain Sources of MSG	**Possible Sources and additives that frequently contain MSG**
Textured protein	Soy extract
The chart above and on the previous page is based on FDA information portal,[94] the book "In Bad Taste: The MSG Symptom Complex" by physician and toxicologist Dr. George R. Schwartz, MD,[95] and the book by neurosurgeon, Dr. Russell L. Blaylock, MD, "Excitotoxins The Taste that kills". [96]	

Unfortunately, the chart above does not include all of the names for this stuff because "new labeling deceptions" [97] are continuing to be invented. For example, there are some other, not as potent ingredients as in the chart above which can serve as a trigger in MSG sensitive people.[98] Some examples include Modified Food Starch, Corn Starch, Rice Syrup, among others. [99]

If you decide to do a web search for hidden sources of MSG, besides the word "Umami", I promise, you will get more than you bargained for. Let me illustrate. The PubChem database, a government website of the U.S. National Library of Medicine, lists over 75 alternative names or synonyms for MSG. [100] Without going into all 75, here are a few of them in no particular order: [101]

- Vetsin
- Ajinomoto
- Zest
- Chinese seasoning
- FEMA No. 2756
- Accent
- AI3-18393
- Ancoma
- L-Glutamic acid, sodium salt
- G0188
- Glutacyl

- 142-47-2
- Glutamate monosodium salt
- Sodium (S)-2-amino-4-carboxybutanoate
- AN-17435
- Natrium L-hydrogenglutamat
- Sodium 5-oxido-5-oxo-D-norvaline
- Sodium hydrogen glutamate

These ingredients are named as something other than MSG. Should I assume that these ingredients are healthy? Shouldn't I? Do you want to sell me the Brooklyn Bridge? I can no longer be fooled!

THE TEA OF PAIN

Approximately four weeks after I quit MSG cold turkey, my headaches were going by way of the Dodo bird, and my brain was clearing. Because my life was turning around in a positive direction, I thought that I knew enough about excitotoxins. After all, I did relatively decent research. Unfortunately, as I was getting better, I didn't pay as much attention to other "disguised" names for MSG as I should have. Oh boy, how wrong I was!

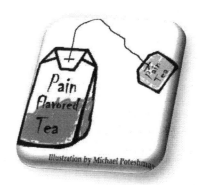

Illustration by Michael Poteshman

On one Sunday afternoon, my younger son and I went shopping to one of our favorite food stores that usually sells a lot of organic and health food. I strongly believed that the majority of items in the store were very healthy. As we walked into the tea isle, there were several thermoses that contained free samples of different varieties of tea from a major manufacturer. One of them was peach flavored, my favorite kind that I haven't had in a long time. I drank four sample cups of this heavenly beverage and it tasted absolutely divine. I also tried cinnamon apple tea. Wow, what a great flavor! It almost tasted like apple juice with cinnamon. I didn't have to add any sweetener to these teas as they were absolutely perfect. My son also had tea, but it was just black tea - without any additional flavors.

We continued to shop in the store for about another hour. As we started to walk towards the register, the back of my head felt like it was squeezed by a vice. I already knew what the symptoms were, and I had a suspicion about the cause. Since I had my usual healthy food for lunch, I knew that my headache could only be caused by foods or beverages independent of my daily meals. I didn't eat or drink anything outside my home besides peach and apple flavored teas, so I asked my son to go back to the tea isle and bring me the packages of these products. To my surprise there was "natural flavor" on the ingredient list. Unfortunately, the manufacturer did not list what this "natural flavor" consisted of. See for yourself:

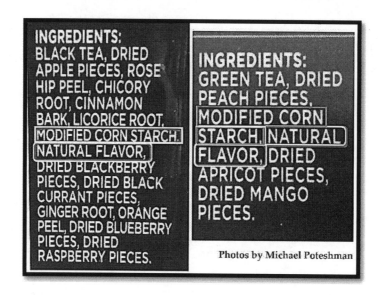

INGREDIENTS:
BLACK TEA, DRIED APPLE PIECES, ROSE HIP PEEL, CHICORY ROOT, CINNAMON BARK, LICORICE ROOT, MODIFIED CORN STARCH, NATURAL FLAVOR, DRIED BLACKBERRY PIECES, DRIED BLACK CURRANT PIECES, GINGER ROOT, ORANGE PEEL, DRIED BLUEBERRY PIECES, DRIED RASPBERRY PIECES.

INGREDIENTS:
GREEN TEA, DRIED PEACH PIECES, MODIFIED CORN STARCH, NATURAL FLAVOR, DRIED APRICOT PIECES, DRIED MANGO PIECES.

Photos by Michael Poteshman

This is where it actually hit me that manufacturers are shoving this "STUFF" into any food or beverage products they can. My biggest gripe was, "how could they put this in the tea?" It's hard to believe that tea would be a suspect! I still don't know whether my reaction was attributed to natural flavor or modified corn starch, [102] because as you saw earlier, these ingredients <u>don't always contain</u> MSG. Perhaps there was something else that wasn't on the label.

As I mentioned earlier, my tea didn't need sugar as it was delicious on its own. Perhaps these teas contained excitotoxin Aspartate which happens to be the amino acid that is present in Aspartame sweetener. But if that were present, why wasn't it on the label?

"Remember also that the powerful excitotoxins aspartate and L-cysteine are frequently added to foods and according to FDA rules require no labeling at all."
(Blaylock, 1998)[103]

I will never know what was in that "almost tea" that made me ill, but a valuable lesson on excitotoxicity and <u>processed beverages</u> was definitely learned.

As we were checking out at the register, my headache was increasing and spreading to the right side of my head while impacting my left eye. I had no other choice but to surrender my car keys to my son who was a novice driver at the time.

Although I recovered a lot sooner than when I had Pho months earlier, I was still in a fairly bad shape. But I pulled through! Once again, my belief (or denial) that processed tea is benign got the better of me. But no more!

After I recovered, my research took a completely new meaning. As I was looking specifically for these substances, I stumbled upon countless articles pertaining to flavor enhancers that used to ruin my life. As usual, I did field research; this time in a big-box grocery store, where I found a plethora of foods that contain these "wonders of modern science." You'll find some examples on the next page:

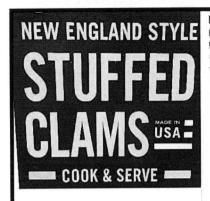

INGREDIENTS: Water, Bread Crumbs (Enriched Wheat Flour (Flour, Malted Barley Flour, Reduced Iron, Niacin, Thiamine Mononitrate, Riboflavin, Folic Acid), Water, Yeast, Partially Hydrogenated Soybean Oil, Salt. Contains 2% or less of the following: Dough Conditioners (Sodium Stearoyl Lactylate, Ammonium Sulfate, Calcium Sulfate, L-Cysteine Hydrochloride, Enzymes, Ascorbic Acid), Corn Flour, Calcium Propionate, Sesame Seeds, Poppy Seeds, Dried Onion, Egg Solids), Textured Soy Protein (Soy Flour), Canola Oil, Clam Meat*, Salt, Garlic, Hydrolyzed Corn and Soy Protein, Spices, Onion, Natural Butter Flavor (Maltodextrin, Salt, Starter Distillate, Paprika and Turmeric), Citric Acid, Red and Green Bell Peppers, Celery, Parsley and Paprika. *Clams from Certified Waters.

Photos by Michael Poteshman

---

2 SANDWICHES

PHILLY STEAK & CHEESE

WITH BEEF STEAK, REDUCED FAT MOZZARELLA CHEESE, PEPPERS, ONIONS & SAUCE IN A

INGREDIENTS: ENRICHED FLOUR (WHEAT FLOUR, MALTED BARLEY FLOUR, NIACIN, IRON, THIAMINE MONONITRATE, RIBOFLAVIN, FOLIC ACID), WATER, BLACK ANGUS COOKED BEEF STEAK GROUND AND FORMED CARAMEL COLOR ADDED (CONTAINS UP TO 14% OF SOLUTION OF WATER, SALT, SEASONING [AUTOLYZED YEAST EXTRACT, MALTODEXTRIN, FLAVORS, BEEF STOCK, SUNFLOWER OIL, SALT, THIAMINE HYDROCHLORIDE, BEEF FAT, SUCCINIC ACID], SODIUM PHOSPHATE, POTASSIUM CHLORIDE, CARAMEL COLOR), REDUCED FAT MOZZARELLA CHEESE (PASTEURIZED PART SKIM MILK, NONFAT MILK, MODIFIED FOOD STARCH, CULTURES, SALT, VITAMIN A PALMITATE, ENZYMES. *INGREDIENTS NOT IN REGULAR MOZZARELLA CHEESE), MARGARINE (PARTIALLY HYDROGENATED SOYBEAN OIL, PALM OIL, WATER, PARTIALLY HYDROGENATED COTTONSEED OIL, SUGAR, MONO- AND DIGLYCERIDES, ARTIFICIAL FLAVOR, SOYBEAN LECITHIN, POTASSIUM SORBATE AND CITRIC ACID [PRESERVATIVES], COLORED WITH ANNATTO AND TURMERIC, VITAMIN A PALMITATE), PALM OIL (WITH SOY LECITHIN, ARTIFICIAL FLAVOR, BETA-CAROTENE [COLOR], CITRIC ACID [PRESERVATIVE]), SEASONING (MALTODEXTRIN, BLEACHED ENRICHED WHEAT FLOUR [WHEAT FLOUR, BENZOYL PEROXIDE, AMYLASE, ASCORBIC ACID, NIACIN, IRON, THIAMINE MONONITRATE, RIBOFLAVIN, FOLIC ACID], BUTTERMILK POWDER, WHEY, NONDAIRY CREAMER [COCONUT OIL, CORN SYRUP SOLIDS, SODIUM CASEINATE, MONO & DIGLYCERIDES, POTASSIUM PHOSPHATE, SILICON DIOXIDE, SOY LECITHIN], NONFAT DRY MILK, CHEDDAR CHEESE [MILK, CULTURES, SALT, ENZYMES], SALT, PARMESAN CHEESE [MILK, CULTURE, SALT, ENZYMES], SUGAR, AUTOLYZED YEAST EXTRACT, SILICON DIOXIDE, SOYBEAN OIL, WHEY PROTEIN CONCENTRATE, DEHYDRATED ONIONS, DISODIUM PHOSPHATE, GARLIC POWDER, METHYL CELLULOSE, NATURAL FLAVOR, ONION POWDER, ANNATTO COLOR, BLUE CHEESE [MILK, CULTURES, SALT, ENZYMES], CITRIC ACID [PRESERVATIVE], XANTHAN GUM, LACTIC ACID, ANHYDROUS MILKFAT, SPICE, CALCIUM LACTATE), ONIONS, 2% OR LESS OF WHEY, MODIFIED FOOD STARCH, GREEN BELL PEPPERS, RED BELL PEPPERS, PARTIALLY HYDROGENATED PALM KERNEL OIL (WITH SOY LECITHIN), ENRICHED FLOUR (WHEAT FLOUR [NIACIN, REDUCED IRON, THIAMINE MONONITRATE, RIBOFLAVIN, FOLIC ACID), SHORTENING BLEND (SOYBEAN OIL AND PARTIALLY HYDROGENATED SOYBEAN OIL), SALT, YEAST, DOUGH CONDITIONER (CALCIUM SULFATE, SALT, L-CYSTEINE HYDROCHLORIDE, GARLIC POWDER, TRICALCIUM PHOSPHATE, ENZYMES), SODIUM STEAROYL LACTYLATE, SUGAR, SOY FLOUR, EGG WHITES. **CONTAINS: MILK, SOY, WHEAT, EGG INGREDIENTS.**

Photos by Michael Poteshman

Chicken Enchilada Suiza

with a sour cream sauce & mexican-style rice

INGREDIENTS: BLANCHED ENRICHED LONG GRAIN PARBOILED RICE (WATER, RICE, IRON, NIACIN, THIAMIN MONONITRATE, FOLIC ACID), WATER, SKIM MILK, ONIONS, CORN FLOUR, COOKED CHICKEN (CHICKEN, CARRAGEENAN, CORN, RED PEPPERS, 2% OR LESS OF TOMATOES (TOMATOES, TOMATO JUICE, SALT, CALCIUM CHLORIDE, CITRIC ACID), BUTTERMILK POWDER, GREEN CHILES, CHEDDAR CHEESE (MILK, CHEESE CULTURES, SALT, ENZYMES, ANNATTO COLOR), MODIFIED FOOD STARCH, APPLE CIDER VINEGAR, CULTURED CREAM, SPICES, GARLIC PUREE, BLEACHED WHEAT FLOUR, GREEN CHILES (GREEN CHILES, CITRIC ACID, SALT, CALCIUM CHLORIDE), SALT, SUGAR, SOYBEAN OIL, JALAPENO PEPPERS, CELLULOSE GUM, MONO & DIGLYCERIDES, AUTOLYZED YEAST EXTRACT, CHICKEN FAT, LIME JUICE CONCENTRATE, NATURAL FLAVORS, TRACE OF LIME, MALTODEXTRIN, JALAPENO PEPPERS (JALAPENO PEPPERS, WATER, SALT, ACETIC ACID, CALCIUM CHLORIDE), WHEAT STARCH, DRIED ONIONS, MEDIUM CHAIN TRIGLYCERIDES, CITRIC ACID, ACETIC ACID, EXTRACTS OF ANNATTO AND TURMERIC COLOR, NATURAL FLAVOR, CALCIUM CHLORIDE. **CONTAINS: WHEAT, MILK INGREDIENTS**

DISTRIBUTED BY NESTLÉ USA.

Photos by Michael Poteshman

Vanilla Ice Cream with Fudge-Covered Toffee Pieces

INGREDIENTS: CREAM, SKIM MILK, LIQUID SUGAR (SUGAR, WATER), WATER, SUGAR, COCONUT OIL, EGG YOLKS, BUTTER (CREAM, SALT), VANILLA EXTRACT, ALMONDS, COCOA (PROCESSED WITH ALKALI), MILK, SOY LECITHIN, COCOA, NATURAL FLAVOR, SALT, VEGETABLE OIL (CANOLA, SAFFLOWER, AND/OR SUNFLOWER OIL), GUAR GUM, CARRAGEENAN.

MAY CONTAIN WHEAT, PEANUTS AND OTHER TREE NUTS.

BEN & JERRY'S HOMEMADE, INC.

Photos by Michael Poteshman

Breakfast Sandwiches
· Sausage, Egg & Cheese ·

INGREDIENTS: WAFFLE STYLE BREAD (WHOLE WHEAT FLOUR, ENRICHED FLOUR [WHEAT FLOUR, MALTED BARLEY FLOUR, NIACIN, REDUCED IRON, VITAMIN B₁ (THIAMIN MONONITRATE), VITAMIN B₂ (RIBOFLAVIN), FOLIC ACID], SUGAR, WATER, SOYBEAN OIL, YEAST, WHEAT STARCH, YELLOW CORN FLOUR, SALT, MODIFIED CORN STARCH, NONFAT MILK, BUTTERMILK SOLIDS, NATURAL FLAVOR, DOUGH CONDITIONER [ISOLATED SOY PROTEIN, MONO AND DIGLYCERIDES, MODIFIED CELLULOSE, SALT, SOYBEAN OIL, SOY LECITHIN], DRIED MOLASSES, NATURAL AND ARTIFICIAL MAPLE FLAVOR, FRUCTOSE, CARROT JUICE FOR COLOR, PUMPKIN JUICE FOR COLOR), FULLY COOKED PORK SAUSAGE PATTY (PORK, WATER, SALT, SPICES, DEXTROSE, SUGAR), SCRAMBLED EGG PATTY (WHOLE EGGS, WHEY, EGG WHITES, NONFAT MILK, SOYBEAN OIL, MODIFIED FOOD STARCH, DICALCIUM PHOSPHATE, SALT, SODIUM BICARBONATE, XANTHAN GUM, GUAR GUM, CITRIC ACID [PRESERVATIVE], PEPPER), PASTEURIZED PROCESS CHEESE (CHEDDAR CHEESE [CULTURED MILK, SALT, ENZYMES], WATER, CREAM, SODIUM PHOSPHATES, SALT, ANNATTO EXTRACT FOR COLOR, PAPRIKA EXTRACT FOR COLOR, ENZYMES).

CONTAINS WHEAT, MILK, SOY AND EGG INGREDIENTS.

Photos by Michael Poteshman

Satisfying balance of great taste, nutrition, and portion size.

Spaghetti & Turkey Meatballs

Spaghetti and turkey meatballs in an Italian-style tomato sauce.

INGREDIENTS: WATER, COOKED ENRICHED SPAGHETTI (WATER, ENRICHED SPAGHETTI [ENRICHED SEMOLINA {WHEAT, NIACIN, FERROUS SULFA THIAMINE MONONITRATE, RIBOFLAVIN, FOLIC ACID}, EGG WHITES, WHEAT GLUTEN, GLYCERYL MONOSTEARATE]), COOKED TURKEY MEATBALLS (TURK MECHANICALLY SEPARATED TURKEY, ITALIAN SEASONING [SALT, DEXTROSE, SPICES, DEHYDRATED ONION AND GARLIC, YEAST EXTRACT, DEHYDRATED BL PEPPER, DEHYDRATED PARSLEY, AUTOLYZED YEAST EXTRACT], SUGAR, SPICE EXTRACTIVES INCLUDING PAPRIKA, CITRIC ACID, DISODIUM INOSINATE A DISODIUM GUANYLATE, NATURAL FLAVORS {MODIFIED CORN STARCH}, NATURAL FLAVORING), TOMATOES, CONCENTRATED CRUSHED TOMATOES, ONION CONTAINS 2% OR LESS OF MODIFIED CORNSTARCH, FLAVORING, SUGAR, PARMESAN CHEESE (PART SKIM COW'S MILK, CHEESE CULTURE, SAL ENZYMES), SALT, OLIVE OIL, SPICES, MONOSODIUM GLUTAMATE, CITRIC ACID, HYDROLYZED CORN PROTEIN, YEAST EXTRACT, OLEORESIN OF PAPRIKA.

Photos by Michael Poteshman

CHICKEN WINGS

BUFFALO STYLE SAUCE

CRISPY BREADED CHICKEN WING SECTIONS WITH SPICY SAUCE PACKETS

INGREDIENTS: SEASONED CHICKEN WINGS (CHICKEN WING SECTIONS, WATER, MODIFIED WHEA STARCH, RICE FLOUR, ISOLATED SOY PROTEIN, SODIUM PHOSPHATES, SALT, WHEAT GLUTE DEXTROSE, SPICES), BUFFALO SAUCE (VINEGAR, CAYENNE PEPPERS, WATER, SALT, NATURA FLAVOR, MODIFIED CORNSTARCH, SOYBEAN OIL, XANTHAN GUM, GUAR GUM, SPICES, CARAME COLOR, EXTRACTIVES OF PAPRIKA [COLOR], GARLIC POWDER), SOYBEAN OIL. **CONTAINS WHEAT, SOY.**

Photos by Michael Poteshman

HONEY BOURBON CHICKEN
Fried chicken strip shaped patties served with honey bourbon dipping sauce, mashed potatoes and corn

INGREDIENTS: FRIED CHICKEN STRIP SHAPED PATTIES (COOKED WHITE MEAT CHICKEN, WATER, ENRICHED FLOUR [WHEAT FLOUR (NIACIN, REDUCED IRON, THIAMINE MONONITRATE, RIBOFLAVIN, FOLIC ACID)], VEGETABLE OIL [PARTIALLY HYDROGENATED SOYBEAN OIL (TBHQ AND CITRIC ACID TO PRESERVE FRESHNESS) AND/OR COTTONSEED OIL], SUGAR, SOY PROTEIN CONCENTRATE, ISOLATED OAT PRODUCT, MODIFIED FOOD STARCH, SALT, SODIUM PHOSPHATE, HONEY, DEXTROSE, NATURAL FLAVORS, SPICE EXTRACT), MASHED POTATOES (RECONSTITUTED POTATOES [MONO AND DIGLYCERIDES, SODIUM ACID PYROPHOSPHATE, CITRIC ACID], MARGARINE [PARTIALLY HYDROGENATED SOYBEAN OIL WITH TBHQ AND CITRIC ACID AS PRESERVATIVES, WATER, MONO AND DIGLYCERIDES (BHT, CITRIC ACID), BETA CAROTENE FOR COLOR (CORN OIL, TOCOPHEROL), VITAMIN A PALMITATE], DRIED DAIRY BLEND [WHEY, CALCIUM CASEINATE, SALT, WATER), HONEY BOURBON DIPPING SAUCE (WATER, HONEY BOURBON DIP MIX [BROWN SUGAR, SUGAR, FRUCTOSE, CORN SYRUP SOLIDS, MOLASSES SOLIDS, MALTODEXTRIN, CARAMEL COLOR, SPICES, GARLIC POWDER, ONION POWDER, TETRAPOTASSIUM PYROPHOSPHATE, CITRIC ACID, ARTIFICIAL BOURBON FLAVOR (WITH RICE OIL, NATURAL SMOKE FLAVOR), HONEY, NATURAL FLAVORS, BOURBON WHISKEY, MODIFIED CORN STARCH, HONEY, SALT, METHYLCELLULOSE, XANTHAN GUM, NATURAL FLAVORS, DRIED EGG YOLKS), CORN, SAUCE (WATER, SUGAR, MARGARINE [SOYBEAN OIL, PARTIALLY HYDROGENATED SOYBEAN OIL, WATER, SALT, WHEY, SOY LECITHIN, MONO AND DIGLYCERIDES, NATURAL FLAVOR, BETA CAROTENE (COLOR), VITAMIN A PALMITATE], SALT, PARTIALLY HYDROGENATED SOYBEAN OIL WITH TBHQ AND CITRIC ACID AS PRESERVATIVES). CONTAINS 2% OR LESS OF: MARGARINE (PARTIALLY HYDROGENATED SOYBEAN OIL WITH TBHQ AND CITRIC ACID AS PRESERVATIVES, WATER, MONO AND DIGLYCERIDES [BHT, CITRIC ACID], BETA CAROTENE FOR COLOR [CORN OIL, TOCOPHEROL], VITAMIN A PALMITATE).

Photos by Michael Poteshman

As you can see, these seemingly benign foods that contain carrageenan, sodium caseinate, autolyzed yeast, gelatin, soy protein isolate, among other wonders that I didn't bother highlighting, are not what you thought they were. If manufacturers could only label these foods for what they really were, at least we would have a choice. But now that you have this information, **you do have a choice**!

"NO MSG ADDED" OR "NO MSG"- WHAT'S THE DIFFERENCE?

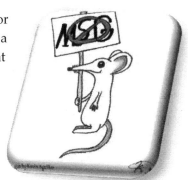

Most of you have seen labels or signs at your local supermarket or at a restaurant that state, "NO MSG ADDED" or "NO MSG." There is a huge difference between the two. The "NO MSG ADDED" only means that pure Monosodium Glutamate wasn't added; hydrolyzed or autolyzed yeast or Caseinate, or other MSG containing ingredients could have been used. [104]   On the other hand, "NO MSG" means that none of these tongue-twisting ingredients including pure MSG were used. [105] Thus, look for "No MSG" labels, as it's much safer.

Now that we know where MSG can be found, let's look at how MSG came to be so widely used.

MSG HISTORY

For centuries, Asian cultures used seaweed called "kombu" to enhance the taste of their dishes. [106] In fact, Kombu was described in a text that was written in 797 AD.[107]

Kombu is usually associated with Japanese dashi soup stock or broth. [108] Our tongues can only sense four primary tastes: sweet, salty, sour, and bitter. "Kombu", whether turned into powder or boiled in broth, provided another taste that's commonly referred to as "umami" or the fifth sense. [109]

In 1908, a Japanese professor isolated the "glutamic acid" out of kombu, which was the component that provided the "umami" flavor.[110] This chemical isolate is also known as MSG or Monosodium Glutamate. Consequently, a multi-billion dollar empire was born. The business was so successful that by 2009 the yearly production of MSG was estimated at two million tons or two billion kilograms; that's over four billion pounds.[111]

The way it has made its way into our food is a story of its own. During World War II, it was discovered that food rations for Japanese soldiers tasted better than rations for American soldiers. [112] It was later discovered that MSG was added to Japanese soldiers' food. In 1948 at a conference, major food manufacturers were introduced to Monosodium Glutamate. [113] [114] MSG was essentially the answer to enhancing the taste of processed foods that were manufactured at the time. As a result, from 1948 all the way through 1968, this substance was added not only to processed foods, but to baby foods.[115] At the time, it was assumed that it was completely safe because it was an amino acid.[116]

In 1957, two ophthalmology residents, Newhouse and Lucas, were conducting a research project where they were studying a degenerative eye disease. [117]As part of the experiment, they fed MSG to newborn mice. They discovered a complete destruction of the nerve cells of the retina of the eyes in these mice; specifically, the visual receptor cells. [118] [119]

In 1968, a neuroscientist, Dr. Olney, used this experiment to study the pathway of the nerve cells from the eyes to the brain. What he found was startling. Not only did MSG destroy the inner layer of the retina, but it destroyed portions of the brain as well. [120] [121]

The damage to the brain resembled the destruction caused by Alzheimer's disease, stroke, as well as hypoglycemia or low blood sugar. [122]

In 1969, Dr. Olney testified at a Congressional hearing about the dangers of MSG. Subsequently, the food industry voluntarily removed MSG from baby food. [123] "But did they really? Instead of adding pure MSG they added a substance known as hydrolyzed vegetable protein that contains three known excitotoxins and has added MSG." (Blaylock, 1998). [124]

Congratulations! You made it through quite a complex chapter. We still have one major excitotoxin to examine, and then we're off to other chapters that will be essential in solving the puzzle of Living Wonderfully.

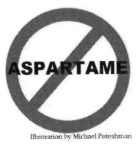

Illustration by Michael Poteshman

*"Regular consumption of artificially sweetened soft drinks is associated with disorders of the metabolic syndrome, including abdominal obesity, insulin resistance and/or impaired glucose tolerance, **dyslipidemia** and high blood pressure."*
(Palmnäs, Cowan, Bomhof, Su, Reimer, Vogel, . . . Shearer, 2014)[125]

Dyslipidemia = elevated LDL (bad cholesterol) or total cholesterol

I want to refresh your memory about my excitotoxin experience that I talked about at the beginning of the book. After I concluded my Pho lunch, I purchased a cup of diet soda in order to put out the crazy tingling sensation in my mouth due to a large consumption of MSG. What I essentially had done is exacerbated my already vulnerable condition. I piled up one excitotoxin on top of another in my already MSG-intoxicated system.

As my diet soda was sweetened with artificial sweetener, it caused additional havoc in my brain. The excruciating headache and disorientation[126] were the contributions from the land of chemistry, or "Aspartame" to be precise!

Because Aspartame and MSG affect the same receptors in the brain, they cause almost identical reaction. [127]

According to the book "Food: Your Miracle Medicine" by Jean Carper, more than 50% of the University of Florida study participants had an increase in migraine frequency after consuming Aspartame. Some experienced symptoms such as reduced vision, dizziness, and instability.[128] These results mimicked mine precisely.

*"Aspartame is a widely used artificial sweetener that has been linked to pediatric and adolescent migraines. Upon ingestion, aspartame is broken, converted, and oxidized into **formaldehyde** in various tissues."*
(Jacob & Stechschulte, 2008)[129]

Formaldehyde = associated with various types of cancer not only in humans but in animals; also an extreme irritant to mucous membranes.[130]

Headaches, disorientation, diminished vision, high blood pressure, impaired glucose tolerance, and shakiness, are not the only symptoms. According to Dr. Mercola, Aspartame hampers diagnoses as it mimics a slew of other ailments such as Alzheimer's disease, Arthritis, Depression, Diabetes, Parkinson's disease, Multiple Sclerosis, among others.[131]

ARTIFICIAL SWEETENERS LINK TO WEIGHT GAIN AND OTHER DISEASES

"Aspartame consumption is implicated in the development of obesity and metabolic disease despite the intention of limiting caloric intake"
(Palmnäs, Cowan, Bomhof, Su, Reimer, Vogel, . . . Shearer, 2014)[132]

What is the primary reason for people drinking diet beverages or eating foods that are sweetened with Aspartame? It is perhaps because there is the word "Diet" on the label. Diet means low in calories or no calories at all." In theory this sounds logical, but is it really? Well, not really. According to the Department of Molecular, Cellular and Developmental Biology at Yale University, there is a connection between the use of artificial sweeteners and weight gain.[133] Not only that, but **artificial sweeteners induce sugar dependence and cravings**. [134]

A study from Purdue University uncovered that drinking sodas with artificial sweeteners (Aspartame, sucralose, and saccharin) was linked to health problems such as **obesity, type 2 diabetes, metabolic syndrome, and cardio vascular disease**.[135] Even when a number of studies were compared, the results were similar:

*"Findings from a variety of studies show that routine consumption of diet sodas, even **one per day**, can be connected to higher likelihood of **heart disease, stroke, diabetes, metabolic syndrome and high blood pressure**, in addition to contributing to **weight gain**."*
(Patterson Neubert, 2013)[136]

In her research, Susan E. Swithers, a professor of behavioral neuroscience at Purdue University, outlined that people who consumed artificially sweetened beverages, **doubled their risk of metabolic syndrome** compared to those who did not consume such beverages. [137] Metabolic syndrome is a disorder of the way your body utilizes energy and storage. This disorder multiplies the risks for cardiovascular disease, stroke, and diabetes.

*"At least daily consumption of diet soda was associated with a 36% greater relative risk of incident metabolic syndrome and a **67% greater relative risk of incident type 2 diabetes** compared with nonconsumption…"*
(Nettleton, Lutsey, Wang, Lima, Michos, & Jacobs, 2009)[138]

The bottom line is that Aspartame may mimic a slew of symptoms as outlined in the previous section. Also, Aspartame, sucralose, and saccharin may be contributing to a bigger waistline in addition to a number of serious diseases as the studies consistently show. [139] [140] [141] [142]

ASPARTAME AND CANCER

A study that was published in the *Environmental Health Perspectives Journal*, as well as in the National Institutes of Health (NIH) publication, outlined the carcinogenic effects of Aspartame.[143] The 7-year, $1,000,000 study was conducted at the European Ramazzini Foundation of Oncology and Environmental Sciences in Italy. [144] Over 1,900 rats were used in the experiment.[145] This sizable study was conclusive in outlining that consumption of Aspartame may cause cancer. [146]

A study published in the National Center for Biotechnology Information of NIH, demonstrates that when Aspartame exposure began during "fetal life", the carcinogenic (cancer) effects are amplified.[147] Depending on dosage of Aspartame used, the results pointed to a significant increase in lymphomas/leukemia in both male and female rats, and mammary (breast) cancer in females.[148]

Should There Be Warning Labels?

So, why are there no warning labels on soft drinks or any other foods or beverages that contain Aspartame? The answer could be much simpler than we may think. The economic impact of aspartame is huge!

"Food companies and consumers around the world bought about $570 million worth of it last year. New regulatory action on Aspartame would also jeopardize the billions of dollars' worth of products sold with it."
(Warner, 2006)[149]

Although it is common knowledge that excitotoxins such as MSG, Aspartame, and others may be harmful, this stuff is still included in many products without warning labels. In all fairness, there are profits and jobs at stake. If this stuff were suddenly removed, a number of food conglomerates built around this substance would suffer greatly, and many people would end up jobless. This is one of the reasons that I try my best not to name any of the processed food manufacturers, restaurants, or fast food chains that use this substance on a daily basis. The good news is that some companies are switching voluntarily to less controversial sweeteners.[150]

I was not the only one who suffered from the effects of Aspartame. Some of the members of my family, including my younger son, did as well. Once this artificial sweetener, as well as MSG, were eliminated from his diet, he stopped having migraine headaches.

How to Avoid This Stuff

As with MSG, the PubChem database, a government web site of the U.S. National Library of Medicine, lists over **160** alternative names or synonyms for Aspartame. [151] Without going into all of them, here are some examples in no particular order:[152]

- NutraSweet
- Canderel
- Methyl Aspartylphenylalanine
- Tri-Sweet
- L-Aspartyl-L-phenylalanine methyl ester
- Dipeptide sweetener
- UNII-Z0H242BBR1
- CCRIS 5456
- Sanecta
- Pal Sweet
- Spectrum2_001706
- BR-47609
- J-502447

In order to avoid Aspartame, read labels very carefully, and question every food choice you make, especially processed foods. All of the sudden, some of the <u>unexplained ailments</u> that you have experienced may just fade away.

I hope that with time, as the trend of "Living Wonderfully" catches on, it will force food producers to practice truth in labeling. I want consumers to decide what we should buy and what we should avoid by just reading a label without hidden names. The good news is that the state of California is considering adding cancer warning labels to products containing Aspartame.[153]

Now that we're finished with the excitotoxin section, we're on to learning about foods that contributed to my former declining health. Indeed, the next section may be considered controversial by some.

SECTION 3. WHAT NOT TO EAT: FOODS TO AVOID

Although there are many foods and food ingredients that we've learned to love and enjoy since we were kids, some may not be beneficial to our health. A number of these foods are truly detrimental. They not only wreak havoc on our system, but literally shorten our lifespan.

This section is one of the most essential, as every item that is outlined below affected my health and the health of my family in a very harmful way. I addressed only the most significant "not to eat" food items to the fullest, as I wanted to alleviate concerns, doubts, and excuse-making. Everything in the forthcoming sections is supported by tangible evidence and studies.

Chapter 4 SUGAR

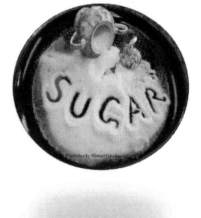

When I was in 11th grade, my social sciences teacher posted a list of different food items on the board. The food items included roast beef, baked chicken, bread, saltine crackers, and a chocolate candy bar. He then asked the class a thought-provoking question, "If you were allowed to eat only one out of these food items, which one would you pick?" He supplied each student with a small piece of paper, and we had to write our answers anonymously. Towards the end of class the teacher tallied up the results. Even though I was only 17, the outcome was not surprising. Over 80% of students picked the candy bar. The next highest number was the saltine crackers, followed by bread. After the teacher read the results, he said that every time he performed this experiment, the outcome was roughly the same, since sugar to a human being is almost <u>like a drug and just as addictive</u>.

You may be wondering what I picked. I was indeed an anomaly, as I picked beef, although my first impulse was to select the option of candy bar. After the class was over, I forgot about this experiment because at the time I worked at an ice cream shop. I actually made it a point to replace my meals with free ice cream during all of my shifts. I have an excuse for this stupid behavior. I didn't know, nor did I care. The sad part is that I completely disregarded this experiment and everything that I knew or read about sugar for the next 30 years.

We really love sugar, not only in the United States, but all over the world. There is an explanation for this phenomenon. It all stems from evolution. The scientific community is claiming that we crave sugar instinctively as our taste has evolved for survival,[154] that is for quick calories, energy, etc. As Dr. Lustig, Professor of Pediatrics at UCSF pointed out, *"When you taste something that's sweet, it's an evolutionary Darwinian signal that this is a safe food…We were born this way"* (Lustig, 2012). [155]

How many times have we heard from one source or another that sugar was not just bad, but very addictive? I've always dismissed these commentaries because I thought, how could one be addicted to sugar? After all, it's not a drug. It's not alcohol or nicotine. It is just sugar that's legal and is sold in every store. So I ate candy, cake, candy bars, doughnuts, and other wonderfully delicious items to my heart's content. Sound familiar?

I recall good times when my kids were trick-or-treating on Halloween. I would eat at least half a dozen of my favorite chocolate candy bars and chase them with diet soda without any problems. It was during my early forties when I began to get headaches after ingesting items that were high in sugar. Although I was aware of this problem, I was craving sugar like there was no tomorrow. So instead of having a whole candy bar at a time, I would divide it in half in order to lessen the severity of headaches. In other words, I was so hooked on sugar that even though I still had headaches, I couldn't eliminate it from my diet. That was until I began my research into Living Wonderfully.

WHY THE ADDICTION?

During the first two weeks of my efforts of trying to get healthy, I usually had the most incredible sugar cravings towards the evening. Unaware of the effects of sugar I know now, I went to the usual places where we kept sweets, but couldn't find any. My wife had purged all of the chocolate, cookies, and candies from the house in order to prevent me from sabotaging my new healthy way of life. I had no idea what exactly was happening to me, but I began to rummage around anywhere and everywhere I could for anything that was sweet. I can only describe my actions as something reminiscent of a drug addict. I literally foraged through every drawer, and when I couldn't find anything sweet, I went to look in my car. Sadly, I found an old piece of candy that fell between the passenger seat and the center console.

Illustration by Kevin Aquilino

With great difficulty, I separated the candy from its stuck-on wrapper. I proceeded to eat this stale piece of something that resembled candy, but lacked smell or flavor. Instead, it only had the flavorless sweet taste because of the years it had been in the car. "Aaaaahhhhh", was the sound that emanated from my mouth when I finally consumed this piece of sugar.

Why did this happen to me? Why would a sane and logical person jump through hoops in order to get his hands on a stale piece of sugar? The explanation is simple. Just like millions of people around the world, I had a sugar addiction. You may be asking if the addiction is real. I can assure you that it's not just real, but exceedingly powerful, as studies consistently show![156] [157]

"It turns out sugar is much more addictive than I think we had sort of realized early on… Sugar activates our brain in a special way. That's very reminiscent of drugs like cocaine."
(Stice, Ph.D., 2012). [158] [159]

According to an article published by the Department of Psychology at Princeton University, sugar dependence was observed through a study of rats that were fed syrup alongside food and water for 12 hours each day.[160] After one month of study, when sugar was removed and then re-introduced, rats showed signs of behavior that occurs after the use of addictive drugs such as morphine, cocaine, etc.

"…'bingeing,' meaning unusually large bouts of intake, opiate-like 'withdrawal' indicated by signs of anxiety, and behavioral depression, and 'craving' measured during sugar abstinence was enhanced responding for sugar"
(Avena, Rada, & Hoebel, 2008).[161]

Eric Stice, Ph.D., a neuroscientist at the Oregon Research Institute, has conducted a non-invasive MRI scanning of the human brain while exposed to sugar, specifically to a "tiny sip of soda." As soon as the soda made contact with the tongue of the human test subject, an increased blood flow was detected in the <u>reward regions of the brain</u>. [162] Furthermore, dopamine was being released in the same manner as if the brain was exposed to <u>alcoholic substances or drugs</u>. [163] When interviewed by Dr. Sanjay Gupta of CBS' 60 Minutes, Dr. Stice explained that by scanning hundreds of people, he discovered that those who ate sweets such as ice cream or other sweet foods, or drank sodas, may **build tolerance to sugar in the same way as drug addicts build tolerance to addictive drugs**.

The more you eat or over-eat sweets, the more tolerance you build. <u>The result is the continuous craving due to dulling of the reward region in the brain.</u>[164]

This was the reason why in the middle of the night I rummaged around my home and in the car in order to find and eat a disgusting piece of stale candy.

SUGAR AND THE HEART

As the old rhyme goes, "Sugar is the thing that makes your heart sing." Knowing what I know now, I have to counter this rhyme with a rhyme of my own, "Sugar is the thing that makes your arteries stick, making your heart sick."
A groundbreaking study by nutritional biologist, Kimber Stanhope, illustrated that calories from added sugar were associated with an increased risk of cardiac disease and stroke only **two weeks** into the experiment.[165]
Furthermore, it was proven that calories from different types of sugar are not the same as what we get from other foods.

"The subjects who consumed high fructose corn syrup had increased blood levels of LDL cholesterol and other risk factors for cardio vascular disease… within two weeks"
(Stanhope, 2012). [166]

When a person consumes foods loaded with "sweet stuff", their liver tries to metabolize as much fructose as it can, but some of the excess gets converted into fat. This transformed fat enters the bloodstream and gets converted into "Small Dense LDL Cholesterol,"[167] [168] which is the most dangerous type of cholesterol. It lodges in your arteries and forms plaque, which is connected to cases of coronary heart disease[169] and heart attacks.

That was alarming, wasn't it? Not as frightening as what is coming up next.

CANCER FERTILIZER

Until I began my research, I had no clue that added sugar had anything to do with cancer or other diseases. It was only when I stumbled upon the 1966 lecture of Otto Warburg, German medical doctor and Nobel Prize winner, that I began to understand the ravages of sugar on the human body. In his study, Dr. Warburg discovered that **cancer cell growth largely depended on sugar.** [170] [171]

Moving on to the present day. Lewis Cantley, Ph.D., a Harvard Professor, and the head of the Cancer Center, pointed out that when sugar is consumed, a spike in the production of Insulin can serve as the mechanism to fertilize a number of cancer types such as breast, colon, among others. [172] It is done through "Insulin receptors" that are located on cancer cells or tumors. Insulin attaches to these receptors, thereby allowing the tumor to begin using glucose for its growth,[173] literally fertilizing these cancer cells.

There are other examples that show how sugar feeds cancer cells and/or cancer tumors, but I believe that the example above paints a very sobering picture. The knowledge of this helped me "kick" my sugar addiction. As this is the book for Living Wonderfully, there is good news!

Studies show that when you limit your sugar intake, your chances for developing cancer are decreased. [174] [175]

If you thought that cancer fertilization is bad, then, as they say in television advertisements, "But wait, there's more!" Indeed, there is a lot more, and it only gets more frightening from here.

SUGAR IS SUGAR IS SUGAR IS SUGAR

I know that I will rattle a lot of cages and irritate a lot of people with this section, but it has to be done. This book is about getting you out of health predicaments similar to what I experienced, and to maintain your good health for the rest of your life. So, grit your teeth; here it comes.

Every time I meet people and start talking about sugar, I hear similar responses. "I know that sugar is really bad for you, but we use honey to sweeten our teas and desserts." "Sugar is really bad for you and honey has a lot of sugar. So we don't use honey, instead we use Agave sweetener because it's not as high in sugar." "I don't use refined table sugar, instead I use natural brown sugar because it's much better than processed sugar." The following excuse is my favorite, "We don't use sugar so we sweeten everything with fruit juices, and instead of sodas we only drink fruit juice."

Some of these excuses are from people who are genuinely oblivious to the effects of sugar in all forms. After all, the information that they get is from televised commercials and advertisements, which by their nature, promote consumption of their products. Some excuses are essentially myths, justifications, and rationalization for the "denials" from people who really want to continue to consume sugar. All I have to say is that I completely understand. I know all about these excuses, because I gave exactly the same justifications over the years, as I desperately wanted to hold onto the sweet and wonderful sensation of sugar. Here's the cold and hard reality, whether we like it or not:

"The body is unable to distinguish between natural sugar found in fruit, honey, or milk, and processed sugar from sugar cane or beet."
(BBC Science, 2013)[176]

Thus, when the body processes sugars, whether obtained from fruit juice, honey, agave-processed sweetener, brown sugar, high fructose corn syrup, or refined white sugar, the results are almost identical. When you consistently ingest these types of sugars, you create a blood sugar imbalance. As sugar hits your digestive system, the pancreas releases the hormone Insulin in order to regulate the glucose that's going to your organs, your muscles, and your brain. The problem is that the more sugar you ingest, the more Insulin will be produced.

This also applies to a <u>high carbohydrate diet</u> as your body very quickly converts carbs to glucose. When Insulin levels remain high, or your pancreas produces continuous Insulin spikes in order to regulate glucose, your body develops Insulin resistance.[177] Such resistance contributes to additional production of Insulin and the downward spiral continues through **heart disease, obesity, diabetes, high blood pressure, strokes, liver disease, and other serious ailments**.[178]

Insulin is not bad. If it's produced in normal amounts, it's actually beneficial. The goodness of Insulin prevents us from dying of glucose intoxication.[179] If it weren't for Insulin, our brain and organs would starve because it influences our organs to absorb glucose that's in our blood.[180] So **the problem is not Insulin but too much Insulin**. We will be discussing this critical subject in "THE MOST POWERFUL COMMON DENOMINATOR" chapter later in the book. For now, keep in mind that when your Insulin levels continue to remain high, **your body begins to use carbs and sugars for energy instead of stored fat**.[181]

PREMATURE AGING

Getting old because of age? Think again. If what we already discussed about sugar hasn't fazed you, I'm certain that a majority of people will take this particular section seriously. Since first impressions come from our appearance, premature aging is not something that any of us desire. What does sugar have to do with aging of the skin? Studies have shown that it's not completely the sun's fault, as sugar is just as much to blame for wrinkles, if not more.

The process known as "Glycation" or production of "Glycotoxins" is responsible for the damage to your skin.[182]

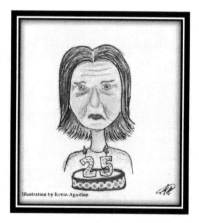

Illustration by Kevin Aguillon

What happens is simple. Sugar that you consume in the form of desserts, foods loaded with carbohydrates, or <u>any foods with a high glycemic index</u>,[b] turn into glucose in your body. Once that happens, the glucose or blood sugar attaches itself to skin protein molecules.[183] [184] As a result, the new destructive AGE or Advanced Glycation End-products, or as they're commonly called, Glycotoxins, are formed.

"It's particularly sour news that the skin proteins most susceptible to glycation are collagen and elastin, the same ones that make a youthful complexion so plump and springy"
(ShapeMagazine, 2013).[185]

Therefore, the more sugar you consume, the more AGEs or glycotoxins are formed. That causes additional damage to your skin proteins that "become stiff and malformed"[186] and not only cause wrinkles, but saggy skin.

The interesting fact is that glycation not only ages your skin, but contributes to other aging conditions such as macular degeneration, cataracts, diabetes, Alzheimer's disease, and atherosclerosis, among others. [187] [188]

Essentially, you don't just age on the outside, you age from the inside out when consuming sugar or any foods that are high on the glycemic scale, which we will discuss in the next chapter.

THE COMPARISON WITH CONSEQUENCES: WHAT ARE THESE SUGAR TYPES?

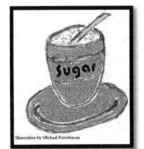

I never knew, or had any interest in learning about different types of sugar. After all, to me, they were sweet and delicious. My eyes were truly opened when I learned why and how these sugar types affected my health. Let's first look at major sugar types:

- **Sucrose** is your everyday table sugar. It is produced mostly from sugar cane or beets. Sucrose occurs naturally in honey, sugar maple sap, dates, etc. [189] It consists of 50% fructose and 50% glucose.[190] Approximately 30% of the world's sugar comes from beets and 70% from sugar cane.[191]
- **Fructose** is found predominantly in fruits, honey, agave, syrups, etc.[192] **High fructose corn syrup or HFCS**, for example, is extracted from corn, and comes in a variety of compositions of fructose and glucose. "The composition of HFCS-55 (55% fructose and 42% glucose) is very similar to that of sucrose (50% fructose and 50% glucose)..." (Storey, Ph.D, 2007).[193]
- **Glucose** is also known as dextrose and is found in fruits, honey, and syrups, just as with fructose. Glucose circulates in the blood of humans and higher animal species, hence the name "blood sugar." It is used in the form of energy, and is absorbed into the blood stream during digestion. It plays an important role in regulating metabolism.[194]

---

[b] Glycemic Index is a chart that shows how certain foods convert to blood sugar (glucose) inside the human body. The glycemic index goes from 0 to 100. **The higher the number, the quicker food converts to sugar**. For example, one slice of white bread is 68, while one cup of bean sprouts is 25. Thus, bread converts a lot faster to blood sugar than bean sprouts. More on the Glycemic Index subject in the next chapter.

The main difference, without going into chemical formulas, is that sucrose is made of two molecules, fructose and glucose.[195] Both fructose and glucose are made of a single sugar molecule,[196] or what we call, simple sugar. If you didn't get that, no problem, as you will learn in the next section if one type of sugar is better than the other.

One thing to remember is that **sucrose (table sugar) triggers production of Insulin**. Fructose in its purest form does not trigger the release of Insulin,[197] but is sent to the liver to get metabolized.

"It is important to understand that fructose does not increase Insulin levels, which is not necessarily good as what it does do is radically increase Insulin resistance, which is FAR more dangerous."
(Mercola, 2010) [198]

IS ONE TYPE OF SUGAR BETTER THAN ANOTHER?

As to which sugar type is better for you, just look at the "Nutrition Facts" labels below and on the next page and judge for yourself, now that you know how your body will react to it. I obtained the majority of these nutrition facts labels from our local supermarket.

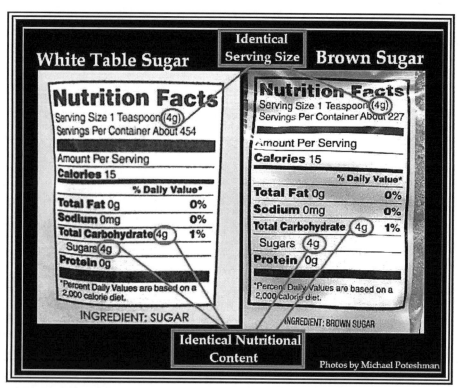

As you can see in the illustration above, the white table sugar and brown sugar are identical. The difference is that brown sugar contains molasses in its native state. Sometimes caramel colors and/or molasses are added back in to make the sugar brown.[199] White sugar is essentially brown sugar with molasses removed.

Although people believe that honey is good for you because it's all natural, the "good for you" part may not be the entire story. As you can see on the photograph below, it is very high in sugar and carbohydrates.

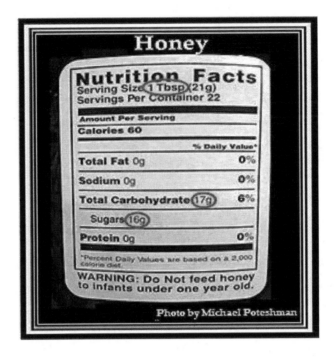

Indeed, honey has beneficial qualities such as antioxidant, antifungal, and antibacterial, but the sugar types that honey possesses are reminiscent of those found in <u>corn syrup</u>. Keep in mind that although honey is a natural product, **it contains high amounts of glucose, fructose, and sucrose**, among other sugars. The fact is, "Sugar accounts for 95–99% of honey…"(Olaitan, Adeleke, Ola, 2007).[200]

*"Honey is a mixture of sugars and other compounds. Related to carbohydrates, honey is mainly fructose (about 38.5%) and glucose (about 31.0%), making it **similar to the synthetically produced inverted sugar syrup**, which is approximately 48% fructose, 47% glucose, and 5% sucrose."*
(Nutritionistic, 2013). [201]

A study entitled, "Consumption of Honey, Sucrose, and High-Fructose Corn Syrup Produces Similar Metabolic Effects in Glucose-Tolerant and -Intolerant Individuals" shows that **body reacts similarly when eating honey, or high fructose corn syrup, or even table sugar**.[202]

Notwithstanding the beneficial elements of honey, as we discussed earlier, direct metabolization by your liver is certain. The extra fructose gets converted into "Small Dense LDL Cholesterol", which is the most dangerous type of cholesterol. It lodges in your arteries and forms plaque, which is connected to cases of coronary heart disease[203] and heart attacks.

If we look at the label of High Fructose Corn Syrup (HFCS) below,[204] we can clearly see that carbohydrate content is almost as high as in honey, but sugars are lower.

Although HFCS is an "isolate" developed in the lab where the extraction of sugar from corn takes place, your body processes it similarly to all other sugars. Some believe that HFCS is really bad for you; some believe it's just like sugar. **Bottom line is that your body processes HFCS in practically the same manner as any other fructose and sucrose products**. In addition, as you saw in the comparison example above, the HFCS comes in a variety of mixtures of fructose and glucose, such as 55% fructose and 42% glucose, etc.[205]

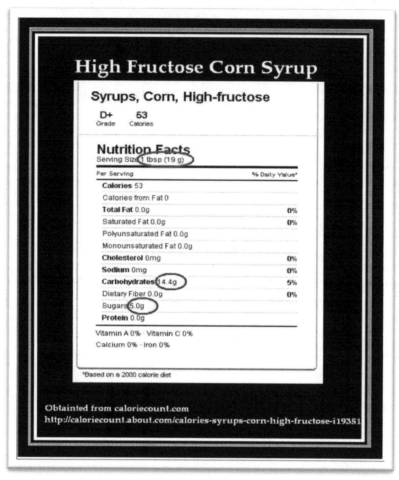

Finally, there is "Agave", with a whopping 16 grams of sugar and 16 grams of carbohydrates per tablespoon, as in the photo below.

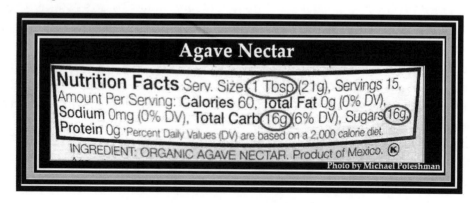

Some believe that agave is a much better sweetener because it is absorbed by your body much more slowly, and therefore does not spike your sugar level in the same way as other sweeteners. Certain people believe that this processed product is a hoax perpetrated upon gullible health conscious people who want to stay fit.

Dr. J. Bowden, PhD., assessed the health value of agave sweetener as "…basically high-fructose corn syrup masquerading as a health food" (Bowden, 2010).[206]

"The American Diabetes Association lists agave as a sweetener to limit, along with regular table sugar, brown sugar, honey, maple syrup, and all other sugars"(Horton, 2014).[207] Furthermore, agave sweetener or "nectar" contains as much as 90 percent fructose which is much higher than what is in high fructose corn syrup. [208] Remember the discussion at the beginning of the sugar segment where the consumption of fructose caused Insulin resistance as well as bad LDL cholesterol to skyrocket, causing heart disease? As such, I will conclude this agave sweetener discussion with the following quote: "*Agave syrup is almost all fructose, highly processed sugar with great marketing*", said Dr. Ingrid Kohlstadt, a faculty member at Johns Hopkins School of Public Health" (Bowden, 2010).[209]

FRUIT JUICES OR WHOLE FRUIT

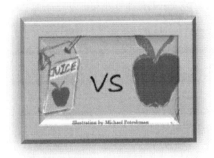

Do you want the good news or the bad news first? I'll give you the bad news first, so that you will be left with good news at the end of this section.

After reading the previous section, you are already aware of what fructose does to your body. Fruit juices primarily contain fructose or fruit sugar and some Vitamin content. Remember that the body treats fructose from high fructose corn syrup and fruit juices in the same manner. Now comes the "but, but, but…" part that I hear every time I talk about juices. "But the fruit juices are full of Vitamins. How can you say that juice is full of sugar? After all, it is a natural sugar that was derived from fruit!"

This is an absolutely correct assessment. Juice is indeed derived from fruits. The difference is in the absorption rate. When you eat fruit whole, the fiber that's in the fruit helps to counteract the typical fast sugar absorption. In other words, **the sugar in fruits is intracellular or is contained within the cells of the fruit, which gets extracted by your digestive system, hence slower digestion.** On the other hand, when you drink a glass of fruit juice, it is precisely the same if not worse than drinking a can of soda as shown in the illustration below, because the fiber has been taken out.

If we look at the label comparison on the next page, the 8 oz. (240 ml) cup of orange juice on the left contains roughly the same amount of sugar as the soda in the center. Continuing with the apple juice nutrition facts on the right, we see a more extreme comparison, as the **8 oz. (240 ml) cup of apple juice actually contains more sugar than the soda in the center**.

The sad part is that my wife and I used to drink this stuff and give it to our kids daily with their lunches at school. Wouldn't this be a recipe for hyperactivity, you may ask? Indeed it might. But we were fortunate that our kids were enrolled in numerous sporting programs after school, and they were able to burn a lot of that sugar.

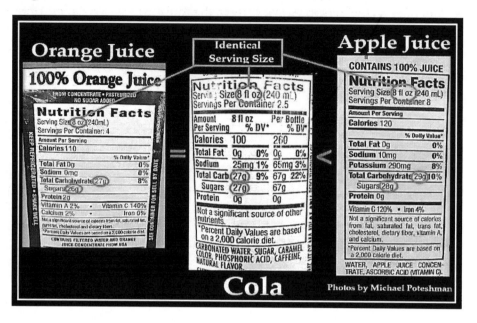

Photos by Michael Poteshman

"These sugars produce a rapid increase in blood glucose levels because they enter the bloodstream so quickly. A child may become more active due to an adrenaline rush produced by this blood sugar spike."
(WebMD, 2014)[210]

As promised, now for the good news. Who said that you can't compare apples and oranges? Well, we can, but only for the sugar and fiber content level as indicated in the picture below.

Looking at apple and orange nutrition information[211] below, we can clearly see that the content of carbohydrates and sugars is quite high.

One Medium Orange	One Large Apple
TotalCarbohydrates...... 19g	Total Carbohydrates..... 34g
Sugars........................14g	Sugars........................ 25g
Dietary fiber...................3g	Dietary fiber....................5g

Nutritional information obtained from:
http://www.fda.gov/Food/IngredientsPackagingLabeling/LabelingNutrition/ucm063482.htm

Illustration by Michael Poteshman

What is different is that dietary fiber sets those fruits apart from juices. "…whole fruits and vegetables also have healthy fiber, which is lost during most juicing." (Nelson, 2014)[212]

It is this dietary fiber which is absent in most of the juices, that keeps you fuller longer. Finally, there is a matter of quantity. How many apples or oranges can a person eat at one time? Well, some people may eat a lot, but they would be in the minority. Depending on the size, it may take two to four oranges to make a cup of juice. That's a lot of sugar!

So, the next time you're with your friends or relatives, and one of them decides to show his or her knowledge when it comes to differences among sugar types, and which are better for you, you will be able to explain that sugar is sugar, no matter in what form it is presented.

Now that you're aware of what sugar is and what it does to your system, we will look at other harms that it can inflict on your body.

THE MYTH OF HONEY AND ORANGE JUICE TO FIGHT COLDS

I couldn't present this short section at the beginning of this chapter because, in most likelihood, you would have booted me out of the room, or in this case, closed the book. I believe that you're now ready for this eye-opener.

Research published in The American Journal of Clinical Nutrition shows that simple sugars can greatly impair your immune system by hindering white cells from destroying foreign bacteria or microorganisms.[213] After I read this research, I understood why I couldn't get rid of "everlasting" colds and allergies.

Besides sucrose, fructose, and glucose, <u>sugar in honey and orange juice</u> are responsible for **"significantly"** **decreasing the capacity of white blood cells to "engulf" bacteria**,[214] thereby impairing the immune system.

Unfortunately, when I had my never-ending colds, I was told to drink orange juice. To add an insult to injury, I followed traditional wisdom, and drank hot tea with honey. The saddest part of this whole situation is that <u>this research has been available to doctors since 1973</u>. Yet, instead of telling my family not to drink sweet beverages and not to consume simple-carb foods, my family was told by doctors to drink orange juice to fight colds, which actually leads to another big problem.

HYPOGLYCEMIA

Hypoglycemia is a term for low blood sugar. Some scientists believe that hypoglycemia is better described as "unstable blood sugar levels."[215] Let's first look at how hypoglycemia is created in healthy or moderately healthy people who don't suffer from diabetes. "This happens in non-diabetic hypoglycemia when the body produces too much Insulin called hyperInsulinism." (Plesman, 2011)[216]

After a person consumes a meal containing high amounts of sugars <u>and/or carbohydrates</u>, blood sugar naturally rises. Once that happens, the pancreas begins to produce Insulin in order to distribute the glucose to all of the organs. Without assistance from Insulin, glucose cannot be absorbed by most of the cells in your body. **The problem arises when more sugar or carbs than required by the body are consumed, resulting in overproduction of Insulin** in order to normalize the amount of glucose in the system. Consequently, because of this overproduction, the blood sugar level drops, resulting in hypoglycemia. That's when something that you've never expected begins to rear its ugly head.

While your body has the ability to utilize energy from fats and indirectly from proteins, your brain uses glucose as its main source of energy. **Hypoglycemia literally starves your brain.**

"When there is a overproduction of Insulin, as is the case in hypoglycemia, the brain will be starved of its source of energy – glucose"
(Plesman, 2011).[217]

Most of the time you won't even notice that hypoglycemia is upon you unless you're having dizzy spells, weakness, heart palpitations, faintness, anxiety, and/or other symptoms.[218] But what happens is very real, as happened to me numerous times.

The consistent rise and fall in the supply of glucose to the brain inevitably affects **your emotional state, your mood, and even your personality**.[219] [220]

The following is hypoglycemia in the making. You eat a couple of slices of pizza, or a big plate of pasta, or even a nice 12 inch sub. You chase this meal with sugary soda. After you finish your meal, you begin to crave sugar, so you eat dessert. The **overproduction of Insulin** occurs due to a rapid conversion of simple carbs in pasta or pizza that you just ate, into blood sugar. As a result, hypoglycemia rears its ugly head. More likely than not, you're still having a sugar craving, so you decide to eat a piece of fruit because consciously you know that sugar in dessert is bad for you.

Unfortunately, you have already consumed too much sugar and simple carbohydrates, and additional fruit just adds more fructose to an already taxed system. **Your body tries to deal with this onslaught by rapidly lowering the glucose level again, with more Insulin.** Then, in about a half hour to an hour, you begin to rummage around again for something sweet, almost as if you were in a drug induced state. The vicious cycle continues through instability in your glucose or hypoglycemia. I just described my actions when I was "Living Dead." I believe that you can recall several episodes from your life when it came to mindless snacking on candy, ice cream, pretzels, chocolates, cookies, or other types of almost foods. Additional causes of hypoglycemia can be found in **Appendix 1** at the end of the book.

Now that you made it through the sugar chapter, let's look at another "Not to Eat" food source where hypoglycemia could be lurking.

Chapter 5 WHEAT

WE LOVE WHEAT!

I've been eating breads, pasta, muffins, doughnuts, cookies, crackers, and other wonderfully delicious foods most of my life. When I got married over 29 years ago, there was a low-fat craze where everyone and their mother was saying that fat was very bad for you because it caused heart attacks. So, my new bride, being a health conscious person that she is, began to research foods with low-fat content. The majority of the foods that she found were wheat based. As a result, we loaded our pantry with "fat-free" pasta, low-fat English muffins, low-fat bagels, cereals, fat-free crackers, and other "stuff" that we deemed healthy according to nutritional experts, doctors, and fat-free alarmists on television.

We also looked at the government food pyramid that advocated breads, cereals and carbohydrate products as the biggest part of the daily allowance. Because we didn't know better, my wife and I regarded ourselves as being smart and frugal, as wheat products were much cheaper than other food items. We were saving a ton of money on our grocery bill and believed that we were eating super healthy foods.

What we had to show for our extremely low-fat, seemingly "healthy" diet is that we began to put on incredible amounts of weight in a very short time. We both blew up like balloons. There were also some adverse health reactions such as an astronomical increase in blood pressure which I never experienced before in my life, as well as elevated blood sugar. We began to cut our portions, but that wasn't helping much. That's when our diet roller coaster began, which we will talk about in later chapters. It wasn't until 20 years later that we grasped the sobering reality that wheat, among other undesirable foods, was literally ruining our health.

WHOLE GRAIN VS THE REFINED STUFF

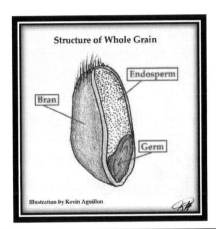

Structure of Whole Grain

Endosperm

Bran

Germ

Illustration by Kevin Aguillon

Let's look at whole grain bread as opposed to something that may say "wheat" on the label. The difference is huge. While "average" white or wheat breads are practically the same on the glycemic index scale, [221] as will be described in subsequent sections, whole grain bread is different. Besides wheat, different types of grains such as buckwheat, millet, quinoa, etc. may be used. Also, the big difference is whether or not the grain was refined. The refining of the grain means **taking out the germ and bran** that contain the most amount of iron, B Vitamins, among other nutrients, minerals, and fiber.[222] [223]

What is left is the endosperm that accounts for the bulk of the seed, which is almost pure starch, and contains very small amounts of nutrients. [224]

After the refining is complete, the flour will have longer shelf life and will have a finer texture. [225] In a nutshell, **that's what goes into your standard wheat bread, pastas, doughnuts, pizza, pretzels, crackers,** and other stuff we love. Unless you immediately exercise, products that are made with refined wheat flour, in many cases, add inches to your waistline because they quickly convert to glucose or blood sugar. Unless you burn this "high octane fuel" quickly by running a marathon, for example, **it turns into fat**. That was one of the big reasons that my wife and I used to put on incredible amount of weight despite our never ending diets and exercise.

BREAD IS A STAPLE FOOD! WHY THE NEGATIVITY?

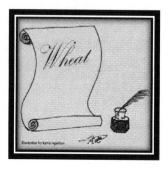

When I start talking to people about the dangers of wheat products, someone always says, "Wheat has been mentioned in the Bible, and wheat bread goes back many centuries. Why is it suddenly so bad for you?"

This is a very good question, and I've been asking that same question myself while doing research for this book.

Indeed, wheat has been a staple food throughout history. Not only that, but some cultures have regarded wheat as sacred. For example, Roman and Greek mythology talk about wheat deities. We know that wheat is an ancient grain that has been around and well respected for almost as long as humans have been on earth. It is undeniable. What changed?

The answer is quite simple. The "daily bread" of today may look somewhat like the bread that was mentioned in the Bible or that was used by our ancestors even a century ago, but it's hardly the same. The wheat of today has been genetically modified from the original "einkorn" wild grass that fed Mesopotamians and other cultures 10,000 years ago.[226] Modern wheat is different and has properties that are poles apart from its ancestor, einkorn.

Through cross-breeding, genetic modification, and "intentional hybridization", by the 1960s and 1970s wheat production had increased by 35%.[227] The dough became pliable, and the bread became lighter and more delicious, a far cry from what our ancestors had to eat. Science didn't stop as modern genetic modifications continued to move forward. The end result is the modern plant known as "semi-dwarf wheat".[228] According to an article published in the Chicago Tribune, Dr. William Davis, cardiologist and author of the book "Wheat Belly", modern wheat possesses destructive properties to a multitude of body functions.[229] He also believes that over 80% of people would benefit from abstaining from wheat; including whole wheat.[230]

Dr. David Perlmutter, a neurologist and author of the book "Grain Brain" has observed through his case studies, that by eliminating gluten, which happens to be a protein in wheat, rye, and barley from people's diets, a multitude of health problems were eradicated.

"I've watched this single dietary shift lift depression, relieve chronic fatigue, reverse type 2 diabetes, extinguish obsessive-compulsive behavior, and cure many neurological challenges, from brain fog to bipolar disorder."
- David Perlmutter, MD- [231]

We will now look at some disconcerting aspects of wheat that may be even more convincing.

WHEAT AND GLYCEMIC INDEX

As food sustains our lives, the evolution of how we digest food comes down to two simple principles. According to the Glycemic Research Institute, **the body has to make a decision to either store food for survival in the form of fat or use the food as energy**.[232] Therefore, the type of food that you consume will determine what your body will do with it.

The evolution of a famine survival instinct is hard wired into us from the day we're born. Therefore, by default, **your body wants to store anything you put in your mouth as fat.** [233]

Foods that are quickly digested and processed by your body for storage generally have the highest glycemic index. [234] Low glycemic foods induce slower release of glucose into your bloodstream because they're metabolized by your body much more slowly. Anything you eat or drink can fall into categories of low, moderate, or high glycemic food items.

In a nutshell, Glycemic Index or GI is a measurement of how fast the glucose or blood sugar rises after a person eats a particular food item.

The glycemic index is a numbering system that looks at how different foods affect the rise of blood sugar level and compares this to the consumption of pure glucose, which has the GI or Glycemic Index of 100. [235] In other words, foods with carbohydrates that break down rapidly into glucose during digestion carry a higher number, while foods that break down gradually result in a slower release of glucose into the blood stream, thus carrying a lower number.

The glycemic index is divided into three categories: [236]
- **High – between 60 and 100** [237] - Wheat or white bread, baked potato, rice, table sugar, etc.
- **Moderate – between 45 and 60** [238] - Carrots, bananas, orange, brown rice, etc.
- **Low – below 45** [239] - Bean sprouts, almonds, peanuts, etc.

Let's compare glycemic index numbers of several foods, as shown in the example below: [240] [241]

Food	GI
Glucose	100
Baked potato (1 Medium or 150g.)	82
White bread - wheat flour (1 slice or 30 g.)	71
Table sugar (2 tsp. or 8.4g.)	63
Quinoa, cooked (1 cup or 150g.)	53
Kidney beans, boiled (1 cup or 150g.)	28
Peanuts (1oz. or 30g.)	18

Based on Data from Glycemic Index and Glycemic Load *Oregon State University Micronutrient Information Center* http://lpi.oregonstate.edu/mic/food-beverages/glycemic-index-glycemic-load#table-1 and Glycemic index and International GI database | *Human Nutrition Unit, School of Molecular Bioscience, University of Sydney* http://www.glycemicindex.com/foodSearch.php

When I first viewed this comparison, I was stunned. If you look at the chart above, white/wheat bread actually has a higher glycemic index than sucrose or table sugar. Recall from the "Sugar" chapter, the type of damage sugar inflicts on your system. Specifically, sugar spikes Insulin levels, leads to development of hypoglycemia, Insulin resistance, etc. **According to the glycemic index, white bread is broken down very quickly and converted into glucose in your body much like sugar, only faster**.

What is the difference between eating a spoonful of sugar and a piece of white or wheat bread? Besides taste, your body will treat bread and sugar in practically the same way!

Perhaps you're about to ask, "How about darker color wheat bread? Doesn't it have lower GI?" No, it doesn't, unless it possesses ingredients such as cracked kernels, nuts, seeds, or other **fibrous** elements that resist quick digestion. Even if you're having whole grain wheat or wheat bread with addition of better grains, <u>wheat should not be on the menu</u> because of its toxic properties as you will read in the next two sections.

WHEAT ADDICTION

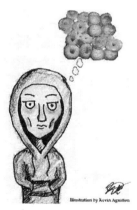

Is it possible to be addicted to modern wheat? Who knew that something as benign as my "ex-favorite" breads, pastas, and other wheat products could actually be addictive? There is evidence that a lot of people suffer withdrawal symptoms when they remove wheat from their diet. I have to say that when I removed wheat from my diet I had cravings galore, especially for carbs.

So what's in the wheat that could make it so addictive? The answer lies in a protein that is contained in wheat: Gliadin.

Illustration by Kevin Aguillon

"Gliadin has the potential to bind to the opiate receptors in the human brain just like heroin, just like morphine…"
(Davis, 2012).[242]

The fascinating thing about the effect of gliadin is that it does not give you the same feeling of "euphoria or pain relief" that you get from addictive drugs. Gliadin just stimulates your appetite so you are prone to consuming more carbohydrates such as breads, cookies, pasta, cake, pretzels, etc.[243]

Because I loved pizza so much, it was quite difficult for me to quit wheat. Where could you buy a whole grain pizza devoid of wheat, containing only quinoa or buckwheat dough? Nowhere! No matter; I had to forego wheat because I knew what it was doing to my body.

So I gave it up, and for the first five days of abstaining from wheat products, my cravings became quite severe. I developed withdrawal symptoms that manifested into irritability, bloating, and anxiety. I wanted to eat every "miserable" food that contained carbs and sugar. Luckily, I knew what was coming when I was giving up this stuff. My expected withdrawal symptoms were practically textbook accurate.[244]

Although my irritability was heightened, especially on the second and third day of abstaining from wheat products, the good news is that while eating the right foods as will be described in the "**WHAT TO EAT**" section later in the book, my wheat cravings completely subsided within a week. Those were a difficult seven days, at times, almost unbearable, but I made it! I no longer crave wheat. Not only that, but my entire family is wheat free.

If you experience withdrawal symptoms after you quit wheat, don't succumb to wanting to have a small piece of bagel or a little spaghetti just to feel contented. It's like a drug addict taking a little cocaine, crack, or other drugs to feel a little better. [245]

Withdrawal is actually good because the body is telling you that you're hooked on this stuff and within a few days you will rid your body and mind of this dependence. [246]

Now that you know exactly what to expect, your journey of abstaining from wheat will be easier.

You may wonder if I still like pizza. Yes I do, but not as much. I tasted pizza recently and in comparison to my awesome meals, the bread part of the pizza had a pasty feel. This is not what I remember when I was gobbling pizza at least three times a week. Because my body is now "clean", I no longer crave bad carbs, like pizza dough that's made out of wheat. So, for those rare occasions when my kids want something different, I make pizza at home from grain-free-gluten-free-wheat-free dough, as seen in the recipe section later in the book.

TOXIC WHEAT

As I kept researching wheat, I uncovered more and more frightening information. The unpleasant surprises were coming out of the woodwork. For example, the definition from an unbiased source piqued my interest. An online medical dictionary had such an intense description for gliadin that my jaw literally dropped:

"gliadin /gli·a·din/ (-din) a protein present in wheat; it contains the toxic factor associated with celiac disease"
(Medical-Dictionary, 2005).[247]

Why didn't I see this 10 years ago? I guess I wasn't interested. We now know that the gliadin in wheat may bind to your opiate receptors and thereby cause addiction. Furthermore, the dictionary defines gliadin as the "toxic factor" associated with celiac disease. Keep in mind that gliadin is a component of gluten. Speaking of gluten:

"Celiac disease is a digestive disease that damages the small intestine and interferes with absorption of nutrients from food. People who have celiac disease cannot tolerate gluten, a protein in wheat, rye, and barley."
(NIH, 2011).[248]

In a nutshell, the body reacts to gluten by attacking its own lining of the small intestine.[249] Once the lining is damaged or destroyed, the body cannot absorb nutrients, leading to a slew of health problems such as osteoporosis, diabetes, anemia, intestinal cancer, and Thyroid disease, among others.[250]

Sometimes you may not even know that you have celiac disease or gluten sensitivity as many people do. The problem is that unless you're directly diagnosed with gluten sensitivity, you never know if wheat is responsible for your ailments. Celiac disease can be diagnosed by conducting a test and looking for antibodies that are celiac disease specific.[251] On the other hand, **it is difficult, and in most cases impossible**

to diagnose if you have a gliadin/gluten sensitivity or reaction. The reason for that is a lot of laboratories only test for one of the wheat proteins.[252] So, even if you are gluten sensitive, you may test negative to this one protein.

"There's no accepted medical test for gluten sensitivity."
(Kam, 2013)[253]

Unfortunately, 30-35 percent of people are gluten sensitive without even knowing it.[254] You may be one of them. The problem with this scenario is that the longer you are exposed to gluten, the more adverse health reactions and autoimmune diseases will continue to develop.[255] So, if there aren't any credible tests for gluten sensitivity, how do we know if we're sensitive to gluten?

Let's look at some of the symptoms associated with gluten sensitivity. Keeping in mind that symptoms vary from person to person.

The symptoms may include chronic inflammation,[256] depressed mood, suicidal thoughts, headaches or migraine pain, angry outbursts, joint pain, fatigue, sluggishness, difficulty concentrating, brain fog, diarrhea, abdominal pains, and cramps or discomfort.[257] [258] Furthermore, gluten sensitive people can develop "...**neuro-psychiatric disorders such as autism, schizophrenia, and depression**." (Lionetti, E., Leonardi, S., Franzonello, C., Mancardi, M., Ruggieri, M., & Catassi, C., 2015)[259]

"Cereal grains contain "anti-nutrients," such as wheat gluten and wheat lectin, that in humans can elicit dysfunction and disease."
(Punder, K. D., & Pruimboom, L., 2013)[260]

Although I was never tested for celiac disease or gluten sensitivity, some of the indicators outlined above have matched symptoms that I experienced. Since eliminating wheat from my diet, I no longer have any of these symptoms.

Perhaps you're wondering about gluten free spaghetti, bread, and other products with gluten removed. The answer is quite simple; the foods that had gluten removed are processed even more, so the nutritional value is further diminished.[261] Not only that, but gluten-free products may contain trace amounts of gluten, which may not be helpful if you suffer from celiac disease[262] or gluten sensitivity.

Furthermore, a lot of the processed gluten free foods are made with preservatives, sugars, and refined oils.[263] Isn't that an interesting phenomenon? As you're trying to eat healthier, you may be eating processed foods that will be further spiking your Insulin levels. Thus, we're back to Insulin resistance, fat retention, and a slew of other problems that manifest as an outcome of Insulin overproduction.

The bottom line, whether you are gluten sensitive or not, genetically modified wheat contains gliadin. I don't have to go any further because by now you know what it's capable of doing to your body. I believe that the following short quote will sum it up:

"Modern wheat is a perfect chronic poison."
- Dr. William Davis -

Once I explain to people what happens to their bodies after wheat consumption, people say "But, isn't whole grain bread better than just whole wheat bread? I still want bread."

Indeed, a lot of people are hooked on wheat or they just love the texture of bread. How can you make a sandwich without bread? I know that you can make lettuce or cabbage wraps, but is there a way to eat bread without the wheat in it? Yes, there certainly is.

As indicated earlier, keep in mind that whole grain bread does not have to contain only whole wheat or any wheat at all. Instead, it can be made by using the "better" gluten-free stuff: millet, buckwheat, quinoa, flaxseeds; also ingredients that do not contain any grain such as almond flour, coconut flour, and even sprouted beans. Although not all whole grains are created equal, they are classified as complex carbohydrates. This is not an "all-you-can-eat bonanza", as even whole grain bread is processed to some extent. Therefore, whole grain bread, depending on its content and glycemic index, may not be as good for you as you think. As far as whole grain bread is concerned, practice extreme moderation.

Keep in mind, even "good" whole grains convert to blood sugar faster than the cruciferous raw vegetables, meats, or nuts.

If you don't want to make bread yourself by using the aforementioned grains, start reading labels very carefully. There are a slew of whole grain breads in practically every store, but the labels can be quite deceiving. The labels may say "Whole Grain", but this can be misleading according to a Harvard School of Public Health (HSPH).[264] The industry's standard "Whole Grain Stamp" actually identified products that were higher in calories and sugar than those that did not have such a stamp.[265]

The last thing you want is added sugar or other stuff that may stimulate Insulin production. The manufacturer wants to make food taste better so you continue to purchase their delicious product. Can we blame the manufacturer if there aren't specific guidelines? Not really.

Scrutinize the nutrition facts, the ingredient list, and anything about the "healthy" products that you are about to purchase and put into your mouth. Seemingly healthy products could not only jeopardize, but even derail your journey to "Living Wonderfully." So, read the labels!

The next item is a true first place challenger of "FOODS TO AVOID":

Chapter 6 HYDROGENATED OIL OR TRANS-FAT

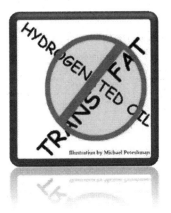

Since honesty is my number one policy, I will get this out of the way first: "Guilty as charged for not only consuming hydrogenated oil myself, but feeding it to my children!" How many **peanut butter** and jelly sandwiches have I made for my kids' lunches? How many times have we gone to a fast food establishment to have fries with our meal? And how many times have we eaten fried chicken, crackers, cookies, popcorn, or even donuts that were loaded with hydrogenated oils? I remember serving a major brand of hot chocolate to my kids, and drinking coffee with creamer that was laden with this stuff. Although not all products as described above contain hydrogenated oils, a great number do. Unfortunately, in the not so distant past I failed to read the labels.

So, why did I include products containing hydrogenated oils on "the not to eat" list? This stuff is quite dangerous and even devastating to your health!

By now you may want to "call me out" on the painful peanut butter subject. I say this because every time I explain to people about hydrogenated oils in peanut butter, I get the same reaction, "What's wrong with my peanut butter? I've been eating this brand since I was a child, and peanut butter is healthy!" "I give it to my kid because it's the only thing that he'll eat." I will fully explain what peanut butter has to do with hydrogenated oils later in this segment. I'm certain that after you finish this section, in all probability, you will not be purchasing peanut butter with hydrogenated oils, let alone any product that's loaded with this "almost food."

Hydrogenated oil is also known as trans-fat. The trans-fat transformation is achieved by adding hydrogen gas to oil. The oil can be vegetable, cottonseed, or soybean, among others. This process is called hydrogenation, hence hydrogenated oil. In order to fuse oil with hydrogen gas, the monosaturated fats are transferred into trans-fats by heating oil and hydrogen gas to high temperatures. As the hydrogen gas is pumped into the oil at high pressure, the catalyst or reactive insoluble metal atoms such as nickel, palladium, and depending on the application, even platinum, are introduced.[266] [267] Without these metals, it would be impossible to fuse hydrogen with oil. The end result is a saturated or trans-fat product that contains molecules that are completely transformed from their initial state. As a result, the stiffness and tackiness of these transformed molecules prevent separation of the product, resulting in extended shelf life by preventing spoilage or rancidity. Essentially, the trans-fats extend shelf life of the products they are added to.[268]

TRANS-FATS AND CHRONIC DISEASES

Why are trans-fatty acids or TFA's bad for you? For one, they promote <u>systematic inflammation in your body while **blocking** chemical mechanisms that battle such inflammation</u>.[269] In addition, they raise bad cholesterol or LDL, and lower good cholesterol or HDL, leading to chronic diseases such as stroke, diabetes, heart disease, etc.[270]

A study of "Trans fatty acids: effects on cardio-metabolic health and implications for policy" concluded that "In both observational cohort studies and randomized clinical trials, TFA adversely affect lipid profiles (including raising LDL and triglyceride levels, and reducing HDL levels), systemic inflammation…" (Micha & Mozaffarian, 2008).[271]

One of the reasons for such phenomenon is that **Trans-fats contribute to Insulin resistance**,[272] but <u>without any consumption of sugar</u>.

TRANS-FATS AND CANCER

Heart disease, strokes, Insulin resistance, and other ailments are only the beginning of the ravages inflicted on the human body by man-made hydrogenated oil. How about this for a headline?

"Trans-fats linked to breast cancer risk in study"
(Reuters, 2008). [273]

The study found that women with a high concentration of trans-fats in their blood have **twice the risk of breast cancer** as women whose trans-fat blood levels were the lowest. [274]

TRANS-FATS, DEPRESSION, AND HEART DISEASE

On March 10, 2011, ABC News revealed a European study that linked trans-fats to depression.[275] The study included 12,000 men and women who were tracked for six years. During that time their mental health, lifestyle, overall health, and diet were tracked. The study revealed that those with a higher intake of "man-made trans-fats" had a 48% greater chance of being diagnosed with depression than those who were consuming less.[276] Researchers who conducted the experiment believed that depression was caused by chronic inflammation as in the cases of heart disease, strokes, etc.[277] Furthermore, people who were evaluated for higher risk of depression consumed trans fats that were "less than 1% of their total calories" (Sass, 2011). [278] As you can see, even a negligible amount of trans-fat is unsafe.

"The daily intake of about 5 g of trans fat is associated with a 25 percent increase in the risk of ischemic heart disease"
(Stender, Dyerberg & Astrup, 2006).[279]

Does this statistic scare you as much as it scared my wife and me? I hope it does. We began by being very discriminating about the foods we were purchasing. The good news is that this "almost food" product is easily avoidable.

KNOWING WHAT TO LOOK FOR

When you go shopping, make certain to read labels carefully as they are a bit tricky. You may find foods that have 0 grams of trans-fat on the Nutrition Facts chart, but the list of ingredients may include partially hydrogenated or hydrogenated oil.

"Because products containing less than 0.5 grams of trans fat per serving can be labeled as having 0 grams trans fat, checking the Ingredient List is important to avoid all artificial trans fat."
(CDC, 2014).[280]

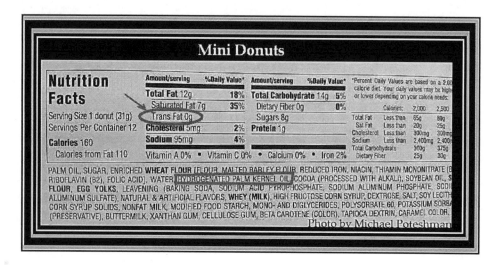

Photo by Michael Poteshman

The picture above clearly stated 0 trans-fat in the Nutrition Facts chart, but look at the list of ingredients. Be very careful with purchasing such products, and especially feeding them to your kids.

How do we avoid these foods? We simply read the labels. As you can see in the examples below and on the next page, some of the ingredients resemble a chemical lab experiment instead of foods or beverages that are fit for human consumption

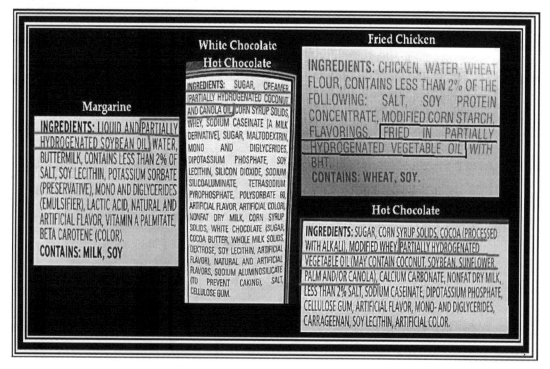

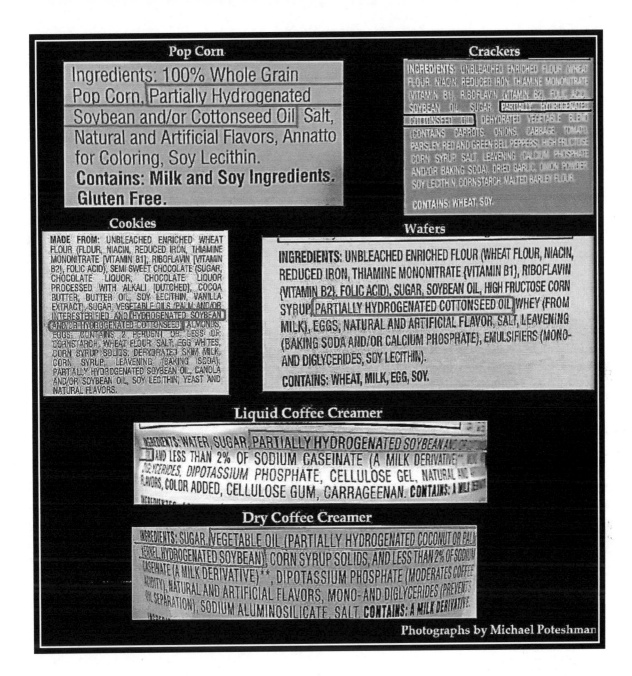

Pop Corn

Ingredients: 100% Whole Grain Pop Corn, Partially Hydrogenated Soybean and/or Cottonseed Oil, Salt, Natural and Artificial Flavors, Annatto for Coloring, Soy Lecithin.
Contains: Milk and Soy Ingredients. Gluten Free.

Crackers

INGREDIENTS: UNBLEACHED ENRICHED FLOUR (WHEAT FLOUR, NIACIN, REDUCED IRON, THIAMINE MONONITRATE (VITAMIN B1), RIBOFLAVIN (VITAMIN B2), FOLIC ACID), SOYBEAN OIL, SUGAR, PARTIALLY HYDROGENATED COTTONSEED OIL, DEHYDRATED VEGETABLE BLEND (CONTAINS CARROTS, ONIONS, CABBAGE, TOMATO, PARSLEY, RED AND GREEN BELL PEPPERS), HIGH FRUCTOSE CORN SYRUP, SALT, LEAVENING (CALCIUM PHOSPHATE AND/OR BAKING SODA), DRIED GARLIC, ONION POWDER, SOY LECITHIN, CORNSTARCH, MALTED BARLEY FLOUR.

CONTAINS: WHEAT, SOY.

Cookies

MADE FROM: UNBLEACHED ENRICHED WHEAT FLOUR (FLOUR, NIACIN, REDUCED IRON, THIAMINE MONONITRATE [VITAMIN B1], RIBOFLAVIN [VITAMIN B2], FOLIC ACID), SEMI-SWEET CHOCOLATE (SUGAR, CHOCOLATE LIQUOR, CHOCOLATE LIQUOR PROCESSED WITH ALKALI [DUTCHED], COCOA BUTTER, BUTTER OIL, SOY LECITHIN, VANILLA EXTRACT), SUGAR, VEGETABLE OILS (PALM AND/OR INTERESTERIFIED AND HYDROGENATED SOYBEAN AND/OR HYDROGENATED COTTONSEED) ALMONDS, EGGS, CONTAINS 2 PERCENT OR LESS: OF CORNSTARCH, WHEAT FLOUR, SALT, EGG WHITES, CORN SYRUP SOLIDS, DEHYDRATED SKIM MILK, CORN SYRUP, LEAVENING (BAKING SODA), PARTIALLY HYDROGENATED SOYBEAN OIL, CANOLA AND/OR SOYBEAN OIL, SOY LECITHIN, YEAST AND NATURAL FLAVORS.

Wafers

INGREDIENTS: UNBLEACHED ENRICHED FLOUR (WHEAT FLOUR, NIACIN, REDUCED IRON, THIAMINE MONONITRATE {VITAMIN B1}, RIBOFLAVIN {VITAMIN B2}, FOLIC ACID), SUGAR, SOYBEAN OIL, HIGH FRUCTOSE CORN SYRUP, PARTIALLY HYDROGENATED COTTONSEED OIL, WHEY (FROM MILK), EGGS, NATURAL AND ARTIFICIAL FLAVOR, SALT, LEAVENING (BAKING SODA AND/OR CALCIUM PHOSPHATE), EMULSIFIERS (MONO- AND DIGLYCERIDES, SOY LECITHIN).

CONTAINS: WHEAT, MILK, EGG, SOY.

Liquid Coffee Creamer

INGREDIENTS: WATER, SUGAR, PARTIALLY HYDROGENATED SOYBEAN AND ... AND LESS THAN 2% OF SODIUM CASEINATE (A MILK DERIVATIVE)... ...GLYCERIDES, DIPOTASSIUM PHOSPHATE, CELLULOSE GEL, NATURAL ... FLAVORS, COLOR ADDED, CELLULOSE GUM, CARRAGEENAN. CONTAINS: A MILK ...

Dry Coffee Creamer

INGREDIENTS: SUGAR, VEGETABLE OIL (PARTIALLY HYDROGENATED COCONUT OR PALM KERNEL, HYDROGENATED SOYBEAN), CORN SYRUP SOLIDS, AND LESS THAN 2% OF SODIUM CASEINATE (A MILK DERIVATIVE)**, DIPOTASSIUM PHOSPHATE (MODERATES COFFEE ACIDITY), NATURAL AND ARTIFICIAL FLAVORS, MONO- AND DIGLYCERIDES (PREVENTS OIL SEPARATION), SODIUM ALUMINOSILICATE, SALT. CONTAINS: A MILK DERIVATIVE.

Photographs by Michael Poteshman

The photos above truly pay tribute to the wonders of modern science. Does the science lab have a place on your kitchen table? Not on mine!

Even though the ingredients are prominently displayed, "Why didn't I see any of this for decades?" Perhaps you're asking yourself the same question right about now.

As promised at the beginning of this section, I'm going to rekindle the discussion about peanut butter. Now that you know about the hydrogenation process and what it does to your body, I believe that you may be more receptive to what I'm about to say. The majority of peanut butter brands include oil that's been hydrogenated or partially hydrogenated in order for the product not to separate, and remain solid or partially solid at room temperature. Peanut butter that has no added hydrogenated oil and has not been emulsified has natural separation of peanuts on the bottom and oil on top. The photo on the previous page represents what "real" peanut butter should look like, as nature intended.

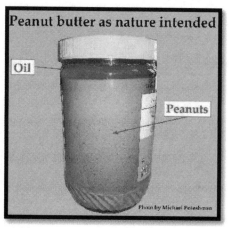

The next time you're shopping for peanut butter at a supermarket, you will notice labels as illustrated below. You may have these peanut butter concoctions in your pantry now:

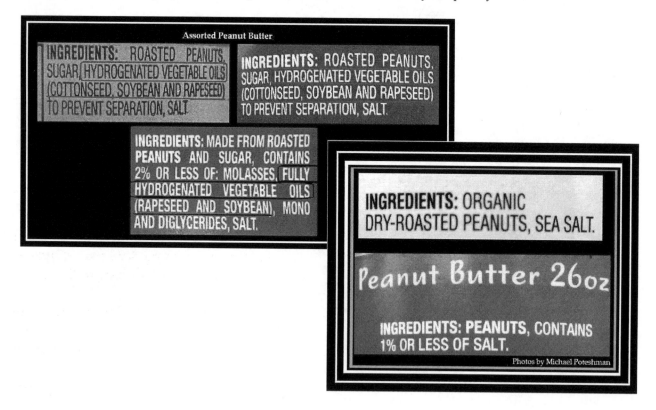

As you can see in the photos above on the left, different jars of peanut butter contain several types of hydrogenated oils. Some may contain partially hydrogenated oil instead of fully hydrogenated as above. Luckily, there is another option that's available in every store, and it is peanut butter without hydrogenated oils, as in the photograph above on the lower right. These products have only one or two ingredients, as they should.

When I uncovered the truth behind hydrogenation, the first thing I did was throw out the remaining peanut butter that we had in the refrigerator. I then purchased the "real" stuff with just two ingredients as in the photos above.

When I brought it home, it had this pesky problem of oil/peanut separation because it contained no hydrogenated oils or emulsifiers. It took a little time to stir the separated peanut oil into the peanut butter, but it was worth it.

When my wife served it to our younger son, the first words out of his mouth were, "What is this stuff? It's not even sweet!" My wife explained to him that this is what real peanut butter is supposed to taste like, and to give it a try for a couple of weeks. We also explained about the hydrogenation process of how this "stuff" is made and what it could do to his body. Interestingly, our son decided to use sliced bananas for sweetness, and has never asked for peanut butter with hydrogenated oils again.

One last point before we conclude this section. When you go to any food establishment, especially fast food restaurants, more likely than not you may be served foods that are prepared with trans-fat. I'm not against eating out; we just need to be vigilant when it comes to what we put in our body. So, don't be shy when questioning the kitchen staff no matter what restaurant you frequent.

Chapter 7 DAIRY

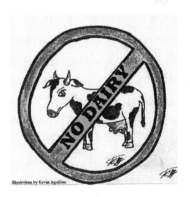

Illustration by Kevin Aguillon

About six years prior to this writing, my wife and I were invited to our friend's house for dinner. After having a nice meal, the hosts served coffee. As my wife was adding milk to her cup, one of the guests, who happened to be a registered nurse, asked my wife if she was aware that drinking milk was "not exactly good for you". My wife and I stared at one another in disbelief. I think that at that time we were both thinking, "What kind of weird question was that?" My wife responded by saying that she wasn't aware of such studies where milk would be bad for you, especially skim milk that contains calcium without any fat. The nurse countered by saying that she was aware of numerous studies that linked milk to health problems and diseases. Furthermore, she said that she would not give cow's milk to her small children because it will affect their health in a negative way in the future. Although both my wife and I disagreed with the lady's opinion, we respectfully listened to her "horrors of milk" stories. We changed the subject the very first chance we got.

As we were driving home from the party, we came to a conclusion that even though we were impressed with the lady's conviction concerning negative effects of milk, we thought that her outlook on dairy products was a bit extreme and even strange. After all, who wants to hear something adverse about a product that you've known all your life as good for you and almost sacred because of your ancestors' precious guidance. Hence, we completely dismissed what she had to say until this research - six years later…

At first I was leery about even starting the research on milk. Since childhood, I was taught that milk is good for you. I remember what my mother and grandmother always used to say, "When you drink milk, you will have strong bones and teeth." Besides that, the television ads and print showcased "Milk does a body good", "Body by milk", or "Got milk?" campaigns. So I was conditioned to not only blindly enjoy milk, but to respect this product for its calcium content and medicinal properties.

As I began to plow through dairy research, a wealth of articles and huge scientific studies were popping up everywhere. These studies revealed sobering evidence when it came to the consumption of milk.

I'm aware that what I'm about to tell you may seem controversial, because milk is as American as apple pie. Nonetheless, I will not tread lightly, as I only present facts. The reason behind such confidence is that every word that you're about to read is backed by scientific evidence that even made my receding hair stand up.

MILK AND BONES

"The higher the dairy consumption, the higher the rate of osteoporosis; the exact opposite of what dairy industry has been telling us for so long."
- T. Colin Campbell, Ph.D. - [281]

A 12-year large scale study on milk and osteoporotic fractures was published in the *American Journal of Public Health*. This study was conducted on a whopping **77,761** women between the ages of 34 and 59, and concluded that drinking milk in higher quantities does not reduce the risk of osteoporotic fractures.[282] Osteoporosis is a progressive bone disease that causes weakening, hollowing, or brittle bones, and may be referred to as "porous bones"[283] as shown in the picture below.

The study also showed that women who drank two or more glasses of milk per day were at a higher risk of having hip and forearm fractures compared to those who drank only one glass of milk per week or less.[284]

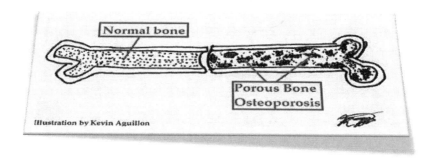

Illustration by Kevin Aguillon

Essentially, the more milk you drink the higher the risk of having osteoporotic fractures. How's that for making your bones strong?

The study was concluded with the following: "These data do not support the hypothesis that higher consumption of milk or other food sources of calcium by adult women protects against hip or forearm fractures." (Feskanich, Willett, Stampfer, Colditz, 1997).[285] What does that mean? It means that drinking milk in larger quantities did not strengthen or protect bones, but actually weakened them by increasing the risk of fractures.

I was stunned, so I had no other choice but to dig around some more in order to find out the reasoning behind bone destruction when consuming dairy. Unfortunately the study above did not address this phenomenon, as it only outlined the negative consequences of drinking milk. What I found was shocking, to say the least. Once I began to go through documentation about the destructive properties of milk, my biases and preconceptions about dairy vanished into thin air. I believe that yours will too.

HOW DOES MILK CAUSE BONES TO WEAKEN?

What causes your bones to weaken, especially when you drink large quantities of milk as outlined in the study above? When you consume milk, your body reacts to Casein, the main protein in milk. As a result of ingesting this animal protein, your system can become acidic. [286] [287] [288] [289] Because your body is smart and self-regulating, it has no other alternative but to put out this "acid fire." What your body does is extract calcium out of your bones in order to put out the fire or counteract the acidic conditions that animal protein has created. [290] [291] [292] Thus, when the calcium is extracted out of the bones in order to neutralize the acid, it causes bones to weaken or increases the risk of fractures. [293]

Here's a sobering conclusion of an Australian study entitled "Case-control study of risk factors for hip fractures in the elderly":

"Consumption of dairy products, particularly at age 20 years, was associated with an increased risk of hip fracture in old age"
(Cumming & Klineberg, 1994). [294]

I was truly surprised to see that the Australian research echoed the rest of the studies. The reason behind my surprise is that unlike U.S. dairy farmers, Australian milk producers are prohibited from using growth hormones or BST/Bovine Somatotropin hormone in order to stimulate milk production. [295] In the past, I thought that hormones and other chemicals were partially responsible for "acidosis", but I was wrong. What this means is **if you drink milk without any added hormones or organic milk, the results are identical**.

DAIRY, GEOGRAPHICALLY SPEAKING

The preceding information prompted me to look deeper into the correlation between hip fractures and geography. I stumbled upon yet another study called "Epidemiology of hip fracture: Worldwide geographic variation." Another Wow!

There is no coincidence that most fractures are experienced by people in countries that consume the most amounts of dairy products: Norway, Netherlands, Austria, Hungary, and Sweden, among other European nations. United States also topped the list, as its population is one of the highest in the world. Meanwhile, populations of Africa and Asia experienced the least hip fractures. [296]

You are correct in assuming that people on these two continents consume the least amount of dairy products. Additionally, the countries listed as the highest in bone fractures have some of the highest consumption and production of cheese.

What is cheese anyway? Technically speaking, cheese is a coagulation of the milk protein – Casein. [297] Keep in mind that **it takes ten parts of milk in order to end up with one part cheese. [298] That's a lot of Casein!**

If you think that what you just read is chilling,   there is much more.

CAN DRINKING MILK REALLY CAUSE CANCER?

"Milk may not grow strong bones, but it does seem to grow cancer cells. Milk increases the hormone called IGF-1 or Insulin-like growth factor, one that is like Miracle-Gro for cancer cells. Dairy products have been linked to prostate cancer"
(Hyman, 2013). [299]

In order to increase milk production in cows, the Recombinant Bovine Somatotropin (rbST) - a synthetic growth hormone is injected into an animal. The way it works is simple. When a cow is injected, the "rbST" raises milk production by increasing the levels of yet another hormone which is called IGF-1 or Insulin-like growth factor.[300] [301] Although some studies link rbST to cancer, others are inconclusive. The rbST still remains controversial for its potential carcinogenic effects.

When I began to read research about milk and calcium, I could not, in a million years, believe that my "ex-beloved" milk had anything to do with cancer. Although in my conscious mind I understood how milk could be causing osteoporosis, subconsciously I did not want to believe that consuming dairy could be linked to life threatening ailments such as cancer. So, I asked myself two questions:

1. "What's in the milk besides "rbST" that's so bad that a person may develop cancer?
2. What if milk is organic and doesn't contain this growth hormone? Can it still be linked to cancer?"

Despite my subconscious reservations, I found my answers in a slew of studies and articles. Hold on to your hats.

LACTOSE AND CANCER

As I sorted through different scientific evidence linking dairy to cancer, I stumbled upon a Swedish study that revealed the strongest evidence linking dairy to ovarian cancer. This was no small study. It was conducted on 61,084 women between the ages of 38 and 76.[302] The study examined the association between ovarian cancer and consumption of dairy products and lactose (sugar in milk).

As researchers examined consumption of lactose, the results became evident. "We observed a positive association between lactose intake and serious ovarian cancer risk" (Larsson, Bergkvist, & Wolk, 2004).[303] Furthermore, women who consumed four or more servings of milk per day had **increased the risk of serious ovarian cancer** than women who drank less than two servings per day. The bottom line: *"Milk was the dairy product with the strongest positive association with serous ovarian cancer"* (Larsson, Bergkvist, & Wolk, 2004). [304] The study went on to conclude: "Our data indicate that high intakes of lactose and dairy products, particularly milk, are associated with an increased risk of **serous ovarian cancer** …" (Larsson, Bergkvist, & Wolk, 2004). [305]

CASEIN AND CANCER

What protein consistently and strongly promoted cancer? Casein, which makes up 87% of cow's milk protein, promoted all stages of the cancer process.
- T. Colin Campbell, Ph.D. -[306]

A study published in "The World Journal of Men's Health" had the following alarming conclusion:

"The milk protein, Casein, promotes the proliferation of prostate cancer cells..."
(Park, S., Kim, J., Kim, Y., Lee, S. J., Lee, S. D., & Chung, M. K., 2014)[307]

Proliferation of cells means the increase of the number of cells. In this case, **the increase of prostate cancer cells**.

T. Colin Campbell, Ph.D., the co-author of the bestselling book, "The China Study" showed a clear connection between dairy, diet, and diseases such as diabetes, cancer, and heart disease, among others.[308] Dr. Campbell and his team conducted a number of studies, one of which involved feeding rats Casein, the main protein found in milk and dairy products. When rats were consuming 20% Casein, the early tumor growth endured, but when the same rats were fed 5% of this dairy protein, the tumor growth got smaller.[309] That's great news! That means that the tumor growth can actually be regulated! [310] That's one of the reasons that my family and I will not touch dairy products.

Note that dairy protein-Casein that may cause osteoporosis, as outlined in the previous section, may also be responsible for cancer growth.

NATURAL HORMONES AND CANCER

As I continued to dig deeper, I discovered more information on what's in milk that may cause cancer. As I was reading a Harvard University article, I had a sudden "aha!" moment. It felt like I should've known this information already, as I understood the science behind milk production, mammary glands, and lactation. I just didn't put two and two together: hormones!

According to the article published in Harvard University Gazette, a physician and scientist at Harvard School of Public Health, Ganmaa Davaasambuu, Ph.D., outlined that there are considerable health dangers posed by hormones in milk. The reason behind such dangers is that milk contains the natural female hormone Estrogen, which is especially concentrated in pregnant cows. [311] [312]

The hormone-dependent cancers such as breast, testicular, and prostate, among others may be linked to consuming dairy products made from cow's milk.[313] [314] [315] [316] [317]

The article also outlined that breast cancer, in particular, has been linked to dairy products such as milk and cheese. [318] [319] [320]

Because cows are either pregnant or have already given birth while being milked, there is a high concentration of Estrogen, the female sex hormone, in milk. [321] [322] Furthermore, the natural Estrogen that is found in cow's milk is **100,000 times more potent** than Estrogen-like compounds found in pesticides. [323]

Dr. Davaasambuu also compared cancer rates in 42 countries. She found that countries like Denmark and Switzerland, where cheese is a national food, had the highest rates of testicular cancer in men between the ages of 20 and 39. [324] [325] [326] In comparison, countries like Algeria, where dairy consumption is low, had the lowest rates. There is a strong correlation between milk and cheese consumption and testicular cancer rates. [327] [328] [329]

Ultimately, this article and several studies that I read, became the convincing "nail in the dairy coffin." My skeptical mind was finally content with the results of my research. I thought that I finally put the dairy issue to rest, but what I found next was equally disturbing.

MILK CONSUMPTION AND ALLERGIES

There are a lot of people who are allergic to milk, and there are some that are lactose intolerant. The difference between lactose intolerance and allergies to milk is vast. Lactose intolerance is when a person is unable to fully or partially digest lactose (milk sugar.) The lactose intolerance symptoms include abdominal pain, gas, bloating, diarrhea, and nausea.[330]

Milk allergies, on the other hand, involve the immune system. What happens after the ingestion of milk or dairy products is that your immune system identifies allergens as harmful and treats them as foreign objects. As a result, you begin to produce the immunoglobulin or (IgE) antibodies in order to neutralize the allergen or milk protein - **Casein**. [331] Casein again? Yes indeed!

Some of the symptoms for these Casein allergies include swelling of the throat, lips, tongue and/or mouth, runny nose, wheezing, hives, skin rash, itching, swelling of the face, and coughing, among other symptoms.[332] People may also experience anaphylactic shock due to the most serious or life threatening allergic reaction called "anaphylaxis." [333]

You may not even be aware that you're allergic to dairy because as you've read above, some of the symptoms may be mimicking other diseases. So, if you have chronic runny nose, for example, quit dairy, and see if the symptom goes away.

DIABETES AND MILK CONSUMPTION

The reason I tackled the subject of allergy in the previous section is to make a point that your immune system treats allergens as harmful foreign proteins. Keeping this in mind, let's look at association between milk and type 1 diabetes. In type 1 diabetes, pancreas does not produce Insulin.[334]

A study from the University of Helsinki, Finland has uncovered that dairy products may trigger type 1 diabetes at an early age. The study is titled, *"Enhanced levels of cow's milk antibodies in infancy in children who develop type 1 diabetes later in childhood."*[335] The study looked at infants who were given formula containing cow's milk. As a result, **infants' immune systems develop antibodies in order to destroy the protein in cow's milk.**[336] **Over time, those same antibodies cross-react and destroy cells in the pancreas that are responsible for producing Insulin.** [337] [338]

The interesting fact about the study is that it pointed out that proteins such as beta-lactoglobulin (BLG) were implicated as risk factor for early-onset of type 1 diabetes. [339] [340]**Those same proteins are absent in human breast milk**, [341] [342] because human breast milk is specifically designed for the human species.

Was that scary or what? Unfortunately while consuming dairy myself and feeding it to my kids, I failed to see the obvious…

WHAT'S WRONG WITH PASTEURIZATION AND HOMOGENIZATION OF MILK?

There is nothing wrong with the Pasteurization and Homogenization processes if you are not aware of what they can do to your body.

As I began my research, headlines like these began to emerge:

- From New York Times – "*Studies Confirm Cholesterol-Heart Attack Link; The Fault in the Milk*"[343]
- From The Weston A. Price Foundation – "*Milk Homogenization & Heart Disease*"[344]
- From US National Library of Medicine National Institutes of Health – "*Milk and other dietary influences on coronary heart disease*"[345]

Just by looking at these and similar headlines, which I did not bother to include, we can determine that somehow milk may be responsible for heart disease.

Let's look at the good and bad aspects of Pasteurization and Homogenization. This will allow you to see a clearer picture, which will make it easier to deal with dairy detractors from the viewpoint of an educated consumer:

PASTEURIZATION

- ❖ The most common method of Pasteurization is heating milk to 161.6°F or 72°C. [346] This process will preserve the shelf life of milk, and it will be able to stay in the refrigerator between two to three weeks without spoiling. [347]
- ❖ I'm certain that you've heard of or seen Ultra Pasteurized Milk, which is basically a method of "sterilization". [348] This process involves heating milk to 275°F or 135°C. The interesting phenomenon is that milk can last between six to nine months. [349]

Bottom line, Pasteurization and Ultra Pasteurization kill many microorganisms, yeasts, molds, and other bacteria in milk that are responsible for spoilage. That sounds good, but there is a caveat. You definitely get milk with a much longer shelf life, but with reduced nutrients, including Vitamin C and enzymes,[350] [351] as the heating process kills some of those as well. Not only that, but as people continue to be exposed to pasteurized milk protein, they may become **more sensitive to allergies**. [352] We already talked about dairy allergies earlier, so I won't go into allergic side effects. We will be revisiting this subject in the "GUT HEALTH" section later in the book.

If the Pasteurization process hasn't fazed you, I believe that what we're about to uncover will.

HOMOGENIZATION

Some of you may remember an old metaphor, "Cream rises to the top". That's what milk fat used to do, in not so distant past. Well, the Homogenization process took care of that. When you go to a store and purchase homogenized milk, even with 4% fat, it will still not rise to the top, but will actually be part of the liquid. How can this be? Fat is lighter than water!

The Homogenization is designed to break up fat molecules at high pressure into extremely small particles, so fat becomes suspended in milk and no longer rises to the top.[353] [354] So, what's the problem of having fat particles suspended in milk? For starters, the homogenization process damages fat molecules. [355]

Donald J. Ross, Ph.D and Kurt Oster, M.D. have conducted research into the Homogenization process, and published a book entitled, "The XO Factor: Homogenized Milk May Cause Your Heart Attack". [356]

According to their book, here's the way it all works. The homogenized milk fat particles or proteins that are usually digested in the stomach can bypass digestion and travel through the bloodstream. [357] The problem with this scenario is these particles also transport a damaging enzyme called Xanthine Oxidase or **XO** through the bloodstream, which can cause damage to the arterial walls, and as time progresses, may develop into heart disease. [358] [359]

Once the arteries are damaged, the human body has a mechanism for healing injured areas, sort of like applying a bandage to a finger cut. In this case, the bandage is in the form of plaque that consists of cholesterol, fat, calcium, among other elements found in blood. Once the arterial walls are inflamed or damaged, the body coats the damage with plague or as many people like to say, cholesterol.[360] As we continue to inflict damage by eating "almost foods" and drinking destructive beverages, the body will continue to accumulate plaque in order to combat additional inflammation. The end result is narrowing of the arteries, [361] and heart disease begins to rear its ugly head.

I have one more thing to add before ending this chapter. Cow's milk is the most perfect, nutritious, delicious, nourishing, and beneficial food for calves! You draw your own conclusion if it's fit for human consumption.

Chapter 8 NITRATES AND NITRITES

I come from a family and culture where the word "salami" is synonymous with the word "happiness." As such, in the past I ate "delicious" processed meats as much as possible. So, what do processed meats have to do with nitrates and nitrites? A whole lot!

Sodium Nitrate is a salty preservative used in processed meats, fish, bacon, hot dogs, salami,

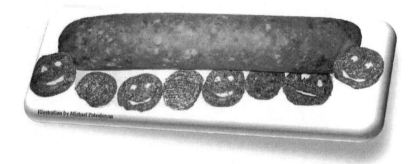

Illustration by Michael Fotenhman

sausage, and poultry to preserve foods from spoiling and to extend their shelf life.[362] It also gives foods cured flavor in addition to preserving and developing its color. [363] [364] [365] Although nitrates and nitrites have very similar chemical formulas, both are used in food. There are other uses for nitrates, such as fertilizer, which we will be discussing later in this chapter.

Once again, I have to invoke my plea: "Guilty as charged!" The amount of processed cold cut meat sandwiches, hot dogs, and sausages that I consumed in the past and fed to my kids in their school lunches was incomprehensible! I'm saying incomprehensible because I'm in possession of information that should be put on warning labels on varieties of processed foods; much like warning labels on cigarettes.   You be the judge.

NITRATES, HEART DISEASE, AND DIABETES

"...researchers from the Harvard School of Public Health (HSPH) have found that eating processed meat, such as bacon, sausage or processed deli meats, was associated with a 42% higher risk of heart disease and a 19% higher risk of type 2 diabetes"
(HSPH News, 2010).[366]

This study was huge, encompassing 1,218,380 individuals from four continents: Europe, Asia, North America, and Australia.[367] [368] The study uncovered that eating processed meats such as one hot dog or one to two slices of deli meats per day, which accounts for around 1.8 oz. or 50 grams, is associated with higher risks for heart disease and type 2 diabetes. [369]

I can remember sandwiches that my family and I used to eat. We were of the opinion that 16 oz. or 453 grams of meats such as corned beef, salami, pastrami, among other processed meats on a sandwich, was not only normal but very desirable.   After all, it's all protein, and it's delicious, isn't it?

It takes less than 2 oz. or 50 grams of processed meat per day to increase your chances for heart disease and diabetes.

NITRATES, NITRITES AND CANCER – FLAVOR OF THE MOMENT

Usually when I discuss the subject of cancer, I hear the following comments: "No one knows when a person will get cancer. People die of cancer all the time. Even the healthiest people that don't drink or smoke die of cancer. It's all hereditary." Indeed, sometimes cancer is hereditary, but only sometimes.

According to the American Institute for Cancer Research, most cancers are not "inherited" but occur as the result of changes to DNA for different reasons.[370]

The DNA changes may occur as a result of eating foods with carcinogens, sugars, trans-fats, etc., and may also be related to environmental factors.   When nitrates are used in protein rich foods such as meats, and are exposed to high temperatures such as frying of bacon, for example, they can be converted into nitrites. [371] [372] [373] [374] Both nitrates and nitrites can react chemically by forming substances identified as "nitrosamines" during the curing process. [375] [376] [377]

"Bacteria convert the nitrates in cured meats to nitrites and nitrosamines, which are potentially carcinogenic to humans"
(Glade, 2008) [378]

Nitrosamines are "known carcinogens." [379] [380] Carcinogens are defined as any substance and/or exposure that can lead to cancer.[381]

Even though some in the business of cured meats may say that nitrates and nitrites are not carcinogenic, I will be presenting hard facts. It will be up to you to decide if you still love your "pastrami" after you've finished reading this chapter.

COLORECTAL CANCER

"Every 1.7 ounces of processed meat consumed per day increases risk of colorectal cancer by 21 percent."
(Weldon & Campbell, 2007) [382]

According to Neal Barnard, MD., President of the Physicians Committee for Responsible Medicine, scientists came to an indisputable conclusion that eating any processed meats containing nitrates and nitrites increases your chance of getting colorectal cancer. [383] [384]

If you only eat one hot dog per day, your risk of getting colorectal cancer increases by 21 percent.[385] [386] That's 1.7 oz. or 50 grams of processed meat per day.

What if you eat <u>two</u> hot dogs per day? You do the math.

As I continued researching diseases linked to nitrates, more information kept popping up. The following sums up what I discovered:

STOMACH CANCER

"Nitrates and nitrites are substances commonly found in cured meats. They can be converted by certain bacteria, such as H pylori, into compounds that have been shown to cause stomach cancer in lab animals"
(American Cancer Society, 2016)[387]

PROSTATE CANCER

"An NIH-AARP Diet and Health Study found a 10 percent increased risk of prostate cancer for every 10 grams of increased intake of processed meats" (Barnard, 2011)[388]

Just to be certain that you get the full impact of the quote above, one hot dog weighs approximately 56 grams or two ounces. You do the scary math...

PROCESSED MEAT AND MORTALITY

When I was eating processed meats and feeding them to my children, I never thought that a person could actually "drop dead" from these delicious foods. It wasn't until I read another large study on nitrates and processed meat that I changed my mind.

In the published research article, "Meat consumption and mortality - results from the European Prospective Investigation into Cancer and Nutrition",[389] authors drew a clear connection between mortality and consumption of processed meats. In the study, 448,568 men and women were examined for cause specific and all-cause mortality. [390] All-cause mortality is defined as early or premature death from any cause.

The results were sobering. *"Significant associations with processed meat intake were observed for cardiovascular diseases, cancer, and other causes of death"* (Rohrmann, S., Overvad, K., Bueno-de-Mesquita, H. B., Jakobsen, M. U., Egeberg, R., Tjønneland, A., et al., 2013). [391] The conclusion of the study was equally as sobering as <u>positive association between processed meat consumption and mortality was observed</u>. [392]

Scientists have estimated that 3.3% of deaths could have been prevented if the study participants ate less than 20 grams or 0.70 oz. of processed meats per day. [393] In reality, 0.70 oz. is smaller than a medium slice of beef bologna which weighs approximately 28 grams or 0.98 oz.[394] Think of how many grams of processed meat goes into a sandwich!

CHILDHOOD AND ADOLESCENT LEUKEMIA

According to the National Cancer Institute, the most common type of childhood cancer is leukemia which has been on the rise along with other types of childhood cancers over the past 20 years.[395]

Can nitrites and nitrates be blamed for these cancers and for the deaths of thousands of children? No one can be 100% certain. Therefore, we can only rely on studies and reliable research to draw the "most likely" conclusion.

"A population based case-control study" of Taiwanese children and teenagers ranging from the ages of 2 to 20 was conducted over a period of 8 years. Out of 515 test subjects, 155 suffered from acute leukemia. [396]

The study concluded that those individuals who ate cured/smoked meat and fish "more than once a week" **increased their risk for acute leukemia by 74%.**[397]

I had to do a double take! An increase of **74%** is huge!

The study also concluded that those children and teenagers who ate higher amounts of vegetables and soy products reduced their risk for leukemia. [398]

ALZHEIMER'S, PARKINSON'S, AND DIABETES

This particular subject left a strong impression on me and my family as I was conducting my research on the most debilitating diseases and their causes. Alzheimer's disease is one of the most devastating forms of dementia; associated with memory loss as well as the loss of intellectual abilities. Parkinson's disease is a debilitation disorder of the central nervous system where movement, sensory, as well as emotional state are affected.

Researchers at Rhode Island Hospital found a connection between Alzheimer's disease, Parkinson's disease, diabetes and the increased consumption of nitrates, nitrites, and nitrosamines found in preserved and processed foods and fertilizer.[399][400] A team headed by Suzanne M. De La Monte, MD, MPH at the Rhode

Island Hospital was able to replicate Alzheimer's disease and link the decrease in production of Insulin and Insulin resistance in the brain with diet trends. [401] [402] In other words, as your brain's main source of energy happens to be glucose,[403] the decline of Insulin literally starves your brain, and different problems begin to rear their ugly heads. How about Type 3 Diabetes? Not too many people have heard of it, but a number of scientist regard Alzheimer's Disease as Type 3 Diabetes.[404]

"We have reasonable evidence that human exposure to nitrosamines is at the root cause of not only Alzheimer's, but several other Insulin-resistance diseases, including Type 2 diabetes, fatty liver disease, also known as NASH and visceral obesity"
-Dr. Suzanne DeLaMonte, Alpert Medical School, Brown University Neuropathologist, Rhode Island Hospital-[405]

Dr. De La Monte pointed out that when foods containing nitrates and/or nitrates are fried, flame broiled, or heated, these chemicals get converted into **nitrosamines – known carcinogens**.[406] [407] [408] **Similar conversion can take place under the acidic conditions in your stomach**. [409]

Dr. De La Monte outlined that "sodium nitrate" listing in the ingredients of foods such as smoked, processed, or preserved meats, processed cheese, bacon, are potentially harmful. [410] [411]

I was especially surprised when I read that beer[412] was one of the items whose consumption should be limited. A high amount of nitrates may be present in a variety of brands in order to extend the products' shelf life.[413]

NITRATES AND DRINKING WATER

"Because nitrate is converted to a very toxic substance (nitrite) in the digestive systems of human infants and some livestock, nitrate-contaminated water is a serious problem"
(Eubank, Carpenter, & Maltsberger, 1998). [414]

Water gets contaminated through soil that has been treated with nitrate fertilizer and from manure and sewage that naturally possesses organic nitrate and ammonia.[415] When it rains, the nitrates are easily carried into the soil and underlying rock. The soil absorbs nitrates through snow melt and irrigation.

Although the Environmental Protection Agency (EPA) sets standards in order to protect public health, nitrates may be present in drinking water. The EPA allows 10 milligrams of nitrates per one liter of water or 10 parts per million.[416] Considering that I drink almost two liters of water during my workout alone, 20 milligrams of nitrates may not be very desirable.

NITRATE-FREE WATER; IS THERE SUCH A THING?

When I begin talking about water with nitrates, there are always a couple of people who say, "We always boil our water, so our water is nitrate and chemical-free." I also encounter others who say, "I have a water filter that removes everything including nitrates out of the drinking water." I only wish that this were true and it was that simple.

Unfortunately, when you boil water containing nitrates, the contamination intensifies, as boiling water "actually concentrates the nitrate." (Eubank, Carpenter, & Maltsberger, 1998). [417]

The claim that water filters remove "everything" is also not true, as <u>filters are utterly ineffective in removing nitrates</u>. [418]

So, how can we avoid drinking water that contains nitrates? There are several ways to rid your water of nitrates and other harmful chemicals. The first one is through a "reverse osmosis" water filter where pressure forces water through a membrane that disallows the undesirable ions or other contaminants to pass through.[419] Although reverse osmosis does not fully purge nitrates out of the water, a reduction of 90% was observed by a study published by the EPA.[420]

Another way is through the "ion exchange system" where ion exchange resin beads are used to reduce the amounts of nitrates and other chemicals such as arsenic from drinking water.[421] The resins trap harmful chemicals by releasing other ions, hence "ion exchange."[422]

The "electro dialysis reversal" is another way of getting rid of nitrates and other chemicals from your drinking water. The electric current is applied to membranes in order to separate undesirable ions.[423] [424]

Where do we get water treated with reverse osmosis, ion exchange, and electro dialysis? There are many facilities that treat water and deliver it to your home and business. Just plug "water treatment services" into your search engine and numerous establishments will pop up. There are systems that you can actually install under the sink in your home. These are a bit costly, but in the long run may prove to be cost effective. In addition, there are water services available in some supermarkets and big box stores where you can bring your own container and fill it up with water.

If for some reason you encounter difficulty when searching for good drinking water, there is another alternative - distilled water. The water distilling process removes nitrates, but there's one caveat. The distillation process also demineralizes water, i.e. removes other minerals.[425] I would only drink distilled water if there weren't any other sources.

NITRATES, VEGETABLES AND FRUITS - REDUCING OR AVOIDING THE BAD STUFF

Let's be realistic: we're constantly exposed to nitrates not only through water and preservatives in food items, but through variety of vegetables and fruits. Yes, vegetables!

It is true that some vegetables are naturally higher in nitrates than others, even organically grown, but vegetables naturally contain ascorbic acid, which partially inhibits the formation of nitrosamines.[426] [427]

The problem arises when soil is treated by nitrate-containing fertilizers.[428] [429] Although plants naturally absorb nitrogen, one of the ways to limit the intake of nitrates is to purchase "organic" fruits and vegetables from a purveyor that you trust. The word "organic" implies that vegetables and fruits have been grown in <u>chemical-free soil and weren't treated with chemical pesticides</u>. We're living in the Internet age. Check your sources and read lots of reviews.

Now for the good news. A study has shown that ascorbic acid or your run of the mill Vitamin C inhibits the formation of nitrosamines in the human body.[430] Now that you have the knowledge of how to reduce nitrosamines formations in your body, you and your doctor can determine how much Vitamin C you need to take. I hope that your doctor is familiar with the study. If not, you can always point to the references section in this book.

My family and I used to love sweet breakfast cereals with their vibrant colors and intense fruity flavors. So, what's wrong with these delicious morsels of "goodness" besides high content of simple carbohydrates and sugar? Coloring!

Although artificial dyes have no food value, food manufacturers recognized long ago that they would sell more foods if they added colors. Vibrantly colored foods appeal to us because we taste with our eyes. We developed that sense from evolution and culture. Although different cultures have dominant color preferences, there is a common denominator. Let's take ripe tomato for example. Historically, through our ancestors we recognized the color red as the color of ripeness and appeal. Thus, as humans we are hard wired by evolution and learned behavior to respond favorably to those visual signals.[431]

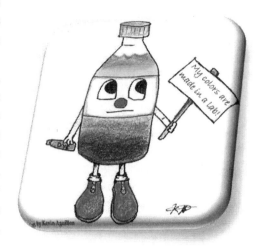

Consider this: how would you like to purchase fresh salmon filet that's gray in color as opposed to pink? Many people believe that gray is an incorrect color for salmon. If you saw a salmon head attached to a gray filet, you might not make the purchase. You would assume that there could be something wrong with the fish as it appears quite unattractive and not what you are accustomed to. Food manufacturers and fish farmers understand your expectations, so you get exactly what you've been accustomed to… pink salmon.

COLORS FOR EVERYTHING

Recently my wife and I went to our local supermarket to purchase some fish for a salad. To our delight, fresh salmon was on sale, but there was something unsettling written on the label: "color added."

So what's wrong with fresh salmon that contains added color? Keep in mind that the flesh of farmed salmon is naturally grey in color.

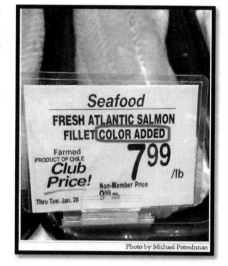

"FDA regulations allow salmon farmers to enhance the pink pigment of fish with artificial chemicals astaxanthin and canthaxanthin…"
(Smythe, 2008).[432]

Both astaxanthin and canthaxanthin can occur naturally. However, when consumed in large quantities, canthaxanthin pigment collects on the retina of the eyes and can potentially cause damage to eyesight.[433] [434] [435] [436]

I'm glad that there was this label because my wife and I ended up not purchasing artificially colored fish. This type of labeling is fairly recent, as not so long ago the California Supreme Court ruled that plaintiffs are allowed to take legal action against store chains that have not disclosed to their customers that salmon was artificially colored.[437]

Let's examine some of the most frequently used food dyes that you may encounter, not only in breakfast cereals or salmon as described previously, but in processed foods and beverages. Fasten your seatbelts:

- FD&C Red #3 (Erythrosine) – According to FDA, this color dye "May no longer be used in cosmetics, external drugs, and lakes" (FDA, 2009).[438] "Lakes" are food dyes that are not water-soluble that can be found in foods containing oils and fats. So, why is Red #3 not allowed to be used in these products? It's prohibited by law because when used in the diet of laboratory animals in high doses, it causes cancer.[439] **Unfortunately, it's allowed to be used in food or drugs that you ingest.**[440] Think about pills with a beautiful cherry-pink hue. According to Catherine J. Bailey, consumer safety officer at FDA, there are approved products that still contain FD&C Red #3.[441] These products include "*soft candy, breakfast cereals, hard candy, juices, meat products, chewing gum, maraschino cherries, icings, cake decorations, cakes, plant protein products, canned puddings and sweet rolls*" (Associated Press, 1990).[442]
- The FD&C Red #40 (Allura Red) – Not recommended for children in the UK [443]
- FD&C Yellow #5 (Tartrazine) and FD&C Yellow #6 (Sunset Yellow)– Banned in Austria, Finland, and Norway[444]

These dyes have few elements in common besides being banned in a number of European countries. These are unfortunately **the most widely used food dyes in the United States, and contain compounds including benzidine and 4-aminobiphenyl.**[445] [446] According to the EPA, both benzidine and 4-aminobiphenyl are known human carcinogens.[447] [448]

"4-Aminobiphenyl is a known human bladder carcinogen and animal studies have reported an increase in bladder and liver tumors from oral exposure"
(EPA, 2000).[449]

In addition, animal studies have shown that when benzidine was administered earlier in life, the cancer potency for this substance was increased significantly.[450] I wish that I had this information before I fed this stuff to my kids in the form of cereal, candies, soft drinks, and other "almost food" items that we no longer consume.

Here are some other approved dyes in the U.S. that you may find in your common processed foods, baked goods, beverages, candies, cosmetics, chips, pickles, shampoos, moisturizers, pet food, and cough syrup:

- FD&C Blue #1 (Brilliant Blue) – Banned in France, Norway, and Finland.[451] On September 29, 2003 FDA released a public health advisory about the toxic effect of this dye: "*The Food and Drug Administration (FDA) would like you to be aware of several reports of toxicity, including death, temporally associated with the use of FD&C Blue No. 1 (Blue 1) in enteral feeding solutions*"(FDA, 2003).[452] Enteral feeding is when a patient is fed through a tube that can be placed in the small intestine, stomach, or nose.
- FD&C Blue #2 (Indigo Carmine) – Banned in France, Norway, and Finland.[453]According to Sciencelab.com, Inc., the data from animal studies has shown that this dye may cause cancer and affect genetic material.[454]

- FD&C Green #3 (Fast Green) – Banned in the European Union.[455] It was found to cause mutagenic affects in laboratory animals and humans, and cause tumors when tested on animals.[456] According to Christopher Gavigan, Board Member - Mt. Sinai Hospital, CA., this dye causes an increase in testicular and bladder tumors in male rats.[457]
- FD&C Red #4 – It is no longer allowed to be used in food or drugs that you swallow. The manufacturers are allowed to use it in drugs and cosmetics that are applied externally.[458]

CHILDREN AND FOOD DYES

"Research has also associated food dyes with problems in children including allergies, hyperactivity, learning impairment, irritability and aggressiveness"
(Columbia Psychiatry, 2010).[459] [460]

In a 2007 British randomized study, researchers found that dyes and preservatives increased children's hyperactivity level.[461] The following is the conclusion of this study: *"Artificial colors or a sodium benzoate preservative (or both) in the diet result in increased hyperactivity in 3-year-old and 8/9-year-old children in the general population"* (McCann, Barrett, Cooper, Crumpler, Dalen, Grimshaw, et al., 2007).[462]

So, before considering Ritalin or some other behavior altering medication for the kid who is naturally hyperactive, please consider the following:

"We see reactions in sensitive individuals that include core ADHD symptoms, like difficulty sitting in a chair and interrupting conversations", says David Schab, M.D., M.P.H., assistant clinical professor of psychiatry at Columbia University and co-author of a 2004 meta-analysis that found food dyes promote hyperactive behavior in already hyperactive children"
(Columbia Psychiatry, 2010).[463]

ARE FOOD DYES SAFE?

It's nice to have colorful and vibrant looking food, but at what cost? There are staunch proponents of artificial dyes who continue to say that these colored chemicals are perfectly safe for everyday consumption. Well, this is what they were saying before the government issued an advisory about the toxicity of FD&C Blue #1 as previously described. Everyone thought that food dyes were safe before the FDA disallowed the use of FD&C Red #4 in foods or ingested drugs.

Let's go back a couple of decades. Over the years, food dyes such as D&C Black #1, D&C Blue #7, D&C Green #7, D&C Orange #3, D&C Orange #14, D&C Orange #16, D&C Red #14, D&C Red #18, D&C Red #35, D&C Green #1, and **many** more were banned in the United States.[464] Before people's health was negatively affected or before these dyes were deemed toxic, I'm certain that proponents were saying that these colored chemicals were perfectly safe.

More recently, according to Forbes Magazine, Yellow #5, **which has been outlawed in numerous European countries**, is under evaluation and testing for links to migraines, cancer, hyperactivity, and anxiety.[465] Out of many colors that were outlawed, only a handful remain, and that handful is currently going through evaluation.

The European Parliament requires warning labels to be used on foods that contain six remaining artificial dyes that are still allowed to be utilized in several parts of Europe.[466]

Not at all surprising, the food companies, including U.S. food manufacturers based in Europe, found a way to avoid putting warning labels on their products. They voluntarily substituted synthetic dyes with natural colors derived from beets, turmeric, annatto, carrots, and saffron.[467] Why did they switch? **Warning labels are very powerful to the consumer and can potentially affect sales in a negative way.** Therefore, food manufacturers are left with very little choice but to switch, even though natural food dyes are more expensive to produce. "Artificial colors often are cheaper, brighter and more stable than natural plant-based colors" (Donahue, 2011).[468]

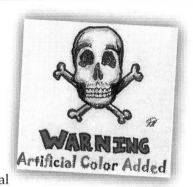

In the United States we don't have warning labels for food dyes, much like we've seen on cigarette packs. I now consider "color added" as a warning label on any food item. Unless I spot labels that state that a food is colored with paprika extract, annatto, or purple cabbage, beet juice, or blueberry juice, among other natural colors, it's a no-no! Otherwise, the only label that my family and I choose is one that clearly spells out, "No artificial colors, artificial flavors, or preservatives added." By the way, if you see a label that states "this food is made with organic ingredients", it does not mean that it was made with "all" organic ingredients. You may just end up ingesting synthetic dyes or other "almost food" stuff.[469]

Chapter 10 ARSENIC IN PORK, POULTRY, WATER, RICE, AND JUICE

When I was a child, I was an avid reader of mystery and detective novels. One of my favorite genres was "whodunit" mysteries. Agatha Christie, Dorothy Sayer, Rex Stout, among other writers have masterfully told elaborate tales by keeping their readers in suspense until the very last minute. Who poisoned the guest of honor? Was it a butler, a cook, or a brother in-law? Perhaps it was the butcher, or the daughter who could have never been suspected of murder?

I will reveal what many of these Victorian authors had in common. The murder weapon of choice for a number of these novels was none other than "Arsenic."

Arsenic is a semi-metallic substance which is tasteless, colorless, and odorless when mixed with foods or drinks.[470] [471] Because it is difficult to detect, it was used by people to kill their adversaries and relatives for inheritance; dating all the way back to the first century.[472] "Inheritance powder" was its nickname. Symptoms of arsenic poisoning resembled many other illnesses that weren't poison related when fed to unsuspecting victims in smaller quantities over time.[473]

By now you may be wondering, what arsenic poisoning or its toxic effects have to do with food. A whole lot! Arsenic has other characteristics besides being a murderous instrument or a substance for getting people sick. When it's fed to pigs, chickens, turkeys, or different types of fowl, it promotes weight gain, adds a more attractive color to meat and animal skin, and contributes to treating parasitic infestation in poultry. [474] The ugly truth is that Roxarsone, an arsenic-based drug, did just that since its approval in 1944 by the FDA.[475] Thus we have been consuming poultry and pork laced with arsenic since 1944. Here's a startling statistic: "*In 2010, industry representatives estimated that 88% of the roughly 9 billion chickens [U.S. Department of Agriculture (USDA) 2012b][476] raised for human consumption in the United States received roxarsone*" (Nachman, Baron, Raber, Francesconi, Navas-Acien, & Love, 2013). [477] On the other hand, arsenic based drugs are prohibited in Europe.

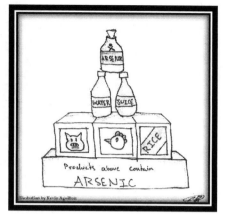

Fortunately for all of us, researchers at Johns Hopkins University have published a study comparing USDA organic chicken meat with standard "run of the mill" chicken meat for the levels of inorganic arsenic (the toxic type.) They uncovered that levels of inorganic arsenic were four times higher than in organic chicken meat.[478] **The use of arsenic based drugs in organic poultry is prohibited by law**. The study concluded that eliminating drugs with arsenic from animal feed could reduce arsenic based diseases in the U.S. population.[479] The following are some examples of arsenic based diseases.

According to the EPA, arsenic has been linked to liver, prostate, bladder, lung, skin, kidney, and nasal passages cancers. [480]

Other effects "*…can include thickening and discoloration of the skin, stomach pain, nausea, vomiting; diarrhea, numbness in hands and feet, partial paralysis, and blindness*" (EPA, 2013). [481] Arsenic is also associated with cases of type 2 diabetes, heart disease, adverse pregnancy outcomes, and cognitive deficits.[482]

A couple of years after the study was published, the FDA banned the use of three out of four arsenic based drugs.[483] So, if the drugs were banned, why am I talking about arsenic toxicity? Well, the remaining drug that was not banned, Nitarsone, which is chemically similar to Roxarson, is alive and doing quite well, as it continues to be utilized.[484] Whether it gets outlawed just like the other arsenic drugs is yet to be seen. If the public outcry is strong and loud enough, we'll see change. But for now, we have an alternative, as you'll read later in the "**WHAT TO EAT**" chapter.

ARSENIC IN WATER

"*Arsenic is a semi-metal element in the periodic table. It is odorless and tasteless. It enters drinking water supplies from natural deposits in the earth or from agricultural and industrial practices*"
(EPA, 2013).[485]

The way this poison gets into our drinking water supply is through minerals that are already present in the soil, as well as agricultural fertilizer such as chicken feces that are loaded with arsenic. [486] There are also less obvious but very significant sources. *"Residues from the decades of use of lead-arsenate insecticides linger in agricultural soil today, even though their use was banned in the 1980s"* (Consumer Reports Magazine, 2012).[487]

Our exposure to arsenic is considerable. The EPA's standard for arsenic in drinking water is 10 parts per billion (ppb).[488] Therefore, government allows some arsenic in drinking water. The problem is that this chemical has a cumulative effect. A piece of chicken here, a glass of water there, a cup of rice, a glass of apple juice; all of it adds up over time.

When I have discussions about this subject, people often say that they don't use municipal water, but only well water. Some even call it "organic water." Unfortunately, they are still vulnerable to arsenic. According to Science Daily, a Dartmouth College New Hampshire study has concluded that levels of arsenic that exceed federal guidelines are **10 times more likely to be found in wells** than in the municipal water supply.[489] I hate to burst the bubble of people who use well for their water needs, but reality is reality.

So, where can you find water without arsenic? The first source you might think of is bottled water. This is what I thought, but after doing a lot of research, not all bottled water is arsenic-free or free of other synthetic chemicals.[490] Sometimes bottled water is just tap water that may have been filtered or poured into bottles completely unfiltered.[491] One of the reasons behind this phenomenon is that FDA relies on state and local government for safety and quality of in-state water.[492] Therefore, some labels are quite misleading,[493] and require due diligence on the part of the consumer. Look up a bottled water company and/or brand name with your favorite search engine, and most of the time you will find honest organizations. If you don't find honesty within a particular company, move on to another brand or other sources.

As far as tap or well water is concerned, keep a couple of things in mind. As with nitrates, you cannot boil arsenic out of the water.[494] In fact, as boiling water evaporates, the concentration level of arsenic will increase.[495] Just as with nitrates, the way to rid your water of arsenic is through reverse osmosis, distillation, ion exchange, and/or ultra-filtration. [496] [497] You can purchase this type of water purification equipment for your home, but if the cost is prohibitive, there may be a number of water services in your area that perform such water treatment. There may also be water service at your local food megastore or supermarket where you can fill up your own container with water that has undergone a purification process.

ARSENIC IN RICE

"Organic rice baby cereal, rice breakfast cereals, brown rice, white rice — new tests by Consumer Reports have found that those and other types of rice products on grocery shelves contain arsenic, many at worrisome levels"
—Consumer Reports Magazine— [498]

Note the very first word in the quote above – **organic**! I had to dig deeper and figure out which type of rice is arsenic-free. To my surprise and amazement, I couldn't find any! The FDA confirmed this unfortunate fact:

"Because arsenic is naturally found in the soil and water, it is absorbed by plants regardless of whether they are grown under conventional or organic farming practices. The FDA is unaware of any data that shows a difference in the amount of arsenic found in organic rice versus non-organic rice"
(FDA, 2013).[499]

Another reason for the arsenic concentration being so high is because the rice plant has to be flooded with water in order to grow. Such "water-flooded" conditions allow arsenic to be easily absorbed by the root system and eventually stored in the grain.[500]

Michael S. Bloom, PhD, an assistant professor at the University of Albany in New York concluded that **rice not only contains arsenic levels that are above and beyond concentration levels in drinking water**, but happens to be a source of exposure to **inorganic** arsenic.[501]

You may be pondering that you've been eating rice all your life and you are not dead. You don't even have thickening of the skin, muscle weakness, damage to liver or kidneys, irregular heartbeat, or cancer.[502] [503] Why not continue eating foods that contain arsenic?

"'Obviously, people don't eat rice and drop dead the next day. You're looking at probably a chronic effect on health,'
says researcher Tracy Punshon, Ph.D, a research assistant professor in the department of biological sciences at
Dartmouth College'"
(Goodman, 2011).[504]

IS BROWN RICE ANY BETTER?

The other day I made one gentleman very upset, as he was explaining to me that although he's in agreement with me about arsenic in white rice, he was certain that brown rice is not only safer but is actually really good for you. He told me that when he takes his family out for sushi, he only orders brown rice. I partially agreed with him because brown rice contains fiber, B Vitamins, and even antioxidants. But if we put it on the scale of good stuff versus ingesting arsenic, we may see an entirely different picture.

Researchers have concluded that brown rice has an even higher concentration of arsenic than white rice since it tends to "converge" in the external layer of the brown rice bran.[505] [506]

So, if you decide to eat any type of rice, how much is safe, or is there such a thing? "Researchers calculated that women who ate just a half cup of cooked rice each day -- the average amount eaten in the study -- would be getting just as much arsenic as if they drank a liter of tap water at EPA's maximum allowable limit for arsenic" (Goodman, 2011). [507] [508]As we discussed in the section above, the maximum allowable limit for arsenic in drinking water is 10 parts per billion (ppb). Therefore, only half cup of rice would be equivalent to 20 ppb. Skeptics who dismiss such information may say, "20 parts per billion is not that much, so eating rice in moderation is not that bad." Let's look at this from a scientific perspective:

In a New Hampshire arsenic study of 229 pregnant women, only 1 gram or **48 grains of rice raised their arsenic level by 1%.**[509] I had to do a double take when I read this outcome. So, if one measly gram of rice increases arsenic level by 1%, how about a half cup of rice that weighs approximately 60+ grams? Scary? You bet! I believe that with this particular number, you are now able to calculate how much rice is safe for you and your family.

There are varieties of rice, grown in different countries that may contain less arsenic. *"Rice grown in the United States, for example, has been shown to have higher arsenic levels than jasmine or basmati rice grown in*

Thailand or India" (Goodman, 2011).[510] That does not mean that we should load up on jasmine or basmati, even though it may contain lower levels of arsenic!

ARSENIC IN APPLE JUICE

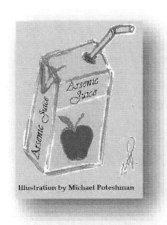

Illustration by Michael Poteshman

I used to give apple juice to my kids all the way through their middle school years. Had I known then what I know now, I would've never dreamed of giving them this stuff, not only because of the high sugar content but because of the high levels of arsenic.

Using an independent laboratory, the televised Dr. Oz Show has investigated claims that there was arsenic in apple juice, which they compared to the EPA's standard for drinking water.[511] As a reminder, the EPA's standard for arsenic in drinking water is 10 parts per billion (ppb).

What they found was quite worrisome; *"...we uncovered that some of the best-known brands of apple juice contain arsenic"* (Dr. Oz Show, 2011).[512] Out of 36 samples from five different brands of apple juice, 10 samples showed arsenic levels above the allowable EPA limit for drinking water.[513] Some of the highest samples for arsenic contained as much as **36 parts per billion**, which is 26 parts per billion higher than what is allowed in water. Here's the web address where you can find results of this study, as well as brand names of the apple juice in question: http://www.doctoroz.com/article/dr-oz-investigates-arsenic-apple-juice

The apple juice samples that registered for arsenic levels that were higher than drinking water may be due to the fact that apple concentrate comes from several countries where arsenic is not regulated in the same way as in the United States.[514] *"In just one type of juice, there can be apple concentrate from up to seven countries"* (Dr. Oz Show, 2011).[515] Furthermore, 60% of apple concentrate that goes into American apple juice comes from China.[516]

"Other countries may use pesticides that contain arsenic, a heavy metal known to cause cancer"
(Dr. Oz Show, 2011).[517]

As I read responses from companies whose juice was investigated by Dr. Oz' Show, there were numerous statements that implied that results of the study were "unreliable at best."[518] Some adjectives that were used implied that communicating to the public that the product is unsafe and had elevated levels of arsenic are "misleading" and "irresponsible."[519][520] I would not expect anything less from these companies as they are protecting their shareholders. What puzzled me is that no law suits were filed against the Dr. Oz show by any of the companies in question, even though these companies believed that information was "misleading." So, I continued my own research and found couple more studies. Here's one example:

Although Consumer Reports Magazine references the outcome of the Dr. Oz show investigation, they conducted their own study where they not only tested apple juice, but grape juice as well. They took into consideration scientific analysis of federal health data, interviewed doctors and other experts, and concluded with the following:

"Roughly 10 percent of our juice samples, from five brands, had total arsenic levels that exceeded federal drinking-water standards. Most of that arsenic was inorganic arsenic, a known carcinogen"
(Consumer Reports Magazine, 2012).[521]

Note the scary wording in the last sentence. To see Consumer Reports' apple and grape juice test results, here is the link where you can download the complete report: http://www.consumerreports.org/cro/magazine/2012/01/arsenic-in-your-juice/index.htm

Looking at both studies we can conclude that not all juice had arsenic that exceeded maximum EPA levels, although some were quite alarming. That's the good news. The bad news is that when you decide to purchase juice, how do you know which type of fruit was used to make that particular batch?

Chapter 11 STEROID HORMONES FOR CATTLE AND SHEEP

Certain hormones are growth-producing which means that animals eat more efficiently and <u>gain weight faster than the livestock that is not subjected to these drugs</u>. [522] [523] [524] Less feed-more weight; what's not to like?

Steroid hormones have been used on beef, cattle, and sheep since their approval by the FDA in the 1950's.[525]

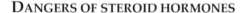

"There are six different kinds of steroid hormones that are currently approved by FDA for use in food production in the US: estradiol, progesterone, testosterone, zeranol, trenbolone acetate, and melengestrol acetate"
(Gandhi, R., Ph.D., & Snedeker, S. M., Ph.D., 2003).[526]

The European Union has banned growth-hormones not only in meat production but also for meat importation into the countries of the European Union.[527] [528] [529]

Some people believe that steroids are delivered into the bodies of an animal through animal-feed or injected intravenously. Not exactly. According to the FDA, steroid hormone drugs that are intended to promote growth are designed in a form of time-release pellets that are injected underneath the skin of the animal's ear. [530] [531] [532] What that means is that 24 hours a day/7 days a week, the hormones are consistently released at a measured rate into the blood stream of an animal.

DANGERS OF STEROID HORMONES

According to Dr. Andrew Weil, steroid hormones may promote prostate cancer in men, increase the risk of cancer of the reproductive system, as well as breast cancer in women.[533]

If that wasn't bad enough, there is also the matter of early onset of puberty in both girls and boys. In an article published in the *Journal of Pediatrics*, the first sentence reads:

"An alarming incidence of premature sexual development has been reported in Puerto Rico during the last 7 years"
(Sáenz de Rodriguez, C. A., MD., Bongiovanni, A. M., MD., & de Borrego, L. C., MD., 1985).[534]

The premature sexual development "epidemic" as described in the title has manifested through "precocious" puberty.[535] Precocious puberty is premature sexual development that begins at the age of 9 in boys and at the age of 8 in girls.[536] The article stated that children experienced premature breast development, premature pubic hair, as well as accelerated pre-puberty breast enlargement in boys.[537]

When different foods that children were eating were analyzed, some meat samples contained "significant levels of estradiol equivalent."[538] Estradiol is the main and the most common form of Estrogen - female hormone.

Another hormone that's worth noting stimulates production of milk in cows. As we discussed in the "Dairy" section earlier, the Bovine Somatotropin (bST) hormone is approved by the FDA in order to increase milk production.[539] This hormone was banned in 1999 by the Council of the European Union.[540] By reading the "Dairy" section earlier you are already aware that milk production increases when cows are injected with Recombinant Bovine Somatotropin (rbST) which increases the levels of IGF-1 hormone known as Insulin-like growth factor.[541] Dr. Mark Hyman believes that IGF-1 works like fertilizer for cancer cells, or to be precise, "like Miracle-Gro for cancer cells" (Hyman, 2013).[542]

The good news is that although this hormone is legal in the United States, many stores stopped carrying milk from cows injected with rbST.[543]

Public outcry takes time and eventually produces results. After all, the public speaks with its wallet. Simple economics tell us that businesses will not carry products that are not selling. Therefore, it trickles down to producers who may have no other alternative but to adjust their practices or suffer the loss of business. There is definitely hope as long as there is an educated consumer.

Chapter 12 ANTIBIOTICS IN MEAT, CHICKEN, SEAFOOD... AND THE CONSEQUENCES THAT FOLLOW

Antibiotics are permitted to be used across most species that we consume.

Most hogs, sheep, cows, chickens, turkeys, fowl, fish, shrimp, and even crabs that are **farmed**, receive antibiotics to treat sicknesses and promote growth.[544] [545]

MEAT AND POULTRY

The use of antibiotics in food has been steadily and alarmingly on the rise in the United States.

The scariest part is that antibiotics given to animals **far exceed those used to treat illnesses of the U.S. human population**.

In 2011, 29.9 million pounds or 13,562,412 kilograms of antibiotics were sold for meat and poultry production.[546] During the same time frame 7.7 million pounds or 3,492,661 kilograms of antibiotics were sold in the U.S. in order to treat human illness.[547]

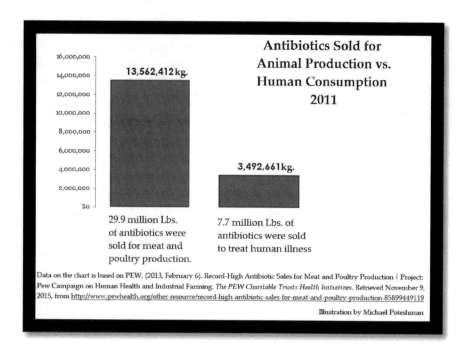

Antibiotics Sold for Animal Production vs. Human Consumption 2011

13,562,412kg.

3,492,661kg.

29.9 million Lbs. of antibiotics were sold for meat and poultry production.

7.7 million Lbs. of antibiotics were sold to treat human illness

Data on the chart is based on PEW. (2013, February 6). Record-High Antibiotic Sales for Meat and Poultry Production | Project: Pew Campaign on Human Health and Industrial Farming. *The PEW Charitable Trusts Health Initiatives*. Retrieved November 9, 2015, from http://www.pewhealth.org/other-resource/record-high-antibiotic-sales-for-meat-and-poultry-production-85899449119

Illustration by Michael Poteshman

Whether we want it or not, **we indirectly ingest antibiotic residue by eating our favorite meat, chicken, or fowl**. Federal standards and regulations specify allowable levels of antibiotic residue after animals have been slaughtered.[548]

One frightening fact is that a **similar class of antibiotics used to treat human sicknesses is used on animals**.[549]

There are potential and ongoing problems, especially with the emergence of "Superbugs", as we will examine at the end of this section.

For now, let's look at something that scared me out of my wits. I believe that you may experience similar horrifying reaction.

SEAFOOD, ANTIBIOTICS, AND OTHER <u>GARBAGE</u>

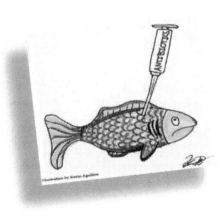

I always knew, from watching television and reading different publications that farmers use antibiotics for cattle and poultry. But who knew that antibiotics could be used on fish, shrimp, or crabs? I never suspected that seafood could be subjected to these and other drugs that were banned in the United States. Here's why.

"About 80% of the seafood consumed in the U.S. is imported from approximately 62 countries..."
(UCDavis, 2008).[550]

Approximately half of the imported seafood comes from fish/seafood farms.[551]   Unlike the ocean with its vast expanse for fish to flourish, farm-raised fish are confined to a closed environment and in many cases, fish pens. In order to avoid mass infections and the spread of disease in closed quarters, fish/seafood farmers use antibiotics or antibiotic-like drugs.[552] Let's just look at one recent horrifying example:

If legal antibiotics in seafood weren't bad enough, amid examination of the seafood imported from China, U.S. inspectors found the illegal carcinogenic antibiotic drug Nitrofuran.[553] In addition, Luoroquinolones were present, which are broad anti-microbial drugs and/or antibiotics that are recognized as unsafe to use in food according to FDA.[554] Known carcinogenic dyes such as malachite green and gentian violet were also found, both of which are illegal to use in food in the United States.[555]

The biggest offenders that perpetrated these drug violations were China, Taiwan, Thailand, Malaysia, Indonesia, India, and Vietnam.[556] Consumers in the United States, Japan, European Union, and Canada were unwittingly victimized by the aforementioned countries.[557]

If inspectors found this horrible stuff in seafood, why worry? In a study, Johns Hopkins' researchers identified U.S. inspections conducted by the Food and Drug Administration as <u>inadequate</u>.[558]

"The study identified a lack of inspection in the U.S. compared to its peers: only 2 percent of all seafood imported into the U.S. is tested for contamination, while the European Union, Japan and Canada inspect as much as 50 percent, 18 percent, and 15 percent of certain imported seafood products"
(Johns Hopkins Bloomberg School of Public Health, 2011).[559]

Only 2% "of all seafood" coming into the United States is being inspected for contamination? Thus, the remaining 98% of un-inspected seafood may or may not have this horrible stuff in it.

Are you willing to take this chance? If your answer is no, then you're on the right track! Consider the following quote from the U.S. Food and Drug Administration (FDA):

"The presence of antibiotic residues may contribute to an increase of antimicrobial resistance in human pathogens. Moreover, prolonged exposure to nitrofurans, malachite green, and gentian violet has been shown to have a carcinogenic affect"
(FDA, 2013).[560]

A pathogen is an organism that may cause disease in another organism, such as the common cold. In this case, the human body may become resistant to fighting different pathogens because of antibiotic residues. A carcinogen is any substance that produces cancer.

ANTIBIOTICS AND FRIGHTENING CONSEQUENCES

"These antibiotics promote faster growth, but this dangerous practice also promotes the development of antibiotic-resistant superbugs that infect about 1.4 million people each year and kill at least 63,000 in North America"
- Michael Roizen, MD., Internal Medicine -[561]

How do these "Superbugs" develop in humans? As discussed earlier, farm animals are given approved antibiotics, similar to what is prescribed to the human population, in order to keep them well or to help them recover from sickness.[562] There is another side benefit to farmers when antibiotics are used consistently in low doses.

What happens truly defies logic, as the animal puts on weight and grows larger while <u>eating less</u>.[563] [564] The business end of this operation makes perfect sense. Less feed equals more meat. Just add a "little drug" to food and water, and voilà – animals stay healthy and generate more meat!

If animals gain weight, what about humans? I will be describing how one can gain weight from the use of antibiotics in Chapter 22, "GUT HEALTH: THE TWO BRAINS PHENOMENON". For now, let's continue with "Superbugs".

The problem is **that antibiotics allow bacteria to adapt and become stronger and more resistant to treatment**.[565] As a result, more potent antibiotics have to be developed and produced in order to combat these "Superbugs."[566] As antibiotic resistant bacteria get stronger and move to the next cycle, a more powerful Superbug emerges and requires an antibiotic that is even more potent. And the vicious cycle continues.

To be fair, the Superbug that flourishes in animals is not the only culprit. The overuse of prescription antibiotics by physicians to treat illnesses that may be overcome without the use of these drugs has also a lot to do with the emergence of treatment-resistant bacteria.[567]

The somewhat good news is that the FDA is working with farmers to remove antibiotics and other drugs <u>voluntarily</u>.[568] **That's right, farmers are practicing self-regulation**. At least this is a start, and I'm hoping that with time, this Superbug producing substance will be banned completely. These drugs have been banned in the European Union since the 1990's.[569] What's taking the U.S. so long???

Chapter 13 ENHANCED MEAT

Two years prior to this writing, my wife and I attended a neighbor's cookout. As both of us were beginning to grasp the reality of processed foods, we asked the neighbor about the type of meat and marinade he was using. He replied that he used only all natural meat and that marinating was out of the question. He told us "Meat speaks for itself and does not require any other ingredients because of such excellent quality." We were in awe when he removed a chicken breast straight from its packaging and placed it directly on his charcoal grill without even a pinch of salt. My wife and I exchanged looks, both thinking how dry and bland the chicken breast would taste. To our surprise, the chicken was not only moist but full of flavor, and for some reason, it tasted salty. But why?

I asked my neighbor if I could examine the packaging of the chicken breast. To my astonishment and horror, I read the following:

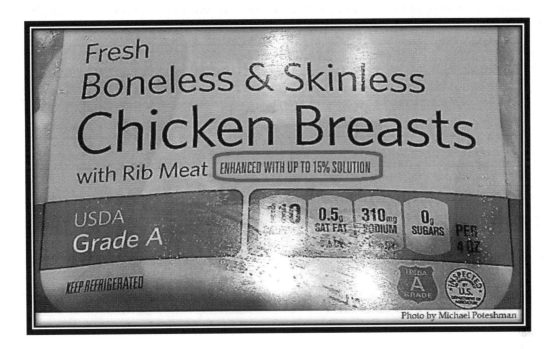

The words that immediately popped out at me were: "ENHANCED WITH UP TO 15% SOLUTION." Solution of what? What exactly was I eating?

The same scenario transpired with his pork loin filet.

This time both my wife and I didn't even want to taste this processed pork, as it contained not only a whopping 25% solution, but natural flavors, spices, and yeast extract, as you can see in the picture below:

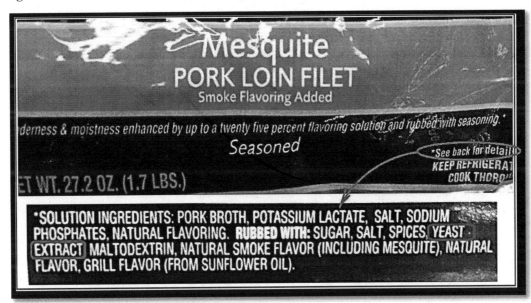

Whatever is in those spices, pork broth, or natural flavors is anyone's guess. After reading the "EXCITOTOXINS" chapter earlier, you can imagine what type of "cocktail" was injected into that pork loin.

I began to dig deeper to figure out more about raw enhanced meats and poultry.

"It turns out that a lot of our meat is enhanced. About 30 percent of poultry, 15 percent of beef, and 90 percent of pork are injected with some kind of liquid solution before sale, USDA says, and it's usually something high in sodium"
(Fulton, 2011).[571]

The interesting wording in the last sentence was *"some kind of liquid solution."* This sounded similar to a lot of processed foods that we discussed in earlier chapters. So I went on the USDA website and here's what I found:

"Enhanced or value-added meat and poultry products are raw products that contain flavor solutions added through marinating, needle injecting, soaking, etc. The presence and amount of the solution will be featured as part of the product name, for example, "Chicken Thighs Flavored with up to 10% of a Solution" or "Beef Steak Marinated with 6% of a Flavor Solution"
(USDA, 2013).[572]

The good news is that manufacturers are mandated to inform the public that meat is enhanced. Unfortunately this government mandate didn't give me too much comfort. Even though ingredients should be displayed, there is no mandate to decipher what is in the "natural flavors or spices." The USDA website, however, gave examples of the type of stuff that foods can be injected with. "For example, pork chops may be packaged with a solution of water, salt, and sodium phosphate (a solution that can add flavor and moisture to leaner meats)" (USDA, 2013).[573] This is why our neighbor's grilled meat tasted salty. Unfortunately it's not the entire story.

After my neighbor's party, I decided to go to the store and find chicken breast or any type of meat with ingredients that were actually listed on the label. I was successful in quickly finding these products. I will give you two examples, although there were many more. Below is a label of the enhanced chicken breast as well as the ingredient list from the back of the package:

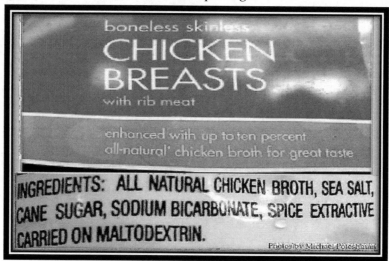

This raw chicken contained not only salt and sugar as well as "all natural broth" without telling you what's in the broth, it contained baking soda which is sodium bicarbonate, and "spice extractives carried on maltodextrin." Wow, what a mouthful!

Maltodextrin is an artificially produced starch that is not found in nature; it can be mildly sweet or nonsweet.[574] According to FDA, maltodextrin is "nonsweet nutritive saccharide polymer" that is made into white powder by partial hydrolysis or a cooking process of potato starch, rice starch, or corn starch.[575][576] So we know what this additive is, but what's in the "spice extractives?" I really have no idea because the components of these extractives are not listed on the label. However, you can see a list of these extractives in the Appendices section at the end of the book. Keep in mind, that's raw chicken we're talking about!

The sad part is that manufacturers don't have to list the ingredients of this stuff. While in the store, I placed a call to a major poultry producer and asked what was in the natural broth and spice extractives. I was told that the company follows all federal and state rules and regulations for their products. I was also told that they didn't have to list ingredients in spices and natural flavors, and everything that was listed is exactly what was mandated by the federal and state government.

While in the same store, I found fresh pork with "12% flavoring solution." Just look at this ingredient list on the back of the package:

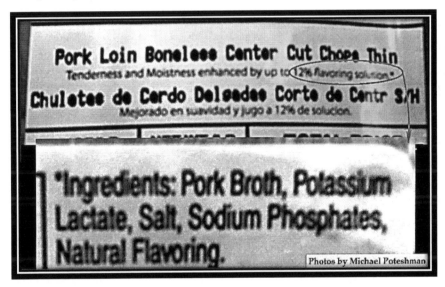

Photos by Michael Poteshman

What's in the pork broth? Your guess is as good as mine, since broth ingredients are not listed. The next ingredient on the list is Potassium Lactate. According to FDA, Potassium Lactate is odorless white solid that is prepared by neutralizing lactic acid with potassium hydroxide.[577] It can be used as humectant in order for the products to retain or preserve moisture, flavor enhancer, as well as PH Control agent which helps to control level of acid in the food.[578] Although FDA finds this ingredient "Generally Recognized as Safe (GRAS,)" it is prohibited from usage in infant formula or infant food.[579]

Besides salt there are Sodium Phosphates. These substances may be used as texturizers for changing the texture and look of meat, as well as a preservative to increase its shelf life.[580][581] Sodium phosphate can also be used as an emulsifier in order to prevent ingredients from separating in processed meats, cheeses, and canned soups.[582] [583] [584] An interesting fact is that sodium phosphate is also used as over the counter drug to treat constipation or purge the colon before a colonoscopy.[585] [586] Although the dosages in meat may be less than in the drugs, according to FDA, a larger than recommended dose of sodium phosphate that is used to treat constipation may cause damage to kidneys, heart, and even cause death. [587]

In addition, gastrointestinal problems such as bloating, nausea, vomiting, and stomach pain, may occur.[588] There are other side effects such as irregular heartbeat, throat tightness, difficulty swallowing and breathing, hives, burning or tingling lips, fainting, rash, hives, swelling of the eyes, face, lips, tongue, and mouth.[589] Although I never had my intestine cleansed with sodium phosphate, I suffered from some of these symptoms in the past. Perhaps these symptoms were the result of eating enhanced meats. Perhaps my condition was exacerbated by all of the other "almost foods" that contained this substance, as well as excitotoxins. Nonetheless, it's all gone by way of the Dodo bird, as we no longer consume this stuff!

"Too much phosphate can be toxic. It can cause diarrhea and calcification (hardening) of organs and soft tissue, and can interfere with the body's ability to use iron, calcium, magnesium, and zinc"
(Ehrlich, 2011).[590]

A final ingredient on the list is "Natural Flavoring." What is in natural flavoring? You may recall the "NATURALLY A COVER UP" section as part of the MSG chapter. This elusive "natural flavoring" is really hard to figure out. At the end of the book you will find some of the possible ingredients that may go into "natural flavoring." Since the immense number of ingredients that are considered natural flavorings is too long to list here, please see "Appendices A, B, C, D, E, and F" at the end of the book.

Whenever I see this natural flavor as an ingredient, I literally run! This is because when I call manufacturers, I cannot get a straight answer beyond, "We're following all state and federal regulations", or in one instance, "We use rosemary." When I ask why not list rosemary instead of natural flavors or spice, I'm told that they're following federal regulations. One customer service representative from a well-known chicken manufacturing facility came up with the most preposterous excuse. She told me that *there wasn't enough space on the back of the chicken package to list all of the ingredients that went into natural flavors.* Manufacturers simply don't have to disclose what's in those natural flavorings.

In an attempt to outline what goes into Natural Flavors or Spices, the USDA has set up a question and answer website. The following excerpt can be used as a refresher that I obtained from: http://www.fsis.usda.gov/OPPDE/larc/Ingredients/PMC_QA.htm

"I. LABELING OF FLAVORINGS
1. Question: What commonly used ingredient may be designated as "flavors", "flavorings", "flavoring", or "flavor?"
Answer: Spices, spice extractives, essential oils, oleoresins, onion powder, garlic powder, celery powder, onion juice, and garlic juice. Spices, oleoresin, essential oils, and spice extractives are listed in 21 CFR 172.510, 182.10, 182.20, 182.40, 182.50, and 184" (USDA, 1995).[591]

These ingredients are listed in several sections of CFR or Code of Federal Regulations. I urge you to at least browse through the Appendices at the end of the book so you can see what these ingredients could possibly be. Some are benign, but there are some that are plain scary! Check out "Natural flavors" and "Spices;" please pay special attention to Appendix F or CFR 184. You may think twice before purchasing products containing these "Natural" ingredients or "Spices."

Chapter 14 SOYBEAN PRODUCTS: THE GOOD, THE BAD, AND THE UGLY

THE BAD AND THE UGLY SOY

Besides dairy, this is one of the most provocative sections of this entire book. Indeed, soy is part of the "**WHAT NOT TO EAT**" section, but only in part. A lot of people swear by soybean products and attribute their good health to the magical qualities of this wonder bean. Others believe that even though there are some benefits to eating soy that's prepared in a certain way, the dangers far outweigh those benefits. So, does consuming soy translate into great health and vigor or is it the opposite? Let's look at this bean that has created a dietary revolution and built some of the world's biggest businesses.

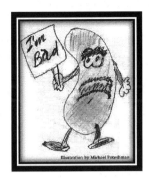

"Israeli manufacturers of soya products were rattled by the recommendation issued by the country's health ministry that consumption of soya products be limited in young children and avoided, if possible, in infants"
(Siegel-Itzkovich, 2005)[592]

Why did the health committee issue such a strong precautionary warning, especially considering that Israel consumes such high amounts of soy products? There are several reasons.

According to an article published by the NIH, research on retrospective human or animal studies shows that consumption of soy may create possible risks for male infertility, higher risk of cancer, among other health related problems. [593]

"Soya contains phytoestrogens that may have some of the effects of the human hormone if consumed in large quantities"
(Siegel-Itzkovich, 2005).[594]

PhytoEstrogens are chemicals that are found in different types of plants such as beans, grains, or seeds that can mimic the **female hormone Estrogen**. Foods made from soybean contain the highest amounts of phytoEstrogens.[595] As you've already read in the "DAIRY" section, higher exposure to Estrogen may increase the risks of breast or other forms of cancer. [596] [597] [598]

Besides the Israeli health committee warnings, is there a proof that soy products are really bad for us? According to an article published by the Harvard School of Public Health, reports have shown that consuming soy protein stimulates growth of breast cancer cells. [599] Other research illustrated that soy products prevent breast cancers from reoccurring.[600]

Several studies show evidence that consuming soy in large quantities could affect memory while others showed benefit.[601] Is the evidence inconclusive? Perhaps. We, as consumers, have to make the final judgment in accordance with the evidence. Let's look at some additional data, specifically at the genetic modification or GMO (Genetically Modified Organism.)

According to the USDA, as of 2013, 93% of all planted soybean acres in the United States were genetically modified.[602]

Although there are proponents on both sides of the issue of gene modification, an interesting section from a WebMD article titled "'Frankenfood' Fears'" piquet my interest. It states that genetically modified foods have been engineered in the laboratory where they would resist drought, herbicides, improve nutritional elements, and even increase food supply.[603] So what's wrong with resisting drought, herbicides and other chemicals? Consider these unplanned side effects:

"Experts say this science, like any other, has no guarantees. Risks include:

- *Introducing allergens and toxins to food*
- *Accidental contamination between genetically modified and non-genetically modified foods*
- *Antibiotic resistance*
- *Adversely changing the nutrient content of a crop*
- *Creation of "super" weeds and other environmental risks"*
  (WebMD, 2015). [604]

GMO SOY, FRUITS, AND VEGETABLES ARE OFF LIMITS

If the GMO explanation earlier has not convinced you, here's a bit of information that convinced my family and me to never eat genetically modified vegetables and fruits, let alone soy. An active ingredient in Roundup herbicide happens to be glyphosate produced by Monsanto.[605] Roundup ready crops are genetically modified to be resistant to glyphosate. While farmers spray the entire crop with Roundup, the weeds die and the Roundup resistant GMO plants remains intact. To an unsuspecting consumer, this may sound like good news, but is it?

Some in the scientific community affirm that glyphosate bonds to minerals in the plants, and as a result prevent such minerals from being available for absorption in our bodies. [606] [607] What that means is that you essentially end up eating some fiber without any or very few minerals being absorbed into your system. [608] Others say that glyphosate "enhances the damaging effects of other food borne chemical residues and environmental toxins" (Samsel & Seneff, 2013).[609] **Not only that, but because glyphosate is considered an antibiotic, it has the power to indiscriminately destroy or alter good bacteria inside your gut.** [610] [611] The problem arises when the good bacteria is destroyed and the bad bacteria takes its place[612] which may lead to slew of gut related problems. We will be discussing these very important life-sustaining bacteria or probiotics in Chapter 22 "**GUT HEALTH: THE TWO BRAINS PHENOMENON.**"

Unfortunately, that's not the only thing that glyphosate may do to your body. How about cancer? As I queried the words "cancer and glyphosate," a slew of headings from numerous law firms began to manifest. Here are two examples of many:

- *"Glyphosate in Roundup® Weed Killer May Cause Cancer."* (Weitz & Luxenberg, 2017).[613]
- *"Monsanto Roundup [glyphosate] weed killer has been designated as a probable human carcinogen by the World Health Organization (WHO). Farmers, farm workers, landscapers and gardeners who use Roundup or other glyphosate products are at risk for developing non-Hodgkin lymphoma and other forms of cancer."* (Baum Hedlund Law, 2017).[614]

The good news is that for the first time, the FDA will begin testing for glyphosate in foods such as eggs, milk, soybeans, corn, among others.[615]

IS ORGANIC SOY BETTER THAN GENETICALLY MODIFIED?

Whether soybeans are organic or genetically modified they share one trait: they contain "**anti-nutrients**."[616] Anti-nutrients are substances that interfere with the absorption of one or more nutrients that your body may require.[617]

One example is "Phytic acid" found in soy that can block the absorption of calcium, magnesium, copper, iron, and zinc in the intestinal tract.[618]   Another scary example is "Goitrogens" that can interfere with Thyroid functions that have to do with the absorption of iodine, which may cause hypothyroidism or inadequate production of Thyroid hormone.[619] [620]

There are other frightening anti-nutrients such as "Trypsin inhibitors" that may interfere with protein digestion, or "PhytoEstrogens" and "Isoflavones" that may block normal Estrogen production.[621]

MORE SOY-RELATED DISORDERS

As I kept investigating soy, I came upon a well-researched book titled "The Whole Soy Story: The Dark Side of America's Favorite Health Food" by Kaayla T. Daniel, PhD, CCN. Some of the facts that she outlined were quite chilling, including predictions of increased cases of heavy metal toxicity, hormonal disruption in infants fed soy based formula, and infertility. [622]   Other disorders which surfaced as a result of numerous studies include: [623]

- Increased risk of heart disease[624]
- Early puberty in children[625]
- Thyroid problems[626]
- Increased risk of cancer[627]
- Infertility in men and women[628]
- Digestive disorders[629]
- Immune deficiency[630]
- Behavioral problems in children[631]

GOOD SOY

Indeed, there is such a thing, as "good soy", which can be beneficial to your health.

There is definitely a way to make soy products safe, as people in Asian countries have been consuming fermented soy for centuries.

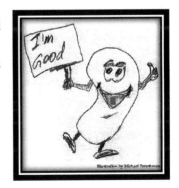

"The soybean did not serve as a food until the discovery of fermentation techniques, sometime during the Chou Dynasty. The first soy foods were fermented products like tempeh, natto, miso and soy sauce"
(Fallon & Enig, Ph.D., 1999)[632]

Unfortunately, the majority of soy products sold in the U.S. stores are unfermented. At one time or another, you may have purchased soy cheese, soy burgers, soy milk, infant formula, soy ice-cream, or even tofu that imitates turkey or chicken meat. I know that I purchased soy products on many occasions because I believed that soy was really good for me.

The reality is, unless soy gets fermented, as **fermentation reduces and in some cases, destroys the anti-nutrients**, caution must be exercised. [633] [634]

Bottom line, enjoy miso in your soup or by itself, relish natto, and tempeh. Just inquire if it's genetically modified or not. According to Dr. Joseph Mercola, the fermented soy products contain Vitamin K2. When combined with Vitamin D, it has the potency to help in preventing heart disease, osteoporosis, different types of cancer, and dementia. [635] That's what I call "Good Soy!"

Chapter 15 **ALCOHOL**

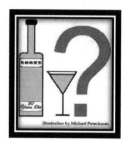

A recurring question that I get most often is about alcohol consumption. Some people believe that hard liquor in small quantities is really good for you. Some believe that wine is the very best thing. Still others believe that beer is superior when it comes to calories and overall health. So, is there such a thing as beneficial alcohol? In order to give a precise answer, this question has to be answered in parts.

BOOZE AND CALORIES

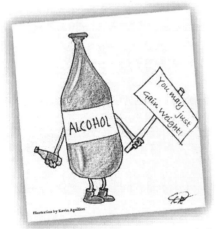

"…Alcohol, whenever taken in, is the first fuel to burn. While that is going on, your body will not burn fat. This does not stop the weight loss it simply postpones it…"
– Dr. Robert Atkins –[636]

Alcohol is the first source of energy that your body will utilize, which means that if you're having a couple of drinks daily, it will be more difficult to rid your body of stored fat until the alcohol is out of your system. The general rule of thumb is the higher the alcohol content, the higher the calories in a given alcoholic beverage. Please don't begin to celebrate just yet, as some alcoholic beverages have calories that originate from carbohydrates and sugar besides containing a modest alcohol content. Thus, we will weigh in (pardon my pun), on three types of alcoholic beverages and their caloric impact: hard liquor, beer, and wine.

HARD LIQUOR

Straight hard liquor contains no carbohydrates, as long as you don't introduce sugary mixes into your drink. Once a mix is introduced, you not only add sugar and carbs to your drink, but in a lot of cases, these mixes are loaded with chemicals. Although straight hard liquor has no carbs, it still contains significant calories.

- Vodka, gin, rum, tequila, whiskey, or scotch with 40% alcohol or 80 proof, have approximately 64 calories per **one ounce** or 28.3 grams.[637]

- Hard liquor varieties that are 100% proof, which translates into 50% alcohol, contain approximately 80 calories per one ounce serving.[638]

What that means is if you have four ounces or 113.4 grams of 80 proof vodka, which is equivalent to about two drinks in many restaurants, you will be packing approximately 256 calories **that your body will have to burn before it can address other calories that you consumed**. You will not be able to burn fat that you're trying to lose until the distilled spirit is out of your system. That's not counting mixes, such as 1 cup or 248 grams of orange juice which contains 20.8g of sugar and 25.8g of carbohydrates. [639] This adds 112 calories on top of the "booze."

BEER

Although beer is much lower in alcohol calories than straight hard liquor, it contains carbs. I recall an old saying that I heard over the years, "This beer is so good, it's like drinking bread." Hence, the carbs...

Some people believe that drinking a 12 oz. bottle of light beer is like having a glass of water. Not true. A 12 oz. bottle of light beer contains approximately 108 calories. [640]

Some people think that light beer is not rich enough in taste. The penalty for drinking regular beer is approximately 36 additional calories or 144 calories per 12 oz. bottle. As for dark beer, some richer beer varieties such as Samuel Adams Boston Lager contain as much as 175 calories per 12oz. bottle,[641] while other brands are as high as 200 calories per serving.

Thus, out of the entire beer variety, although calories vary from one label to another, light beer would have the least calories.

WINE

One theory is that if you drink two glasses of red wine per day, you will lose weight. Not true. As red wine contains approximately 21 calories per ounce, with an average serving of 5-6 oz., you would still be consuming as much as 126 calories per glass.[642] Dry white wine has less calories, with approximately 100 calories per 5 oz. serving. [643] Dessert wine is loaded with calories because of the sugar, and a 5 oz. glass will have as much as 235 calories. [644]

Dry white wine would be the best choice for your waistline if you decide to drink it.

WHICH ALCOHOL TYPE IS BETTER?

According to the American Cancer Society, one alcohol type is no better than another. The **Ethanol** that's present in all alcoholic beverages is responsible for the increased risk of breast cancer, cancers of the mouth, throat, esophagus, liver, voice box, colon, and rectal cancer. [645]

It is not the alcohol type that is a concern, but the amount of Ethanol that's being consumed.[646]

"Ethanol is a type of alcohol found in alcoholic drinks, whether beer, wines, or liquor (distilled spirits). These drinks contain different percentages of Ethanol, but in general a standard size drink of any type — 12 ounces of beer, 5 ounces of wine, or 1.5 ounces of 80-proof liquor — contains about the same amount of Ethanol (about half an ounce)"
-American Cancer Society -[647]

Although there is some discussion about the benefits of red wine, there are also **calories, chemicals, and alcohol, among other undesirable substances in it**. We will be discussing the "bad" in any alcoholic beverage in the next section.

For the sake of full disclosure, there is a hypothesis that moderate alcohol consumption is associated with better health in "some people."[648] The key phrase here is "some people." Others may have problems while drinking even small amounts of alcohol. But when it comes to cancer, you're putting yourself at a higher risk, even at moderate or less than moderate amounts.[649] [650] "Thus, as the amount of alcohol consumed increases, the risk of developing cancer increases."(Rehm & Shield, 2014)[651]

Moderate alcohol consumption is approximately one drink per day for women or two for men, with one drink considered to be 1.5 oz. of 80 proof hard liquor, or 12 oz. of beer, or 5 oz. of dry red or dry white wine.[652]

Once again, I have to disclose that various articles indicate that there may be some benefit to the heart when drinking alcohol in moderation.[653] On the other hand, alcohol may be bad because it increases the risk of gastrointestinal bleeding,[654] and may have negative effects on hormones in addition to many other alcohol related complications, as will be discussed in the next few sections.

Also, if you don't drink, don't start drinking for the sake of health. **The same health benefits can be achieved through exercise and awesome food**, as will be described in detail in the "WHAT TO EAT" chapter. Keep in mind that alcohol may only benefit some people, and you may or may not be one of them. Furthermore, such "benefits" may **only be temporary**, considering a multitude of complications that you will read about in the next section.

So, what should one drink while "Living Wonderfully?" We don't live in a vacuum, and from time to time we enjoy attending social functions with co-workers, friends, or family. Just keep in mind, **when you consume _any_ alcohol, your body burns calories from alcohol first, which neglects all of the other calories and fat stores until the alcohol is used up.** Thus, if you must have a drink at a social function while trying to normalize your weight, choose an alcohol type and serving size with the least amount of calories. Also be mindful of preservatives and other chemicals.

The chart below outlines the alcohol calories with examples of serving amounts:[655]

Calories in Selected Alcoholic Beverages

Beverage	Approximate Calories Per 1 Fluid Oz[a]	Example Serving Volume	Approximate Total Calories[b]
Beer (regular)	12	12 oz	144
Beer (light)	9	12 oz	108
White wine	20	5 oz	100
Red wine	21	5 oz	105
Sweet dessert wine	47	3 oz	141
80 proof distilled spirits (gin, rum, vodka, whiskey)	64	1.5 oz	96

Obtained from:
http://www.health.gov/dietaryguidelines/dga2005/document/html/chapter9.htm

[a] Source: Agricultural Research Service (ARS) Nutrient Database for Standard Reference (SR), Release 17. (http://www.nal.usda.gov/fnic/foodcomp/index.html) Calories are calculated to the nearest whole number per 1 fluid oz.

[b] The total calories and alcohol content vary depending on the brand. Moreover, adding mixers to an alcoholic beverage can contribute calories in addition to the calories from the alcohol itself.

As you can see from the chart, the least amount of calories is in a 1.5oz serving of hard liquor. So, if hard liquor is not your "cup of tea", so to speak, the next choice would be a 5 oz. glass of white wine. It goes up from there.

People usually ask me about my drink of choice when attending social functions. First and foremost, while your body is in the process of normalizing itself on a "Living Wonderfully" routine, it's better to abstain from any alcohol, otherwise weight loss will be postponed. For those social functions that I attend, and have no other alternative but to show that I'm part of the group, I usually make one of two choices:

1. A 1 oz. – 64 calorie straight shot of tequila or vodka "nursed" for an extended period of time, or
2. A 1 oz. shot of the aforementioned liquor, poured in a tall glass of club soda with a couple of slices of lemon or lime in order to "stretch" the drink.

That way, I'm not regarded as antisocial (in some circles,) and I'm not consuming excessive calories. It's not the calories I worry about, it's the alcohol itself. Once again, when drinking alcohol, it's quite easy to derail your body from burning fat, as it takes your system some time to snap back to the business of burning what's necessary as opposed to <u>empty alcohol calories</u>.

Bottom line:

"There is no evidence that any particular form of alcoholic beverage (beer, wine, or distilled spirits) confers greater health benefits than any other"
-Prof. David J. Hanson, Ph.D., Potsdam University-[656]

ALCOHOL-INDUCED "OUT OF WHACK" HORMONES

As I was explaining to one of the members of my audience about alcohol's caloric implications, a gentleman replied with the following: "Big deal, 128 calories! I can burn them off during one swift walk around the block." Indeed you could, I said, but you need to consider other implications. Alcohol essentially places your body in an "out of whack" or an unbalanced state.

When you drink alcohol, the production of the hormone Leptin, which determines whether you're full or still hungry, is suppressed.[657][658] Thus, your body is not only forced to burn alcohol calories first as illustrated earlier, but by disrupting the Leptin production, your appetite gets out of whack, and you **eat more without being satisfied**.[659] You read it correctly: alcohol "screws" with your hormones. That's a double whammy on your system. **Besides not addressing your stored calories, you add additional calories due to suppressed Leptin production, which triggers a voracious appetite**. As you're trying to get healthy and lose weight, alcohol, <u>in any form</u>, may sabotage your newly found health. Until Leptin production is normalized, you will continue to stay hungry and may not be able to properly keep yourself in check due to lowered inhibitions that alcohol elicits.

Another reason for your body being off-balance when drinking alcohol is due to the way your liver tackles its effects. **Alcohol is considered a toxic substance by your liver**, which begins metabolizing it immediately in order to excrete it in the shortest amount of time possible.[660]

"That means your liver puts other metabolic jobs on hold, and the easiest thing for it to do is <u>store away calories you've just consumed</u> from food as body fat"
(Cabot, 2013).[661]

15-99

When I talk about the subject of alcohol, some people find it difficult to fully comprehend the damaging effects of alcohol on the digestive system and the problems that follow. Let's take this one step at a time as we get to the bottom of this very important subject.

Drinking alcohol causes growth or overgrowth of certain bacteria in the intestines, which are categorized as Gram-negative. For example, E. coli bacteria belongs in a category of Gram-negative. Although Gram-negative bacteria are always present in your gut, additional growth of these bacteria takes your gut out of balance, and causes an accumulation of a toxin called an endotoxin.[662] Excessive amounts of endotoxin in the blood stream can cause inflammation, injury to the liver, abnormal blood clotting, among many other symptoms.[663] [664] [665] [666]

"Endotoxin appears to play a central role in the initiation of alcohol-induced tissue/organ damage and its role is most convincing for liver injury."
(Purohit, Bode, Brenner, Choudhry, Hamilton, Turner, 2008)[667]

In addition, the Gram-negative bacteria, as well as your own cells in the liver, will convert Ethanol from your favorite alcoholic beverage into a toxic chemical called Acetaldehyde as a byproduct.[668] [669] Besides being a known carcinogen (substance that causes cancer,)[670] Acetaldehyde wreaks havoc on your gut.

Acetaldehyde makes it easier for the toxins produced by the bacteria to pass through your intestines. [671] Although the endotoxins have a difficult time passing through your intestinal walls on their own, **alcohol essentially causes holes in the gut (permeation of the intestines)** [672] **to become big enough for the molecules of bacterial toxin to fit through**. [673] As a result, these toxins wind up in your blood stream and will eventually end up in your liver. This directly causes liver damage and may induce **injury to other organs**.[674] These toxins then cause a slew of enzymes/hormones to be released throughout your body, which cause direct liver damage. [675] To add insult to injury, this liver damage in turn, may produce more hormones that make your intestines EVEN MORE permeable (bigger holes) to the toxin which caused the damage in the first place. [676]

The liver then produces a hormone called TNF-α which can make it even easier for the toxins to **pass through your intestines and into the blood stream**, thus creating a vicious cycle of toxins and hormones amplifying the damage to the entire body. [677]

Let's summarize this not-so-easy-to-grasp concept in layman's terms.

Drinking alcohol causes bacterial growth, which causes bacterial toxin, which causes damage to the gut by making holes (permeation of the gut,) which causes damage of the liver, which then goes back to the gut and to the rest of the body, over, and over again, as you continue to consume alcohol.

Sorry to be a buzz kill; pardon the pun.

OUT OF WHACK THYROID

As I was working on this chapter, by a sheer coincidence, my wife informed me that one of her co-workers was diagnosed with insufficient Thyroid hormone production or hypothyroidism. Please keep in mind that the hormone producing Thyroid gland that is located in the neck, <u>influences most metabolic processes and regulates many genes in your body</u>.[678] In the case of my wife's co-worker, she was chronically tired, depressed, and had very low energy to move through her day. In a subsequent conversation, her co-worker mentioned that in order to unwind after a long and difficult day at the office, she had a couple of glasses of wine before going to bed. She had her wine daily, including weekends, for approximately five years.

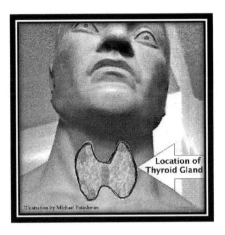

Location of Thyroid Gland

Illustrations by Michael Potashman

No one knows exactly why my wife's co-worker came down with hypothyroidism and depression. We do know, however, that she was consistently having several glasses of wine after work. As such, the Ethanol in her wine may have been responsible for hypothyroidism, as **Ethanol is toxic to the Thyroid gland, including the endocrine system**, as studies consistently show.[679] [680]

"The fact that alcohol causes direct cellular toxicity on thyroid cells, thereby producing Thyroid suppression and reducing Thyroid volume, is well established."
(Balhara & Deb, 2013) [681]

You are already aware from the previous section that alcohol "screws" with your hormones, so here's a small refresher as it relates to other destabilizing functions of your body when drinking alcohol:

"These alcohol-induced hormonal dysregulations affect the entire body and can result in various disorders such as stress abnormalities, reproductive deficits, body growth defect, thyroid problems, immune dysfunction, cancers, bone disease and psychological and behavioral disorders."
(Rachdaoui & Sarkar, 2013)[682]

As to her problem with depression, the answer, in this specific situation, couldn't be simpler, as published in the *Journal of Thyroid Research*:

"Patients with Thyroid disorders are more prone to develop depressive symptoms and conversely depression may be accompanied by various subtle thyroid abnormalities."
(Hage & Azar, 2012)[683]

It is only logical to assume that if one fixes the initial Thyroid condition, the depression may go away. So, what ended up happening to my wife's co-worker? She saw a doctor and was prescribed a drug to treat the symptoms without getting to the root cause of the problem. The side effects of this drug included headaches, weight changes, and from time to time, uneven heartbeat. She was also prescribed an antidepressant, the side effects of which will be discussed in Chapter 19, "MEDICINE IS MY FRIEND-MEDICINE IS MY FOE". Unfortunately she had no idea what caused her Thyroid problem and depression in the first place, and neither did her doctor. We will also be addressing the subject of prescription medications in Chapter 19.

ESTROGENIC EFFECTS

Both women and men are affected by the Estrogenic effects of different types of alcohol.

"Plants used to produce alcoholic beverages contain Estrogen-like substances (i.e., phytoestrogens). Observations that men with alcoholic cirrhosis often show testicular failure and symptoms of feminization have suggested that alcoholic beverages may contain biologically active phytoestrogens."
(Gavaler, J., Ph.D., 1998).[684]

Just to refresh your memory from the previous chapter, phytoestrogens are chemicals that are found in different types of plants such as beans, grains, seeds, and that can mimic the **female hormone Estrogen.** Foods made from soybean contain the highest amounts of phytoestrogens.[685]

Just to give you an example of how potent these phytoestrogens are, I have to mention Hops, the flowers of the Hop plant that are used to brew beer in order to give it bitterness, aroma, and stability.[686] The reports of the disturbances in the menstrual cycle of female Hop workers may be linked to Estrogenic substances in hops. [687]

How about a study of healthy males that clearly showed significant elevation in Estrogen after consuming beer or wine.[688] The interesting phenomenon is that blood samples were taken between five and ten hours after drinking. [689] Why are these findings significant? These findings are significant because increased Estrogenic activity may feminize males by growing breasts and reducing the male hormone – Testosterone, which may also lead to weight gain and even obesity.[690] [691] Unfortunately, these are not the only symptoms of increased Estrogenic activity in a male body. How about Erectile Dysfunction or ED?

"Erectile function is adversely affected by Estrogen exposure in early penile development, and exposure to estradiol in the mature penis leads to increased vascular permeability with increased ED. ED from increased estradiol exposure is independent of Testosterone level."
(Ramasamy, Schulster & Bernie, 2016)[692]

But you might say that you don't drink beverages made with Hops or work in the Hop fields. The sad reality is people with alcohol dependence may develop several types of sexual dysfunction. Here is a straightforward result of one of many studies that I read.

"Seventy-two percent had one or more sexual dysfunction, the most common being premature ejaculation, low sexual desire and erectile dysfunction. The amount of alcohol consumed appeared to be the most significant predictor of developing sexual dysfunction."
(Benegal & Arackal, 2007)[693]

We can safely assume that the more you drink, the higher the chances of developing sexual dysfunction.

As you've read in the "**DAIRY**" chapter earlier about wonders of hormones, Estrogen in particular, in the case of alcohol, may affect the way the female body metabolizes this hormone. The grim reality is **women who drink alcohol have higher levels of Estrogen than those who do not drink**.[694] [695] Keeping in mind that increased concentrations of Estrogen are implicated in different types of cancer, including lung,[696] and breast cancer in particular,[697] here's the reality of <u>less than one drink per day</u>.

Analysis from the 53 studies that involved over 95,000 women who did not have breast cancer and more than 58,500 women who suffered from the disease, drew a definite conclusion. Breast cancer risk was increased by <u>over seven percent</u> when consuming only 10 grams or 0.35 ounces, which is <u>less than one drink</u>.[698]

A more recent study conducted by the University of Oxford, Cancer Epidemiology Unit, showed even a greater breast cancer risk of <u>12 percent</u> when consuming 10 grams or 0.35 ounces or alcohol.[699] This particular study was significant, as it involved over 1.2 million middle-aged women.

But a lot of the doctors recommend two glasses of wine per day to keep you healthy. This study showed that there was no difference whether women "drank wine exclusively" or indulged in other types of alcohol. [700]

Some, as in a case of my wife's co-worker, are having more than one drink per night. You can only imagine how she multiplied her chances for not only breast cancer, but for "out of whack" hormones, as well as the Thyroid gland. How's that for two glasses of wine per day to keep you healthy? Talking about Estrogen in wine and other types of booze.

"Biochemical analyses have identified several phytoestrogens in the congeners of bourbon, beer, and wine."
(Gavaler, J., Ph.D., 1998).[701]

Congeners, which may include phytoestrogens as we discussed earlier, are substances other than Ethanol in a given alcoholic beverage. Congeners also affect the taste and aroma of many alcoholic beverages. The bad news is that even though congeners account for a very small quantity, many of them are potentially **toxic**.[702]

Besides everything that you just read in this section, the male reproductive system is affected in a very negative way by not only lowering Testosterone, but can alter the sperm to the point that it may affect fertility. [703] [704]

"Alcohol use is associated with low Testosterone and altered levels of additional reproductive hormones"
(Emanuele, M. & Emanuele, N., 2001)[705]

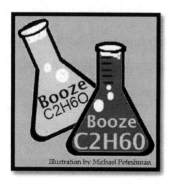

Illustration by Michael Poteshman

There is another very important factor to consider about the type of alcohol you may decide to consume. As we discussed earlier, ingredients in alcohol such as nitrates added to several beer types may lead to numerous of health problems. Many wine and beer brands have added sulfites, which are preservatives that depress bacterial growth.[706] Although the FDA banned the use of sulfites in raw fruits and vegetables, such as apples and lettuce in 1986, sulfites are used in beer and wine, processed foods, such as canned vegetables, potato chips, pickled onions, dried fruits and vegetables, bottled soft drinks, baked goods, as well as cordials. [707] [708] Sulfites are also used in the processing of corn sweetener, beet sugar, gelatin, food starches, etc. [709] Sulfites are added to many pharmaceuticals that include bronchodilators, injectable antibiotics, local anesthetics, injectable corticosteroids, and eye drops, among others. [710]

"The addition of sulphite additives to beer and wine is permitted in most countries, and although the use of sulphites in fresh salads, fruit salads, mincemeat or sausage meat, is illegal in many countries, it may occur illegally."
(Vally & Misso, 2012) [711]

According to the FDA, one out of 100 people is sensitive to sulfites, and out of that number, 5% suffer from asthma. [712] Sulfite sensitivity includes a slew of symptoms. Here are some examples:

- Pulmonary – asthma symptoms such as shortness of breath. [713] [714]
- Gastrointestinal - diarrhea, abdominal cramping, nausea. [715]
- Dermatological - skin problems such as rash, itchiness, or hives. [716]
- Cardiovascular - chest pain. [717]

Although the cause for the sulfite trigger is not yet known, sensitivity to sulfites can manifest at any time during a person's life.[718] The human body may respond mildly or the reaction can be "life-threatening." [719]

There is another matter related to red wine. In the past, when I drank more than two glasses of red wine, I usually got migraine headaches. When doing research, I stumbled upon multiple studies outlining a naturally occurring substance in red wine called "Tyramine". Red wine contains some of the highest amounts of this element besides soy sauce, aged cheese, beer on tap, fermented meats, and aged chicken livers.[720] Experts are still assessing tyramine and headache triggers.[721] There is one explanation: "...tyramine can cause nerve cells in your brain to release the chemical norepinephrine. Having higher levels of tyramine in your system -- along with an unusual level of brain chemicals -- can cause changes in the brain that lead to headaches" (WebMD, 2012).[722]

As the saying goes, "Choose your poison very carefully!" Keeping in mind everything outlined above, if I had to, I would only choose 1 shot of high quality multi-filtered distilled alcohol. The varieties could include premium vodka or tequila, or other high quality distilled alcohol without added sugar, chemicals, or preservatives.

Better yet, abstain from alcohol altogether, which will not only help with your waist line, but may prevent the **depletion of several vitamins** such as Vitamins B1, B6, B9, B12, and Vitamin A.[723][724][725] The consumption of Ethanol may affect the way you <u>absorb, metabolize, and store</u> these very important nutrients.[726] You will also reduce the chances for "out of whack" hormones, as well as Thyroid gland that influences most metabolic processes and regulates many genes in your body.

Chapter 16 PROPYLENE GLYCOL

"Propylene glycol is a synthetic liquid substance that absorbs water. Propylene glycol is also used to make polyester compounds, and as a base for deicing solutions. Propylene glycol is used by the chemical, food, and pharmaceutical industries as an antifreeze when leakage might lead to contact with food."
-ATSDR - Agency for Toxic Substances and Disease Registry-[727]

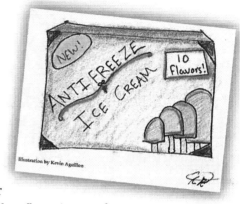

Illustration by Kevin Aguillon

Let's talk about everyone's favorite - ice cream. Ever since I was a child, I knew that ice cream had three major ingredients: milk and/or cream, eggs, and sugar. There is also flavoring such as strawberry, vanilla, or any other "deliciousness" that may be added. As I never read labels in the past, I consumed my share of ice cream with interesting ingredients.

For all of you ice cream and frozen yogurt lovers, be aware that propylene glycol (PG) is added to a number of your favorite brands:

INGREDIENTS: LIGHT ICE CREAM: NONFAT MILK, SUGAR, CORN SYRUP, MILK FAT, WHEY, MALTODEXTRIN*, PROPYLENE GLYCOL MONOESTERS, CELLULOSE GEL, MONO AND DIGLYCERIDES, CELLULOSE GUM, LOCUST BEAN GUM, GUAR GUM, POLYSORBATE 80, CARRAGEENAN, NATURAL AND ARTIFICIAL FLAVOR, CARAMEL COLOR, ANNATTO (FOR COLOR), VITAMIN A PALMITATE. WAFER: BLEACHED WHEAT FLOUR, SUGAR, PALM OIL, CARAMEL COLOR, DEXTROSE, HIGH FRUCTOSE CORN SYRUP, MODIFIED CORN STARCH, BAKING SODA, SALT, COCOA, SOY LECITHIN. *NOT IN REGULAR ICE CREAM.

INGREDIENTS: LIGHT ICE CREAM: NONFAT MILK, SUGAR, CORN SYRUP, MILK FAT, WHEY, MALTODEXTRIN*, PROPYLENE GLYCOL MONOESTERS, CELLULOSE GEL, MONO AND DIGLYCERIDES, CELLULOSE GUM, LOCUST BEAN GUM, GUAR GUM, POLYSORBATE 80, CARRAGEENAN, NATURAL AND ARTIFICIAL FLAVOR, CARAMEL COLOR, ANNATTO (FOR COLOR), VITAMIN A PALMITATE. DARK CHOCOLATE FLAVORED COATING: SUGAR, COCONUT OIL, CHOCOLATE LIQUOR PROCESSED WITH ALKALI, COCOA PROCESSED WITH ALKALI, MILKFAT, SOYBEAN OIL, SOY LECITHIN, VANILLIN (ARTIFICIAL FLAVOR), VANILLA. NOT IN REGULAR ICE CREAM.

INGREDIENTS: MILKFAT AND NONFAT MILK, SUGAR, CORN SYRUP, PECANS (PECANS, COTTONSEED OIL, BUTTER, SALT), SWEETCREAM BUTTERMILK, WHEY, CONTAINS LESS THAN 2% OF MONO- AND DIGLYCERIDES, GUAR GUM, CELLULOSE GUM, PROPYLENE GLYCOL MONOESTER, CARRAGEENAN, NATURAL FLAVORS, MOLASSES, ANNATTO (COLOR), CARAMEL COLOR, VITAMIN A PALMITATE. CONTAINS: MILK, TREE NUTS (PECANS).

Churned BUTTER pecan ICE CREAM LIGHT
BUTTER pecan LIGHT ICE CREAM WITH REAL pecan PIECES
120 2 60
Photos by Michael Poteshman

16-105

Some brands, including those claiming to be healthier alternatives such as low-fat or even fat-free, use this stuff in addition to other manmade chemicals.

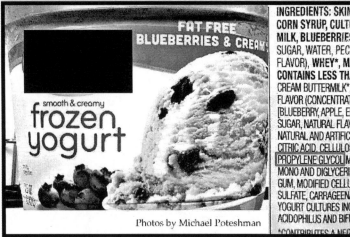

INGREDIENTS: LOW FAT ICE CREAM: MILK, SKIM MILK, SUGAR, POLYDEXTROSE, RASPBERRY FLAVOR BASE (RASPBERRY SEEDLESS PUREE, WATER, SUGAR, RASPBERRY JUICE CONCENTRATE, MALTODEXTRIN, PROPYLENE GLYCOL, ETHYL ALCOHOL, CITRIC ACID, NATURAL FLAVOR, CAROB BEAN GUM, RED 40 AND BLUE 1, GUAR GUM), MALTODEXTRIN, CELLULOSE GEL, MONO & DIGLYCERIDES, CELLULOSE GUM, CARRAGEENAN, POLYSORBATE 80, VITAMIN A PALMITATE. COATING: COCONUT OIL, SUGAR, CHOCOLATE LIQUOR, COCOA PROCESSED WITH ALKALI, SOYBEAN OIL, SOY LECITHIN, ARTIFICIAL FLAVOR, PGPR.

Photo by Michael Poteshman

Photos by Michael Poteshman

INGREDIENTS: SKIM MILK, SUGAR, CORN SYRUP, CULTURED SKIM MILK, BLUEBERRIES (BLUEBERRIES, SUGAR, WATER, PECTIN, NATURAL FLAVOR), WHEY*, MALTODEXTRIN, CONTAINS LESS THAN 2% OF SWEET CREAM BUTTERMILK*, BLUEBERRY FLAVOR (CONCENTRATED FRUIT JUICE [BLUEBERRY, APPLE, ELDERBERRY], SUGAR, NATURAL FLAVOR, CITRIC ACID), NATURAL AND ARTIFICIAL FLAVOR, CITRIC ACID, CELLULOSE GEL, PROPYLENE GLYCOL MONOESTER, MONO AND DIGLYCERIDES*, CELLULOSE GUM, MODIFIED CELLULOSE, CALCIUM SULFATE, CARRAGEENAN, LIVE ACTIVE YOGURT CULTURES INCLUDING L. ACIDOPHILUS AND BIFIDOBACTERIUM. *CONTRIBUTES A NEGLIGIBLE

Ice cream or frozen yogurt are not the only places where you'd find this chemical. You typically find it in the radiator of your car, specifically in the antifreeze! It can also be found in deicing solution for airplanes.[728]

"Antifreeze typically contains ethylene glycol as its active ingredient, but some manufacturers market propylene glycol-based antifreeze, which is less toxic to humans and pets."
- EPA.gov-[729]

If propylene glycol is "less toxic", it must be OK to eat??? Well, let's get a bit deeper into this stuff, and then draw our own conclusions, as we're examining food grade PG.

The DOW Chemical Company, one of the producers of this chemical, outlined the uses for PG.[730] Here are some examples:

- Solvent and carrier for colors, flavor formulations for the processed foods and beverage[731]
- Softening agent for cork seals and other food contact items[732]

- Preserves moisture and stabilizes prepared vegetables, fruit, as well as bakery goods, but not in Europe. [733]

As you can see, you find PG in a lot of processed food and bakery goods. Europe, on the other hand, has limited its use as you saw above.

This chemical, not found in nature, has made its way onto the list of "Direct Food Substances Affirmed as Generally Recognized as Safe"[734] (GRAS) along with numerous chemicals that you'll find in Appendix F at the end of the book.

The FDA can only deem this chemical safe if it's used in the specific amounts. Here are some examples:

- 2.5 percent for frozen dairy products[735]
- 5 percent for alcoholic beverages[736]
- 24 percent for confections and frostings[737]
- 5 percent for nuts and nut products[738]
- 2.0 percent for all other food categories [739]
- 97 percent for seasonings and flavorings[740]

So, if you decide to indulge in cake with frosting or candies that may contain a whopping 24% of PG, processed nuts, ice cream, seasonings or flavorings on your steak or chicken, or other foods that contain propylene glycol, you may just go over the safety zone. In addition, this stuff has a lot of uses such as dough strengthener, emulsifier, flavor agent, moisture preserver, stabilizer and thickener, and texturizer.[741] Scary? You bet!

After researching volumes of information, I found that 25 mg. of propylene glycol per kilogram (kg) or 2.2 lbs of body weight is considered "acceptable" by the World Health Organization.[742] Does that mean that it is acceptable for a 185 lbs. or 84 kg. person to consume approximately 2 grams or 0.071 ounces before being affected? Let's dig a little deeper.

TOXICITY OF PROPYLENE GLYCOL

"Propylene glycol is manufactured by treating propylene with chlorinated water to form the chlorohydrin which is converted to the glycol by treatment with sodium carbonate solution. It is also prepared by heating glyercol with sodium hydroxide"
(FDA, 2013).[743]

So, what happens if you consume PG in unsafe doses? I found my answer on the "Toxic Substances Portal" on the website of the Agency for Toxic Substances and Disease Registry, which is a part of Centers for Disease Control or CDC. A screen shot on the next page is from their website:[744]

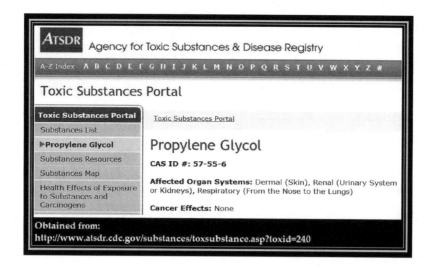

The good news is that PG does not cause cancer as you can see on the screen shot above.[745] The bad news is that it may affect skin, urinary system or kidneys, or respiratory system from the nose to the lungs.[746]

This information was echoed by the IPCS or International Program for Chemical Safety - Chemical Safety Information from Intergovernmental Organizations:

"It is primarily a CNS depressant in high doses. On rare occasions, stupor and unconsciousness occurred after parenteral administration. After chronic exposure, seizures in man and renal and hepatic damage in animals have been described"
(Szajewski, 1991).[747]

Here's the translation for some of the terminology in the quote above:
- CNS depressant - Central Nervous System psychological depressant
- Hepatic damage - damage of the liver
- Renal damage - damage of kidneys
- Stupor - reduced or impaired level of consciousness[748]
- Parenteral administration - injection or infusion, but not through the mouth
- Chronic exposure - continuous exposure

You think that was disconcerting? There is definitely more. Before I present another quotation from the "Summary of clinical effects" for propylene glycol section of the INCHEM website, here is translation for the upcoming terminology:
- Ocular exposure – exposure of the eye(s)
- Hyperaemia – excessive accumulation of blood in an organ(s) or part of the body[749]
- Lactic acidosis – "…is when lactic acid builds up in the bloodstream faster than it can be removed. Lactic acid is produced when oxygen levels in the body drop"(MedlinePlus, 2012)[750]
- Cardiac arrest - stopping of the heart

…And now the quote:

"Ocular exposure causes mild ocular irritation with hyperaemia; chronic or prolonged skin and mucous membranes exposure may also cause irritation; gastrointestinal disturbances, nausea and vomiting have been observed after ingestion.

Rapid intravenous injection of preparations of drugs containing propylene glycol as a solvent (in significant amounts) may cause unconsciousness, arrhythmias and even cardiac arrest.

Chronic exposure may cause lactic acidosis, hypoglycaemia, stupor, and seizures; renal and hepatic damage have been observed only in animals"
(Szajewski, 1991).[751]

Since this substance is found on the "Toxic Substances Portal", it's only logical to assume that Propylene Glycol is is toxic. As you can see, this substance can be found in many products including a number of processed foods, cosmetics, shampoos, hair conditioners, soaps, and even medicines. Be aware that when you use PG in cosmetics or other products described above, you may be absorbing it through your skin.

"When you put shampoo or conditioner onto your scalp, the 20 blood vessels, 650 sweat glands, and 1,000 nerve endings soak in the toxins"
(Mercola, 2010).[752]

Propylene Glycol can be present in your pantry or bathroom under different names such as 1,2-propanediol, 1,2-dihydroxypropane, methyl glycol, and trimethyl glycol. [753]

Let's look at this stuff from a logical perspective. In the morning, you may have a little PG pastry, in the afternoon you may have a couple of fruits and vegetables that were treated with PG for stability, then perhaps an ice cream bar. And don't forget makeup as well as shampoos and conditioners that that you may be using on daily basis. Do you know for certain that you're using this stuff in safe doses? What about symptoms that you cannot explain?

Knowing what you know now, products that containing PG can be easily avoided by reading labels. A better alternative is to purchase natural products that don't contain this substance; yes, even your ice cream. There are more and more manufacturers that avoid using propylene glycol. All it takes is a quick search on the Internet, and you'll get plethora of choices.

Even though propylene glycol may be toxic in high doses to humans and animals as outlined above, it has its uses. I especially appreciate this substance in the radiator of my car so my coolant does not freeze during the winter.

This concludes the section on major "NOT TO EAT" foods, or foods that contain toxic substances. There are definitely more "NOT TO EAT" foods; actually a lot more. I believe that with this section you now have the foundation on how to avoid them. So, before purchasing any food, do a simple one-word query in your favorite search engine, and I can promise you, you'll get a plethora of results. Some may be conflicting. Ultimately, you will be able to determine whether you want to put this item into your body or leave it on the store shelf. You can also email me, and I'll do my best to respond to your issue in the question and answer blog. **Remember, "Your body is your temple;" why would you put garbage inside the place of worship?** You would not!

Now that we are done with "WHAT NOT TO EAT" section, let us look at the doctor's prescriptions for low-fat or fat-free "stuff".

SECTION 4. UNCOVERING MYTHS AND WIDELY DISTRIBUTED UNTRUTHS ABOUT FAT, DIETS, MEDICINE, VITAMINS, GUT HEALTH, REVERSAL OF HEART DISEASE, SLEEP, INSULIN, AND HOW TO EAT TO LIVE

Chapter 17 LOW-FAT-FAT-FREE-CHOLESTEROL-FREE MYTHS

In the late 1980s, dietitians and health professionals jumped on the low-fat bandwagon. I regretfully recall the miserable years of suffering and eating tasteless and disgusting "cardboard-tasting almost foods", because my doctor recommended that I go on a low-fat and fat-free diet. When I did, things turned from bad to worse, with higher weight, higher blood pressure, and a more miserable outlook on life. Why did my bad condition worsen by eating supposedly healthier alternatives such as low-fat, fat-free, and cholesterol-free foods?

"Why hasn't cutting fat from the diet paid off as expected? Detailed research shows that the total amount of fat in the diet isn't really linked with weight or disease"
-South Denver Cardiology-
(Collins, MD & Buckley, RDN, CDE, 2015)[754]

It's the complete opposite from what we've been told! When the manufacturers recognized the "low-fat" or "fat-free" craze, they were only too happy to give the public what it wanted. It's always good business to oblige the customer, as this leads to greater monetary rewards. Manufacturers began to substitute fat with sugar, as well as different carbohydrate elements. [755] In order to mimic the satisfying texture and flavor of fat, manufacturers also added something "very special:" thickeners, chemicals, and flavor enhancers in order to adjust consistency and taste.[756]

The photographs below show a chemical smorgasbord of starches, sugars, MSG and its derivatives, among other wonders of modern science in so called "lite" or "low-fat" foods:

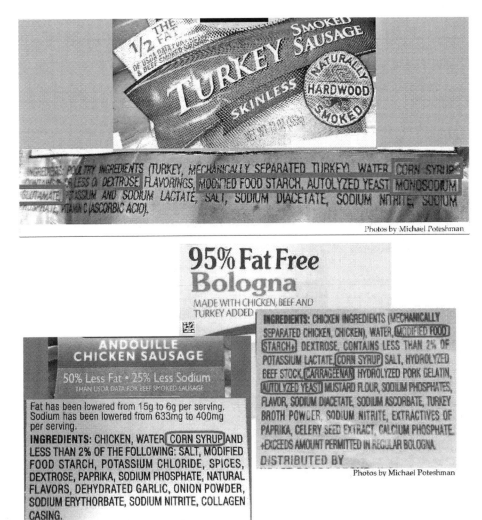

Photos by Michael Poteshman

No wonder I was gaining weight and feeling worse by the minute! Knowing what I know now, I should never have put anything remotely resembling this "almost food" stuff inside my body. What frustrated me even more is when I realized that sugar and corn syrup were used to adjust the taste of fat-free foods.

Sugar is absolutely fat-free, even if you eat two pounds of it, it will still remain fat-free!

What it does to your body is beyond scary. But we have already established the alarming effects of sugar in the "SUGAR" chapter. Interestingly, the products containing these "chemical wonders" and sugars are given names such as "lite", "low-fat", "fat-free", among other healthy-sounding names. A lot of times these "almost foods" may not be low in calories, but quite the opposite.

In the days of "Living Dead", I used to eat a lot of cheese, and purchase low-fat varieties which were not only high in calories but contained a slew of chemicals, sugars, or corn syrup. I now understand why so called low-fat or fat-free cheese had peculiar labels such as "cheese food" or "cheese product."

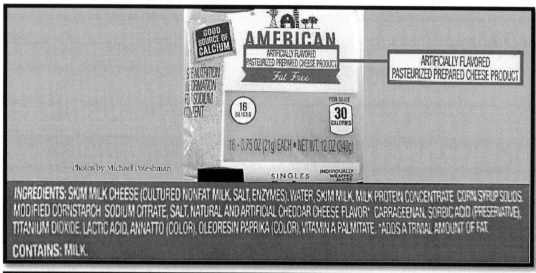

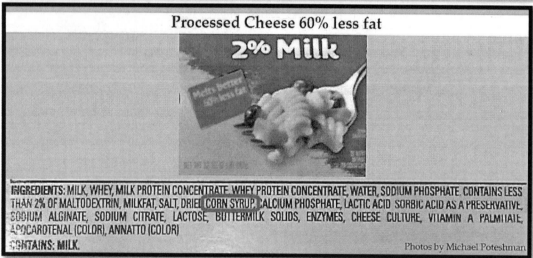

According to Keri Glassman, MS, RD, CDN, author of the book "The New You and Improved Diet", there has to be only 51% cheese in "cheese food."[757] **The rest can be preservatives, coloring, whey solids, and emulsifiers, in addition to other additives and flavor enhancers.**[758] These preservatives and other "wonders" make you put on and hold on to more weight instead of getting rid of it! [759] [760] Even if we disregard high calories, as you will read in the "Food Detox and resulting weight loss" chapter, **your body tends to hold on and not release fat when you consume foods that are loaded with chemicals and toxins.**

FATS ARE ESSENTIAL

"Fats supply energy and essential fatty acids and serve as a carrier for the absorption of the fat-soluble Vitamins A, D, E, and K and carotenoids. Fats serve as building blocks of membranes and play a key regulatory role in numerous biological functions"
– USDA –[761]

There are not only good fats, but some fats are essential to our lives. Let's look at cholesterol, for example. I always heard that cholesterol was bad. First of all, not all cholesterol is bad, and second of all, <u>it is extremely necessary</u>.

"The body uses cholesterol as the starting point to make Estrogen, Testosterone, Vitamin D, and other vital compounds"
(HSPH, 2002).[762]

Thus, **we must consume fats not only because they are important for our existence, but also because <u>if you don't consume enough of them, you may remain hungry and unsatisfied</u>**. The type and quantity of fat is another matter, as we will examine next.

THE BAD, THE SATURATED, THE GOOD FATS, AND CHOLESTEROL

If Harvard School of Public Health or South Denver Cardiology and its doctors are satisfied that fats aren't linked to diseases or weight gain, why are we worried about fats?

BAD FATS

Hydrogenated oils are bad fats. These trans-fats were part of "**WHAT NOT TO EAT**" chapter. Remember the discussion about foods with added trans fats such as peanut butter, margarine, many baked goods, potato and corn chips, and French fries? Recall that **consumption of these "really bad fats" may lead to heart disease, different forms of cancer, type 2 diabetes, inflammation, among other ailments**. Thus, you are already familiar with their devastating effects on the human body.

CHOLESTEROL

As we discussed earlier, cholesterol is extremely necessary for our existence and is the starting point for Vitamin D, phosphorous and calcium metabolism, in addition to playing an important role in making hormones such as Estrogen, Testosterone, substances that help you digest food, as well as detoxification of foreign substances out of the liver.[763] Yet, the 2010 USDA Dietary Guidelines for Americans recommended eating less than 300 mg/day.[764] Considering that one large egg contains approximately 186 mg of cholesterol means that if I ate two eggs, I would be breaching the 300 mg threshold by 72 mg. Because of my research since I began to "Live Wonderfully", I've been consuming between two to four organic eggs on any given day, while maintaining textbook perfect cholesterol numbers, despite my doctors' advice to the contrary.

Three years later, a report came out that confirmed yet again that everything I was "preaching" and doing holds true. I took the following excerpt out of the advisory report to the Secretary of Health and Human Services and the Secretary of Agriculture:

" Previously, the Dietary Guidelines for Americans recommended that cholesterol intake be limited to no more than 300 mg/day. The 2015 DGAC will not bring forward this recommendation because available evidence shows no appreciable relationship between consumption of dietary cholesterol and serum cholesterol… Cholesterol is not a nutrient of concern for overconsumption."
-USDA Scientific Report of the 2015 Dietary Guidelines Advisory Committee-[765]

What that means is that the 2015 Dietary Guidelines is not recommending any type of a limit to consuming dietary cholesterol. They explain their decision by pointing out that there was no considerable relationship between dietary cholesterol and cholesterol that is found in blood (serum cholesterol). Isn't that interesting? They went from recommending measly 300 mg/day to **no limitation**! Wow!

Although all of the credible dietary cholesterol studies were conducted years earlier, I'm glad to see that the advisory committee consisting of many doctors and health professionals finally consented to the studies.

As you continue to read this book, you may find that something that may seem controversial at the time, may not be as controversial years or even decades later, as illustrated clearly by this report.

SATURATED FATS

In doing research, I came upon several reputable sources that were clearly against all forms of saturated fats. But knowing what I know now, despite these sources, I could not, in good conscience, name these fats "bad." There are some really healthy and even beneficial qualities to consuming them.

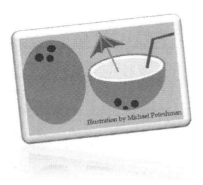
Illustration by Michael Peteshman

Not all saturated fats are created equal. For decades, professionals have been saying that coconut oil was bad for your heart because of its high saturated fat content. There is still a controversy brewing in the health community. The fact is, coconut oil contains lauric acid - a form of saturated fat which promotes good HDL cholesterol.[766] [767] [768] Coconut oil is mostly comprised of medium chain triglycerides (MCT), which are much easier for the body to process than your typical long chain triglycerides (LCT) that are found in other sources of fat.[769] [770] [771] [772]

Some in the health community preach that coconut oil is bad for the heart, and also is the cause for weight gain because of its fat content. Based on the evidence that I uncovered, this argument is completely blown out of the water. Consider a study entitled, *"A coconut extra virgin oil-rich diet increases HDL cholesterol and decreases waist circumference and body mass in coronary artery disease patients."* [773]

Just the name of the study alone asserts that coconut oil increases good cholesterol and promotes weight loss. The conclusion is equally as powerful, especially that the study was conducted on mostly elderly patients with coronary artery disease, who **lost the weight and increased their good cholesterol**. [774] What that means is that even though some in the health community believe that coconut oil is bad for cardiovascular system and promotes weigh gain, this study rips their argument to shreds.

Talking about weight. Consider a study on women that shows that consuming coconut oil helps to reduce **"abdominal obesity"**.[775]

How about another study entitled, *"Weight-loss diet that includes consumption of medium-chain triacylglycerol oil leads to a greater rate of weight and fat mass loss than does olive oil"*.[776] The conclusion was equally as exciting, even though we know that olive oil has beneficial qualities.

"In conclusion, the results of this study show that a weight-loss diet that incorporates moderate amounts of MCT oil leads to greater losses of body weight and fat mass than does consumption of an equivalent amount of olive oil."
(St-Onge & Bosarge, 2008)[777]

Once again, coconut oil is mostly comprised of medium chain triglycerides or MCT's.

There are more studies that show the benefits of coconut oil, but I believe that you get the picture. The fact is that unrefined extra virgin coconut oil does not produce an Insulin spike unlike sugars, simple carbohydrates, or even whole grains. More on that in Chapter 24 where we will be uncovering how Insulin affects our entire existence.

Draw your own conclusion about whether you want to consume or stay away from coconut oil. My family and I enjoy it tremendously while maintaining healthy cholesterol numbers, unlike what was preached to us over the years of low-fat/ fat-free/ cholesterol-free misery at the doctor's office! We add extra coconut oil to **all of our meals** in order to maintain satiety.

Besides coconut oil, here are some examples where you can find saturated fat; some are good, and some are not:

- Milk, cheese, butter, cream, ice-cream or other dairy products (not skim or fat-free). You already know about dairy products as part of the "**WHAT NOT TO EAT**" chapter
- Lard, for as long as the animal was grass fed with an ample supply of Vitamin A.[778] Therefore, grass fed organic would be my only choice in order to obtain fat soluble vitamins from this and other types of fat
- Meat with fat "marbling" or fatty cuts. Once again, meat has to be organic and grass fed
- Poultry with skin; grass fed and organic
- Palm oil or palm kernel oil - "… also consists of vitamins A and E, which are powerful antioxidants. Palm oil has been scientifically shown to protect the heart and blood vessels from plaques and ischemic injuries. Palm oil consumed as a dietary fat as a part of a healthy balanced diet does not have incremental risk for cardiovascular disease." (Odia, Ofori, & Maduka, 2015) [779]
- Eggs –approximately 2.6 grams of unsaturated and 1.5 grams of saturated fat [780] in one large egg, mostly in the yolk. Pasture raised organic is the key, as yolk in the organic eggs contains the highest amount of protein when compared to conventional eggs.[781] Furthermore, eggs from pasture raised hens contain higher Vitamins A, E, and Omega-3 fatty acids.[782]
- Stick margarine is one of those foods that may contain trans fats and other undesirable ingredients,[783] thus I would consider it an "almost food" that I would not eat myself or feed to my kids
- Fully or partially hydrogenated oil, or any type of trans fat is off the menu, as you've read in "**WHAT NOT TO EAT**" chapter

How do we distinguish between foods that contain saturated fat, while keeping in mind mixed opinions and studies?

According to 2010 USDA Dietary Guidelines for Americans and USDA Scientific Report of the 2015 Dietary Guidelines Advisory Committee, less than 10% of your daily calories should come from consuming saturated fats.[784] [785]

From time to time, I enjoy a fatty cut of meat. The interesting phenomenon is even when I breach the 10% guideline for saturated fat, which happens more often than not due to the consistent use of unrefined organic coconut oil, two to four eggs per day, I still maintain exceptional blood cholesterol numbers. In fact, my cholesterol figures are better now than when I was in my twenties.

As you've witnessed USDA's complete reversal on consumption of dietary cholesterol earlier, perhaps years down the road or even sooner, we may see a reversal of saturated fat consumption guidelines.

WHY NOT JUST CUT OUT MEATS?

I'm often asked, "Why not cut out meat, chicken, or other animal products altogether?" This is certainly your prerogative. I, however, believe in "taste" and not cutting out something that I really enjoy. Especially something that's not part of the "**WHAT NOT TO EAT**" list.

I also advise taking another very important factor into consideration. Vitamin B12 exists mainly in different types of meats including organ meats, fish, eggs, dairy, [786] [787] and in the fermented soy product-tempeh.[788]

The function of Vitamin B12 is vital not only for metabolism, but also for forming red blood cells and for maintaining the central nervous system.[789]

Equally as important is Vitamin K2, that none of my doctors have ever mentioned or recommended throughout my years of "Living Dead."

Vitamin K2 works with Vitamin D3, and is responsible for taking calcium out of arteries or soft tissue where it does not belong, and distributing it into your bones and teeth[790] where it does belong. **What that means is that it promotes cardiovascular and bone health while lowering the chances of heart disease, arthritis, and osteoporosis.** [791] [792] Without Vitamin K2, you may end up with calcium plaguing in the arteries.

Because we are on the saturated fats section, you've already guessed that the best sources for Vitamin K2 are grass fed (not grain fed) organic beef, organic chicken, organic egg yolks, organic organ meats [793] such as goose liver, among other foods that I was warned against by my doctors. That's right, all of these foods are high, and in some cases, very high in saturated fat and cholesterol. Even though I consume them daily, my cholesterol numbers are textbook perfect!

If you're a vegan, you can find this important Vitamin in natto, [794] a fermented soy product. Check with your doctor or credible nutritionist if natto will provide sufficient amount of Vitamin K2 for your dietary needs. Also, fermented vegetables such as sauerkraut contain Vitamin K2, but not in the same quantity as animal products or natto.

Now that you have all of the variables, you make a choice if you want to eat meat, or cut it out completely. There is nothing wrong with becoming a vegetarian or a vegan, as long as you can get all of the necessary Vitamins and minerals from other sources. Keep in mind that it's best to get most of the necessary Vitamins from food and not through supplements.[795]

Also, if you're a meat eater and decide to cut all of it out, you may be creating a deficit within your psyche where you might enter dangerous dieting territory. That's where cravings for something that you have taken out of your diet will begin to occupy your life. There's more on this subject in the section called "D#@t - A four letter word" in the next chapter.

GOOD FATS

I don't want to suggest that you should run to the store and get these ingredients and wolf them down in large quantities. As you will learn in "WHAT TO EAT" chapter, these ingredients will be used as a complement to your "Living Wonderfully" meals. Let's begin.

UNSATURATED FATS

"Unsaturated fats, which are liquid at room temperature, are considered beneficial fats because they can improve blood cholesterol levels, ease inflammation, stabilize heart rhythms, and play a number of other beneficial roles. Unsaturated fats are predominantly found in foods from plants, such as vegetable oils, nuts, and seeds."
- Harvard School of Public Health - [796]

Unsaturated fats are comprised of monounsaturated and polyunsaturated fats:
- Monounsaturated fats have one carbon in the molecule. [797] These fats stay liquid at room temperature, but begin hardening under cold conditions.[798]
- Polyunsaturated fats have more than one carbon in the molecule, but unlike monounsaturated fats they typically don't harden when chilled.[799]

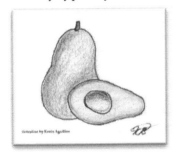

Monounsaturated fats can be found in foods such as avocados, olive oil, olives, sesame seeds, pumpkin seeds, almonds, hazelnuts, and sunflower oil, among others.[800] In addition, these fats contain Vitamin E, which happens to be an antioxidant. [801]

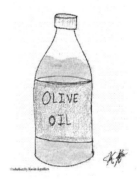

Polyunsaturated fat sources are well known, especially Omega-3 fatty acids. The Omega-3 is found in fish such as salmon, catfish, mackerel, trout, tuna, herring, among other fatty species of fish,[802] as well as, shellfish.

According to analysis of multiple studies, when eating between one and two servings of fish per week that are high in Omega-3 fatty acids, the risk of dying from heart disease is reduced by 36%.[803]

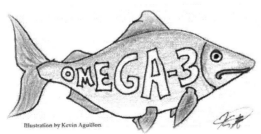

Other sources of Omega-3 polyunsaturated fatty acids are found in walnuts, chia seeds, flaxseed, and even in oils that I do **not** recommend, which are soybean and canola.[804]

Another polyunsaturated fatty acid not as well known by many is Omega-6 which is found in vegetable oils such as safflower, soybean, cottonseed, poppy seed, among other oils.[805]   One thing to remember is to limit your intake of Omega 6 because it may cause inflammation, which leads to multiple health problems and chronic diseases.[806] [807]   Therefore, **it's more desirable to consume a higher ratio of Omega 3 fatty acids to Omega 6,** [808] or the ratio of 1:1 at the most.

Enjoy your fatty fish and seafood as discussed above, flax seeds or flax seed oil, and limit your intake of safflower, sunflower, corn, cottonseed, peanut, among other oils that are high in Omega 6 fatty acids.

There you have it: not all fats are bad. In fact, you just witnessed that a lot of fats not only extremely good but are essential for your health.

Now that the low-fat-fat-free-cholesterol-free prescriptions from our doctors are not what they're cracked up to be, let's delve into the prohibitive diet routine and how it affects us physically and mentally.

Chapter 18   DIETS-SHMIETS: DO THEY REALLY WORK? ANY OF THEM?

The short answer is no. Unless you're a superwoman or a superman, diets cannot be sustained. There are exceptions to almost every rule and some may claim that a particular diet really works. Unfortunately, I have never met a person who was able to sustain a specific diet plan for a prolonged period.

D#@T - A FOUR LETTER WORD

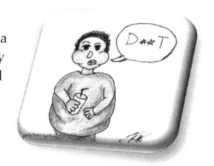

When I think about the word "diet" or hear something about a diet, it makes me cringe and shiver. I don't believe that I'm the only person who regards **diet** as an unsavory four letter word. Our learned experience tells us that a diet consists of poor-tasting food, small portions, and suffering; **lots and lots of suffering!** Many of you are familiar with stories, or have experienced yourself that once you go on a diet, and lose X number of pounds, you dread this "dietary" existence. As my new diet of the month always began on Monday, I was automatically switched into the prohibitive "diet mode."

That meant that I couldn't eat certain foods, and if I did, I skipped meals to make up for added calories. Sound familiar? I know firsthand about self-defeating strategies and creating scenarios which thwart attempts of getting healthier. There is no shame in admitting it. Even if I didn't jeopardize my own diet, there is no possible way that I could have succeeded.

The majority of "diet plans" are destined for failure. Once you go off the specific dietary routine, you regain just as much or even more weight than before you began that particular diet.[809] [810]

Resulting weight gain is due to binging on prohibited foods or backfilling the portion size that was literally "seized" from you during the calorie counting nightmare.

To prove my point, let's look at a couple of examples of the recent diet trends. Drum roll please... Food paring, shake diet, coffee diet, green tea diet, coconut milk diet, eating less diet or perfect portion diet, grapefruit diet, or the all protein diet by the late Dr. Atkins. These diets promote different approaches to weight loss, and in some cases, healthier living. They all have the same common denominator: <u>taking something away,</u> whether it is a "prohibited" food item or two to three quarters of your meal altogether.

Some of these diets may take away nutrients that your body is starving for, thereby leaving a nutritional void. As a result, you begin to crave nutrients that a particular "diet of the month" is lacking.

"Fad diets may be unhealthy. They may not provide all of the nutrients your body needs"
(Win, 2014)[811]

There is no way that a human being can exist on these types of dietary plans; perhaps for a little while, but not permanently! I was one of the "robots" who listened and abided by doctors' recommendations. I also followed advice on television shows and what I read in nutritional books and articles. The information was scattered and chaotic as the diets were alternating from one TV show to another. Unfortunately, I blindly believed that a particular diet would actually be beneficial if I tried it.

I ended up being on many different diets, starting with Dr. Atkins, and continuing with South Beach, High Carbohydrate, Soy Milk, Grapefruit, and Cabbage Soup diet, among others. All produced some positive result, but only at the beginning. Because I knew that I needed to stay on a particular "diet of the month", I forced myself to either eat the recommended foods at the recommended time intervals, or abide by the prescribed number of calories. All were wildly unsuccessful and <u>unsustainable</u>!

The only marginal and consistent short term success I had was on Dr. Atkin's diet, at the age of 36. On Atkin's I ate low carbohydrate foods in the form of red meat, poultry, cheese, eggs, bacon, fish, sausage, scrapple, ham, and other proteins. After six months of eating these foods, while being partially starved of carbs, I went on a four-month "after-diet" carbohydrate binge, which resulted in 35 pounds weight gain. I actually gained more weight than I lost initially on this diet plan. The rest of the diets only lasted two to four months. Once again, I always gained more weight than I lost.

Speaking to others and doing research before this book was conceived, my wife and I concluded that stories like ours were universal. There are very few diet reviews or experiences that indicate that any diet really works long term and is sustainable. There is a clear reason for such unsustainability.

WHY ARE DIETS UNSUSTAINABLE?

Throughout my life, my dieting results have been very consistent: feeling hungry, dissatisfied after every meal, and experiencing overwhelming food cravings. Why do we have cravings while on all of these diets? The answer is simple. Please recall our earlier discussion. If any diet or even non-diet foods contain excitotoxin MSG, you may begin to not only crave sugary and starchy foods, but due to the altered production of hormone Leptin, your appetite may get out of control. On an All Protein diet you can eat protein, but few carbs, so you're craving carbs the entire time. On a High Carb diet, you're eating carbs and little protein, so you're craving protein. You also want to eat more carbs because of the insulin spikes, which we will be discussing later. On portion size diets, you're eating less than you normally would, as you must count calories or "points." **The portion size diet is extremely difficult because your stomach possesses stretch and density receptors[812] that have to be triggered.**

When the stretch and density receptors are barely activated by tiny food portions, you're constantly hungry and dissatisfied with your meal.

We will be discussing in later chapters how "Eating Wonderfully" activates your stretch and density receptors to signal to your brain that "you're stuffed to the gills." For now, let's continue with why diets are unsustainable.

Some of the large diet enterprises offer counseling when you start feeling low and dissatisfied as you are getting ready to get off this "dietary torment." Operators on the phone are trained to help you with staying on these torturous plans. How crazy is that? Eventually, you get sick and tired of tiny portions, "feel good" operators, and dieting altogether, and can't wait to get off this exhausting way of life.

My wife was one of the victims of these diet plans. She spent thousands of dollars on pre-portioned foods, and regularly spoke to a motivational counselor as part of the plan. The irony is that before ending her diet suffering, she eventually began to double up on the tiny portions that were prescribed. Approximately three months before she quit this particular diet, I observed some success, so I decided to join in her weight loss misery. I asked her to double her order so we could lose weight together.

Within one month I began to eat four pre-plated meals as opposed to one. Don't get me wrong, besides being convenient, the food tasted relatively good. But there was so little of that food that I had to quadruple my portions. After a while we realized that we spent so much money on so little food that we reverted back to the old way of eating, which was cheaper and more plentiful. We went to a supermarket frozen food section and realized that we could get almost the same nutritional value as the pre-portioned TV dinners but at a fraction of the cost. The saddest part was our realization that the diet didn't really work unless one stuck to eating bird-sized portions. We didn't even need to binge on food, as we actually ended up gaining the initial weight after we spent an absurd amount of money.

Dissatisfaction with diets completely envelops your life, as you're always weighing pros and cons between eating and staying on the dreadful "diet of the month."

"We found that the average percentage of people who gained back more weight than they lost on diets was 41%... In each of the studies, a third to two-thirds of the subjects gained back more weight than they lost."
-Traci Mann, PhD, UCLA- [813]

The body is consistently craving nutrients that are missing in a particular diet plan, while such plans direct you to eliminate the necessary nutrients in part or as a whole.

Bottom line, we cannot fool nature and millions of years of evolution. Here's how it works.

PRINCIPLES BEHIND WEIGHT LOSS AND WEIGHT GAIN

First and foremost, one must understand the nature of weight loss and weight gain. Second, one must realize that even people with faster metabolism must abide by the same principles as everyone else in order to lose weight. You are no different than your skinny neighbor or overweight cousin! Therefore, one principle that governed our weight control has been consistent throughout ages, but only in part:

"One must burn more calories than one takes in to lose weight at any age"
-University of Maryland Medical Center- [814]

Sounds sad and unfair, doesn't it? It certainly does, because I followed that motto for decades, and as a result, I kept gaining weight and saw my body in decline. So, how are we now losing weight effortlessly since we're NOT starving, eating huge portions, and when we leave the table, we feel stuffed to the gills with food?

The good news is that **not all calories are created equal**! As we discussed earlier, when you consume good fats that are very high in calories such as organic unprocessed coconut oil, avocados, or even extra virgin olive oil, your body responds more favorably as compared to consuming sugar, simple carbohydrates, and different types of processed foods that may be much lower in calories. A lot has to do with the release of **Insulin**, which in part directs how your body stores fat. Here's this "Insulin" word again…

The rest of the answer of how we're eating huge portions and retaining ideal weight is coming up later in the book. For now, it is imperative that you understand your body's potential and the way it operates in order to keep you healthy before you're able to "Eat Wonderfully."

There is something that exists within us that we call, "storing food for the winter", or in terms of evolution, "storing food in case of famine."

Throughout human history, it was very difficult to get food, and especially pure sugar, as it was reserved for influential people of different societies. As a result, the bodies of our ancestors began to adapt and store fat for times when famine was imminent. Humans were hunters and gatherers, and existed on very little food but were quite physical in acquiring it. Hunting, cultivating crops, or harvesting fruits and vegetables involved substantial physical activity.

Over millennia, the <u>bodies of our ancestors adapted to live on very few calories while being able to perform immense amounts of physical activity</u>.

Even during times of plenty, while our ancestors were stuffing their faces, they continued to burn calories by performing physical activities of hunting and gathering. So what changed? Our bodies remained the same as our ancestors', but we began to enjoy a sedentary way of life and indulge in high-calorie/**low-nutrition food**.

DIET, THE CENTER OF YOUR UNIVERSE

Consider the following scenario. You've been feeling especially sluggish, tired, sleepy, and frustrated because you're putting on some unwelcome pounds. You experience escalation in blood pressure and brain fog. Finally you decide to do something about it.

While sitting in traffic, you hear yet another diet commercial on the radio. The announcer talks about shortened life span due to the increase in weight, and an absolutely perfect new diet plan is being offered at a discount. Naturally, you decide to try this new approach.

When you make it home after a long day, you talk to your loved ones who are supportive of your new diet. After all, you're trying to improve your life. You're pumped up, and ready to conquer this war on fat. You wait for the perfect moment and a perfect day, as my wife and I always waited until Monday. And then it happens - this phenomenon that happens to millions of people on <u>all diets without exceptions</u>.

You begin the very first day on this "shiny new" diet with planning your eating schedule, what snacks you are going to have and when, and even what you're going to eat tomorrow. Finally, the first week has passed, and you're doing seemingly well. You even dropped 5 pounds and it was relatively easy. That's how it always happens <u>on practically every single diet</u>.

Now comes the weekend. People in your family and your friends are indulging in different types of food. But because you're disciplined and committed to your new diet, you're not touching any of it. Even when you're offered a bottle of beer, you say, "This particular brand of beer has too many calories." You say that you would rather not have any; at least until you lose some weight.

You're very pleased with yourself. You go home, and the evening comes, and the cravings begin. You try to ignore the cravings, but they are too strong. So you decide to have a little piece of something that's not part of this particular diet. You say to yourself, "a little piece will not make a huge difference." Once you have this little piece, you decide to have another piece, and then another. Since you already had a few pieces, why not just enjoy something that you truly love? So you indulge. You promise yourself that you will start anew on Monday.

Monday comes, and you go back on a regimen. Once again, you're preparing and planning meals, forecasting your perfect time to eat including timing your snacks that this new diet allows you to have. Some of the foods included in your new diet are the ones that you may hate. However, being a disciplined person, and staying committed to this particular diet, you continue to eat these "*&%$☺^@ foods" with great disdain. Although a particular diet food may not be your favorite, you begin to obsess about every kind of food. [815] I know I did. It sends shivers down my spine every time I recollect those horrific decades of dieting.

What's even crazier, you begin to observe what people in your office are eating. All of the sudden, your **dieting becomes the center of your universe**. To illustrate my point, I was so obsessed with food while on a diet that I began cooking for others, but I was not eating any of the food myself. I was only deceiving myself, thinking that I was still on the diet and was able to cook and not eat. In reality, I felt miserable, dissatisfied, and was hanging on every possible calorie I could muster. Sometimes I would dream about food in my sleep. When I woke up in the morning, I began to dread the prescribed diet food and the subsistence that it offered.

Looking back at the way I behaved while dieting, now seems bizarre. Even in meetings at work I was talking about food. When I wasn't on a diet, I usually ordered donuts on Fridays for my staff members, and had one or two myself. However, when I was in the midst of dieting, I was ordering donuts for my staff almost daily so "I could enjoy the smell, and just eat a crumb or two." That's what I was telling my team while watching them devour doughnuts.

The interesting phenomenon is that after I went off these diets, I was ordering a dozen doughnuts for myself, and would eat them in my office throughout the day, as opposed to one to two doughnuts during the non-famine phase. Once I was back to my overweight self, I resumed ordering donuts on an occasional basis, and only eating one or two during meetings as I'd done before the dreadful dieting.

I'm certain that a lot of you can relate to my bizarre dieting behavior. Some of you may think this was a bit extreme, as each person reacts differently to the restrictions that various diets impose. We can all agree that as soon as you go on a diet, something changes within your psyche and begins to affect your behavior in a negative way. It is because your body and your mind initiate "famine management."

Famine management begins by turning down your metabolism to a lower point so you can retain more calories. As a result, all you think about is food.

"When you keep to a reduced-calorie diet, your body makes metabolic adjustments that make it harder and harder for you to lose weight…Your body becomes very efficient, and you have to eat less and less to continue to lose weight. If you had the will to go on a diet, the fact that it steadily becomes less and less effective makes it even harder to stick to it"
-Traci Mann, PhD, UCLA-[816]

Even in diets that advocate that you eat frequently but in smaller portions, the food cravings in a lot of people are heightened because of restrictions. I recall six miserable tiny meals that I had to eat. Although some swear by it, for me and my wife, the "eating often diet" lasted the shortest amount of time. I have to invoke this "Insulin" word again. The fact is, eating six meals per day, **consistently stimulates Insulin production, which makes it difficult to lose stored fat**. More on that in the Insulin chapter.

As you continue to stay on a diet, you become more anxious, and in some cases, depressed due to a void in your life—food. Although you may see some weight loss, your mind is affected in a very negative way as you may also become serotonin deficient.

Some people may experience a drop in serotonin level while dieting.[817] Serotonin is a "happy neurotransmitter" that is responsible for mood balance among other functions such as sleep, sexual desire and function, memory, etc. [818]

"Dieting in general tends to lower serotonin in the brain and this can cause depression in susceptible people"
(McDonald, 2009). [819]

As you continue to chug along on these restrictive diets, in time your self-esteem begins to slump, and anxiety begins to kick in with a vengeance.[820]

ALL DIETS COME TO AN END

There is a holiday celebration around the corner and we're invited. We tell ourselves that we'll just "taste" some of the delicious foods that hosts have prepared, and then resume our diet the next day. After all, some diet gurus advocate that "You should have at least one day off per week from a diet in order to enjoy yourself, so you should taste everything, but don't overeat." Unfortunately, those gurus never told us about MSG, chemicals in food, among other Insulin spiking/fat storing/health damaging properties of different "almost foods". We follow gurus' advice and begin to taste. But instead, while we taste, we begin to overindulge as if we were ingesting our last meal.

All of a sudden our mood heightens, and we feel great. We begin to relax because of the lie that we told ourselves about restarting this dreadful diet on Monday. Our body and mind feel terrific when we're finally consuming food that may contain nutrition that the body was lacking, and also we're eating foods that we were craving for months.

So you eat, and you eat, and you eat until you are completely over-stuffed. In fact you ended up eating almost the amount of food that's equivalent to what you consumed during the entire dieting process. But you feel content, since there is little to no guilt as you're feeling relieved from the suffering that you endured in the past couple of months! Perhaps you feel some guilt, but it goes away very quickly. All of a sudden the world seems brighter, and the birds start chirping, and everything is wonderful. The only problem is that you are back to putting on pounds at a much faster rate because you are now in the binging mode. It's almost like an alcoholic falling off the wagon.

Two years prior to writing this book, I was at the gym, doing my best to stay somewhat fit. I was speaking to a gentleman who went through a twelve-step alcohol rehabilitation program. He was 10 years sober. He started telling me about the excuses that he came up with when he was craving alcohol. He said that one morning, before leaving the house to go to work, while tying his shoes, his shoelace broke. This was his excuse for drinking the entire day because in his mind, this particular day started so poorly. The next day when he was leaving the house, he tied his shoes, and the shoelace did not tear. He said that this was his reason to celebrate that his shoelaces were intact. As a result he drank for the next two weeks. When he came back home after binge drinking, his wife left him.

Perhaps we don't think that craving and binging on food are as severe as drugs and alcohol, but judging by the example above, we can clearly see that my "bizarro" behavior of consuming a dozen doughnuts when coming off a diet is somewhat equivalent. You may have similar experiences of this ridiculous self-deceit. At one point or another, we made every possible excuse to ourselves and others in order to justify the need for eating foods that will eventually make us gain more weight.

Some diets last longer, some not as long. The bottom line is:

"Diets Don't Work Long-Term"
(DeNoon, 2007).[821]

ENTER THE LIVING WONDERFULLY LIFESTYLE

The Living Wonderfully approach has absolutely nothing to do with dieting. Many who have experienced this lifestyle have declared that it's an anti-dieting movement. I tend to agree.

Your body is never starved for nutrients and is actually thriving instead of hanging on to every calorie it can muster. The cravings suddenly go away, and you are no longer thinking about food, as it's no longer the center of your universe. Not only that, but the weight and fat loss occur naturally as a result of the improved health, and not the other way around.

You are already aware that cutting out the necessary high calorie fats is the thing of the past. Because I do not want to spoil the extremely pleasant surprises, as you continue to read on, you will be uncovering other facts and incredible evidences that will put all of the calorie-counting diet horrors that you experienced in the past to rest.

You will not be starving for calories, and your "happy neurotransmitter" serotonin does not decrease, as in most diets. Instead, you begin to experience contentment and happiness that you haven't felt in years or even decades, as in my case, and in the cases of many, many others who have hopped aboard the Living Wonderfully train.

As you continue to perfect your new lifestyle, you suddenly become full of life as a result of the improved sleep, sharpened memory, increased energy, and for some of us, improved sex drive. Instead of using a cliché of a lifestyle, I call it "Your new and significantly improved way of life". You begin to Live Wonderfully, every single day for the rest of your new and healthier life, without the necessity of dieting nightmares of the past!

Now that you are aware of foods that wreak havoc on your system, the importance of fat, and the way your body responds to restrictive dieting, let's look at other doctors' prescriptions; literally.

Chapter 19 MEDICINE IS MY FRIEND – MEDICINE IS MY FOE

"When diet is wrong, medicine is of no use.
When diet is correct, medicine is of no need."
-Ayurvedic Proverb-[822]

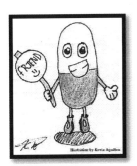

I did a lot of soul searching before I was able to present this chapter. The reason it was so difficult is that I truly respect the noble profession of medicine. I'm also a fan of the incredible advancements in therapy and diagnosis that modern Western medicine has achieved. Please understand that I'm not a "psycho" who thinks that all medicine is bad; only some aspects. Let's put it plainly; the information that I'm about to present may appear controversial, but it is factual and is backed by credible evidence. Readers may draw their own conclusion after finishing this chapter.

I firmly believe that the medical industry should do what it was designed to do: help people who are in serious trouble. Broken bones need to be set properly, and appropriate pain medication should be administered if pain is severe. If a person requires surgery in order to live a productive life, surgery must be performed. If a diagnosis is required, Western medicine has exceptional equipment to do so. If there is a "real" infection, then antibiotics should be prescribed.

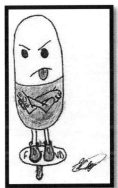

I'm not in any way, shape, or form "anti-medical industry crazy." What I am against is the medical industry practice of keeping people dependent on **liver-toxic**[823] [824] [825] medications for prolonged periods of time. I used the phrase "liver-toxic" several times throughout the book for a reason. Just look at the statistics.

"Worldwide, the estimated annual incidence rate of drug-induced liver injury (DILI) is 13.9-24.0 per 100,000
*inhabitants. **DILI is one of the leading causes of acute liver failure in the US**."*
(Suk & Kim, 2012)[826]

This was my experience for almost a decade and a half. **Such methods concentrate on <u>treating symptoms</u> rather than diagnosing and resolving the underlying cause**. The result is a sicker patient.

Here's a sobering preview of how some factions of the medical industry are treating our symptoms, and in effect slowly destroying our bodies and shortening our lives.

The medical business is like any other business which has to be profitable or at least break even in order to survive. Doctors, pharmacists, drug company personnel, researchers, technicians, and even animal handlers who look after research animals need to earn a living. Their jobs are necessary in order to produce new and revolutionary medical treatments. All is done with the objective of making sick people well.

I don't have a problem with people making money. That's what puts food on the table. But there isn't too much money to be made if everyone were to suddenly become healthy. Doctors would not be able to prescribe cholesterol or blood pressure medication if patients' cholesterol and blood pressure were normal. Surgeons would not be able to perform coronary bypass surgery if arteries weren't blocked. Psychiatrists would not be able to prescribe anti-depressants if patients were happy and full of life. The medical business would wane, because **there is no money in health, only in illness.** There is no way for the medical industry to profit from healthy people, as healthy people may only visit a doctor once a year for their "physical." That's what I'm experiencing now, at 53 years of age, where I visit my doctor once a year or less. Looking at the past 15 years, I was a profit center for different doctors and for the pharmaceutical industry. As a result, I existed on different toxic medications that caused other symptoms where additional liver-toxic medications were prescribed to treat secondary side effects.

"And so the story goes, one drug causing symptoms that demand another drug. That's what doctors learn about in medical school: drugs. They don't learn about diet and nutrients, so it seems that all they know how to do is prescribe drugs."

-Carolyn Dean, MD, ND-[827]

Here's a small glimpse of the "profit center" that I used to contribute to: "Statins are the best-selling drugs in the United States, with $14.5 billion in combined sales in 2008" (AboutLawsuits, 2010).[828]

CIRCULAR DESTRUCTION: THE BEGINNING

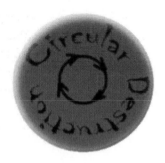

In today's society there is a pill for everything. There is a pill for headache, a pill for cold symptoms, a pill for sleep, a pill for losing weight, a pill for gaining weight, a pill for erection, a pill to reduce blood pressure, and a pill to increase blood pressure. The list goes on and on. Many people think the way I used to: "Why worry about eating healthy? I'll visit my doctor and he'll prescribe medicine that will fix all of my health problems." Unfortunately, this type of attitude backfires as it backfired on me.

Living through chemistry instead of "Living Wonderfully" eventually takes a toll on the health of unsuspecting patients who trust doctors to heal them. But do we really get healed? Well, I personally experienced this so called "healing."

"... It has been estimated that for every dollar spent on ambulatory medications, another dollar is spent to treat new health problems caused by the medication" (Kohn, Corrigan, & Donaldson, 2000).[829]

Yes, we're talking about side effects!

How did we get to this point? We got to this scary place by consuming foods and beverages that you read about in the "WHAT NOT TO EAT" and "EXCITOTOXINS" sections. These include simple carbohydrate foods, foods high in sugar, hormones, trans fats, nitrates, arsenic, antibiotics, and other health-destroying, carcinogenic chemicals. After years of consistently consuming this stuff, the **standard ailments** include high blood pressure, elevated cholesterol, blocked arteries, type II diabetes, and higher incidences of cancer.

This is where Circular Destruction begins.

BLOOD PRESSURE MEDICATION

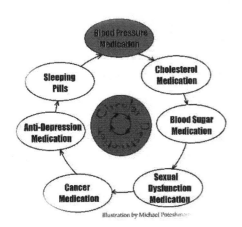

Illustration by Michael Poteshman

You go to the doctor and he/she finds that your symptoms include pounding headaches and dizzy spells.

The doctor measures your blood pressure and determines that it's elevated. The doctor sends you out for a blood test which reveals that your LDL, or bad cholesterol level, is high and your HDL, or good cholesterol, is low.

The doctor prescribes drugs to treat symptoms, but the root of these problems still exist.

When you have high blood pressure as I used to have, you may get a prescription of ACE inhibitors with diuretics (water pill). Appendix II at the end of the book lists generic and brand names of these prescriptions. Perhaps you recognize some of the ones that you're currently taking or have taken in the past. These drugs help to dilate blood vessels so the blood pressure is reduced. In theory this sounds good, but in reality, these ACE inhibitors have a slew of side effects. More drugs are then prescribed in order to lessen the consequences of taking this stuff in the first place.

So I don't put you to sleep, I'll just summarize the side effects for ACE inhibitors in one sentence. Taking this stuff may lead to impotence, depression, kidney failure, gout, mental confusion, fatigue, blurred vision, loss of vision, impaired kidney function, pancreatitis,[830] among many other undesirable side effects.

Alternatively, doctors may prescribe beta blockers and water pill if they feel that there may be complications with ACE inhibitors. Please see Appendix III at the end of the book where you may recognize some of these drugs by name.

Beta blockers reduce heart rate. Blood pressure is reduced by dilating blood vessels. That sounds good as well, but the side effects?

"It's known that diuretics (or water pills, like hydrochlorothiazide) and beta-blockers (like Atenolol) can also cause erection problems."
(WebMD, 2017)[831]

Because there are too many side effects to list, let's sum it up. Taking this stuff may lead to the reduction in testosterone and sexual disfunction,[832] kidney failure, impotence, heart failure, heart block, depression, hallucinations, confusion, nausea, stomach cramps, rash, visual disturbance, dry mouth, among other side effects.[833] "Beta blockers may cause low or high blood glucose and mask the symptoms of low blood glucose (hypoglycemia) in patients with diabetes" (Ogbru, 2013).[834]

CHOLESTEROL/STATINS MEDICATION

Illustration by Michael Poteshman

Now that you've gotten your blood pressure prescription, you can bet that your doctor will prescribe a statin drugs in order to combat your high LDL cholesterol.

If you haven't taken one, you're familiar with some of the names of these medications as they're heavily advertised on radio and television. Here are some examples: atorvastatin (Lipitor), rosuvastatin (Crestor), pravastatin (Pravachol), simvastatin (Zocor), fluvastatin (Lescol), lovastatin (Mevacor).[835] I was on one of these drugs for a number of years.

So what's wrong with lowering your cholesterol with these drugs? Nothing, if you are not concerned with side effects. For one, statins work in the liver as they **block the enzyme HMG-CoA which is responsible for production of cholesterol**.[836]

Since statins suppress one of the liver functions, there may be a possibility of moderate or **severe injury to the liver**.[837] [838]

Not only that, but statins commit the biggest robbery of the essential nutrient Coenzyme Q10 or CoQ-10, as statins block production of this nutrient. [839] CoQ-10 is responsible for the **energetic support** (mitochondrial health) of the **heart, liver, kidneys, pancreas,** and other organs.[840] So, why is CoQ-10 so important? Well, because studies clearly show that deficiency in this nutrient may be linked to cardiovascular disease, **heart failure**, neurological disorders such as **brain dysfunction**, as well as, **kidney failure**, **muscle weakness**, **chronic pain**, among others. [841] [842] [843]

I was faithfully taking statins without knowing what side effects were lurking in the background. One study showed that statins decreased heart muscle function[844] (**weakening of the heart muscle**). Here's the conclusion of the study: "*Statin therapy is associated with decreased myocardial function…*" (Rubinstein, Aloka, & Abela, 2009).[845] Myocardial refers to heart muscle or muscular tissue of the heart.

For years I was having unexplained **muscle aches and pains** (myalgia) **and muscle weakness**, but I never attributed these terrible discomforts to statin use. After reading documentation pertaining to the statin drug that I took for years, it was clearly noted, "*Uncomplicated myalgia has been reported in atorvastatin-treated patients… Myopathy, defined as muscle aches or muscle weakness…*" (Pfizer Ireland Pharmaceuticals, 2007).[846] Furthermore, FDA has expanded its advice on the risks pertaining to **muscle injury** of statin interactions with other drugs. [847] [848] There is a distinct possibility that my muscle pains and weakness[849] [850] of the past were caused by the CoQ-10 deficiency as a result of taking statin medications.

Talking about muscles. While following my doctors' advice when it came to exercise and taking statins, for some reason, I did not see much improvement in my muscle tone. Well, there is a big reason for that! How about this for a headline:

"An important new study suggests that statins, the cholesterol-lowering medications that are the most prescribed drugs in the world, may block some of the fitness benefits of exercise, one of the surest ways to improve health."
(The New York Times, 2013)[851]

A study from the Division of Cardiology at Duke University Medical Center entitled "Simvastatin impairs exercise training adaptations" showed that these drugs **don't just decrease the fitness of the muscles, but also of the heart and lungs.**[852]

There are other, just as potent side effects, some of which I suffered from while taking this stuff. **Memory loss and confusion** are side effects that have to be listed on the statin medications label according to the FDA.[853]

…And here's a big one – connection related to **diabetes**.[854] Once again, the FDA mandates statin manufacturers to include information on the label pertaining to the **increase in blood sugar**, as well as effect of statins on diabetes. [855]

I was very excited to find a study that gave an explanation why no matter how much I exercised and dieted, and did not touch any sweets, my blood sugar numbers were constantly elevated. I will summarize and translate this study's conclusion.

It makes no difference whether you are young or old, or if you have diabetes or not, <u>statin use is associated with an **increase in blood sugar**</u>.[856]

A Canadian population based study that evaluated Ontario residents, and echoed by other studies, showed that statins were implicated in the **increased risk of developing new diabetes**.[857] [858]

*"More than 20 million Americans take statins. That would equate to **100,000 new statin-induced diabetics**"*
(Topol, 2012).[859]

Another study that was published in the medical journal "Lancet", analyzed the results of 13 studies of statins' side effects. It was concluded that 9% of people who used these drugs were at a higher risk of incidents of Type 2 diabetes.[860]

There is another side effect that has impacted me greatly in the past. How about **Insulin resistance**? Yes, yet another study showed that taking statin drug **increases Insulin resistance significantly**![861] We will be talking about Insulin and Insulin resistance, and how it affects your entire existence in Chapter 24.

Lastly, we see the increased number of class action law suits by major law firms due to inadequate warning labeling of statin drugs:

*"The Lipitor lawyers at Saiontz & Kirk, P.A. are reviewing potential product liability lawsuits for users of the popular cholesterol drug who have been diagnosed with diabetes…Statins have been linked to a number of serious health problems and side effects, including **muscle injury, kidney problems, and diabetes**…"*
(Saiontz & Kirk, P.A., 2014)[862]

The good news is that I no longer have any symptoms as described above, as I am off the statin induced nightmare. What a relief!

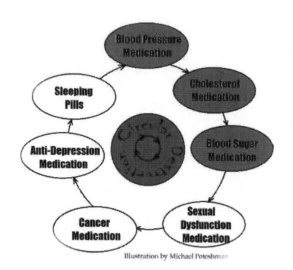

Illustration by Michael Poteshman

If you're not alarmed by now, you most likely will be by the end of this chapter. I still don't know how I survived the onslaught of chemistry on my system. Keep in mind that this is only the beginning of "Circular Destruction" as there is a lot more to follow.

So you've got the usual package of beta blockers or ACE inhibitors with water pills to ease your blood pressure, and statins to reduce cholesterol. You go home and begin taking this stuff only to realize that all of a sudden you have some of the symptoms that we just discussed.

You decide to go back to your doctor and complain about your new symptoms.

The doctor measures your blood sugar and it seems to be elevated, so he prescribes a blood sugar lowering drug or combination of drugs. Perhaps you recognize some of these: Metformin, Januvia, Avandia, Actos, or Dymelor.[863] You thought that your doctor solved all of your problems and then, all of a sudden, your blood sugar medication causes new side effects.

Let's examine some of the side effects of two of the more often prescribed drugs, Metformin and Actos. Incidentally, my late mother was on Metformin for years as her condition continued to deteriorate.

Here are some side effects, as there are many more. Metformin may cause impaired liver functions, muscle pain, difficulty breathing, lightheadedness or dizziness, weakness, irregular heartbeat, heart palpitations, electrolyte disturbances, and reduced level of Vitamin B12, among other side effects.[864] [865] [866] [867] [868] Scary? When taking Actos, another blood sugar lowering medication, one of many side effects is even scarier: how about the increased risk of **bladder cancer**? [869]

The FDA, in a "Safety Announcement", notes that if you took Actos (pioglitazone) for longer than 12 months you may have **40% increased risk for bladder cancer**.[870]

Your doctor evaluates these new symptoms caused by blood sugar medication, and may prescribe drugs to address the symptoms. For example, for heart palpitations the doctor may prescribe higher dose of Beta Blockers in order to slow down the increased heart rate.[871] You already know what these are, so I won't go into "gory" details. As you can see, a vicious circle has been completed.

Alternatively, the doctor may prescribe calcium blockers to treat arrhythmia.[872] Side effects may include swollen legs and feet, dizziness, nausea, tachycardia or **rapid heartbeat,** and a slew of other side effects. Wasn't the whole point to take these drugs in order to normalize the heartbeat? *"Some side effects can make an arrhythmia worse or even cause a different kind of arrhythmia"* (NHLBI, 2011).[873] The circular destruction of your system continues its vicious cycle, but now with more destructive intensity!

CIRCULAR DESTRUCTION INTENSIFIED

One of the many side effects of statin medication and beta blockers that is worth mentioning is impotence and/or erectile dysfunction or ED. According to a 2009 study by Université de Toulouse, France, statins may not only exacerbate erectile dysfunction but may "**induce**" it.[874]

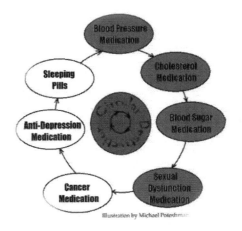

I thought that this was a relatively new study, and that's why <u>my doctors never cautioned me about these side effects</u>. Unfortunately, I was wrong.

The Oxford University Press published a review in 2002, seven years prior to French study. The name of the study is unambiguous: "Do lipid-lowering drugs cause erectile dysfunction?" [875] The conclusion is clear: *"The systematic review procedure was applied successfully to collect evidence suggesting that both statins and fibrates may cause ED"* (Rizvi, Hapmson, & Harvey, 2002).[876] Fibrate drugs are designed to lower blood triglyceride levels. Although this was published while I was taking these drugs, my doctors, for some reason, failed to mention this nugget of information. Interesting? Isn't it?

While taking these statin drugs, all of the sudden you're experiencing ED. You go to your doctor and complain. Your doctor wants to help the way he knows how, and suggests medicine to help with this "ailment." So he prescribes Viagra or Cialis, or the equivalent. These drugs may help with ED, but at what cost?

As I queried side effects of these drugs, I was bombarded with overabundance of results with headings like these:

- From Fox News – *"Erectile dysfunction drugs linked to skin cancer?"* (Martinez & Samadi, 2014)[877]
- *"Study Shows Viagra Users 84% More Likely to Develop Melanoma"*(Sokolove Law, n.d.)[878]
- From CBS News - *"Viagra may increase melanoma risk, study finds"* (Firger, 2014)[879]
- From NBC News – *"Viagra May Boost Risk of Deadly Skin Cancer, Study Finds"*(Aleccia, 2014)[880]
- *"Melanoma Victims May Be Owed MILLIONS by Pfizer, the maker of Viagra®"* (Litster Frost Injury Lawyers, n.d.)[881]
- *"Sildenafil Use and Increased Risk of Incident Melanoma in US Men A Prospective Cohort Study"* is the name of the study published in JAMA Internal Medicine Network publication of the American Medical Association in June, 2014.[882] Sildenafil citrate is a drug sold under the names Viagra and Revatio. [883]

This particular side effect may not only require cancer medication, but may require chemotherapy among other unpleasant procedures.

Although skin cancer is a substantial side effect, there are many others. Here are some examples:

Hearing loss or sudden hearing decrease, vision loss in one or both eyes, muscle pain, urinary tract infection, rash, back pain, abnormal and/or blurred vision, headache, upset stomach, anxiety, stuffy or runny nose, dizziness, among other side effects. [884] [885]

FEELING DEPRESSED? YOU'RE NOT ALONE!

As you're continuing to take statin drugs, you may find yourself sitting in the corner and wallowing in your own desperation and anxiety. A number of publications and credible studies, show that there is a relationship between statins and depression.[886] There are also articles stating that statins actually help people who are depressed.[887] Here's what the British publication, *Daily Mail,* had to say about these claims:

> *"The study, published in the Cochrane Library, which reviews drug trials, also points out that the vast majority of trials have been carried out by **drug companies who may play-down any possible risks**. Some patients taking statins have **suffered from short-term memory loss, depression and mood swings**"*
> (Borland, 2011).[888]

The Drug Safety Case Reports publication outlined that the use of statins may increase the risk of personality, behavior changes and/or "serious psychiatric evens" in some people.[889] The name of the study is also unambiguous: "Mood, Personality, and Behavior Changes During Treatment with Statins: A Case Series".[890]

Let's move on to meds that doctors may prescribe in order to combat your newly acquired depression.

There are a number of antidepressants that your doctor may prescribe. The list of side effects is long, and in some cases redundant. So we will begin with examples of the scary stuff first, and then outline a couple of examples that are a bit less frightening.

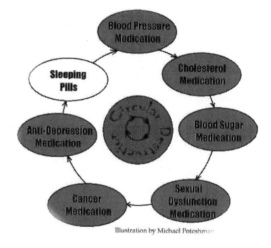

In 2007 The Food and Drug Administration (FDA) proposed that producers of **all antidepressant** medications update their black box labeling to include a warning that taking of these drugs may increase the risk of suicidal thoughts or behavior, also known as "suicidality."[891] The group that's at risk is young adults between 18 and 24 years of age.[892] Isn't the whole point of these drugs to fight depression?

Unfortunately, this sounds too familiar! Not only the 18 to 24-year age group is susceptible to such thoughts and behavior. After my mother had her first heart attack in her late 40s, her doctor prescribed Prozac. Her exact words still resonate in my mind: "I feel like throwing myself out the window." As soon as she discontinued taking this antidepressant, her suicidal thoughts subsided within days. Luckily, she took only three doses.

It's hard to concentrate on any single antidepressant because a lot of the side effects are redundant. I'll pick an arbitrary and common anti-anxiety medication that's frequently prescribed: Xanax, also known as Alprazolam. Some of the side effects include: depression, thoughts of killing oneself, memory impairment, tiredness, weakness, difficulty concentrating, difficulty with coordination, irritability, slurred speech, and dizziness.[893]

Here are a couple more examples that we can add to our circular destruction list:

- **Sexual dysfunction**[894] [895]– *"Troubles in the bedroom range from lack of sex drive to impotency"* (Alprazolam.org, 2014).[896] Please recall our discussion earlier about ED drugs prescribed on top of other drugs. In this case, the problem may be compounded if more ED medication is prescribed, and more side effects may manifest. <u>Another circle of destruction is completed.</u>

- **Weight gain.**[897] [898] Now that you put on additional weight, your blood pressure and cholesterol level may increase, or other cardiovascular problems may manifest. Supplementary **drugs to combat blood pressure or to deal with additional problems as a result of the weight gain will be prescribed.** <u>Another vicious cycle is completed.</u>

- **Trouble sleeping** is also on the list of more common side effects associated with Xanax.[899] Insomnia raises the risk for elevated blood pressure, higher risks of depression and other psychiatric disorders,[900] among other ailments that we have already addressed. Thus, <u>we have completed yet another vicious cycle of circular destruction</u>.

CAN'T SLEEP OR COMPLETION OF ANOTHER VICIOUS CYCLE?

So, you go to your doctor and complain that you can't sleep. Consequently, your doctor may prescribe sleeping medication.

Let's look at several side effects of one of the most commonly prescribed sleeping drugs, Ambien:

- Worsening of depression and suicidal thoughts.[901] How about that? Didn't we just finish our discussion on anti-depression medication?

- Abnormal changes of behavior or thinking – *"Some of these changes included decreased inhibition (e.g. aggressiveness and extroversion that seemed out of character), bizarre behavior, agitation and depersonalization…"* (Sanofi-Aventis, 2014).[902]

- *"FDA Drug Safety Communication: Risk of next-morning impairment after use of insomnia drugs; FDA requires lower recommended doses for certain drugs containing zolpidem (Ambien, Ambien CR, Edluar, and Zolpimist)"*(FDA, 2013).[903]

- Cardiovascular side effects that include palpitations and increased blood pressure.[904] [905]

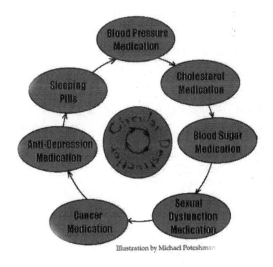

Illustration by Michael Poteshman

There you have it: depression that may require additional antidepressants, heart palpitations that may require additional heart medication, and increased blood pressure that may require additional blood pressure medications.

The circular destruction never stops because it is a circle, a vicious cycle that has no end until the day of demise, or until one decides to "Live Wonderfully" instead of living through pharmaceuticals!

We only touched on this subject as there are many more circular destruction scenarios for different types of medication. Therefore, before giving any drugs to your kids, or taking drugs yourself, please use the power of the Internet, and query the name of the medicine you intend to take. You will be able to weigh pros and cons with your doctor from the perspective of an educated consumer. The best doctor will listen and understand your concerns.

Next we'll look at what my doctors should have been prescribing instead of liver-toxic stuff that was slowly poisoning my body and mind. Oops, sorry, forgot, ☺ you can buy Vitamins over the counter; no need for prescription. But wait, there's a big caveat.

Chapter 20 VITAMINS AND MINERALS – FACT OR FICTION?

Whenever I went to see my doctors, they never offered any discussion about the role that Vitamins played in keeping me healthy. Instead I was prescribed higher doses of statin drugs for cholesterol as well as blood pressure lowering medications. As a result, I kept getting worse and worse while blindly trusting my doctors.

What are these things called Vitamins and minerals? As simple as this question is, most people get it wrong. The correct answer is: Minerals are substances that come from the earth and are absorbed by plants during their lifecycle.[906] Vitamins are considered organic and are made by plants and animals.[907] Humans absorb Vitamins and minerals from plants and from the animal meat that we consume.[908]

Are these substances really that important? You bet! Without these incredible life-saving substances I would have never recovered after 15 years of being in decline and taking more prescribed beta blockers that had nutrient-depleting effects! Let's look at the proper and not so proper ways to deliver these incredible elements into our bodies.

SUPPLEMENTS ARE SERIOUS BUSINESS

As with a multitude of fads, our Western culture always gets on a bandwagon. First we had high carb diets that made a lot of people fat, then we jumped on a pure protein fad, and everyone got tired of it very quickly. Later we jumped on the low-fat/fat-free mania, and it made matters worse. I'm the prime example of this madness. Now a lot of the gurus are saying to load up on supplements because most of us have some sort of a deficiency. I don't completely disagree with this assessment, as most of us are deficient in some way as I used to be. However, supplements are not a complete solution. Wouldn't it be great if we just took a supplement pill or a multivitamin capsule and completely forgot about tough nutritional requirements? Unfortunately our complex internal and external systems do not operate that way.

First and foremost, do you really know what Vitamin or mineral you are deficient in, and how much you really need to take, if any? Health gurus say that you need to take Vitamin supplements daily. The problem with this scenario is that if you're taking Vitamins and minerals that your body has enough of, especially some "mega-doses", you're running a risk of Vitamin overdose. Yes, there is such a thing!

WHAT VITAMINS ARE YOU TAKING AND FOR WHAT PURPOSE?

"Too much Vitamin C or zinc could cause nausea, diarrhea, and stomach cramps. Too much selenium could lead to hair loss, gastrointestinal upset, fatigue, and mild nerve damage"
(Nierenberg, 2014).[909]

Vitamin intake is especially uncertain when you're eating fortified processed foods with different Vitamins added. Breakfast cereal, Vitamin water, and even orange juice are some of the foods that are fortified with Vitamins and minerals.[910] When you decide to consume these foods and take an additional multi-Vitamin supplement, you may reach a Vitamin overload.

"Any ingredient in a multiple Vitamin supplement can be toxic in large amounts, but the most serious risk comes from iron or calcium"
(MedlinePlus, 2011)[911]

But a lot of the health gurus would say that you'd just "pee out extra Vitamins and minerals." Indeed, an oversupply of certain <u>water soluble</u> Vitamins can be excreted from your system through urination. Others are not as easily expelled. For example, taking over 2000 mg/day of Vitamin C on a regular basis may cause a slew of problems; *"Such doses may acidify the urine, cause nausea and diarrhea, interfere with the healthy antioxidant-prooxidant balance in the body…"* (Johnson, L. E., MD, PhD., 2012).[912]

WEIGHT GAIN?

Can one actually gain weight from taking too many supplements? The answer is a big yes! How about certain B Vitamins or B Vitamin complex?

*"…ecological studies have shown that increased B vitamin consumption is strongly correlated with the prevalence of **obesity and diabetes**."*
(Zhou, 2014).[913]

Do we really know how much Vitamin B we consume when we eat processed foods that are fortified with B Vitamins, and in addition taking Vitamin B complex supplements? Although Vitamin B complex supplements usually contain six or more B Vitamins, the amounts or doses in a single supplement may vary. Therefore, you may be having more B vitamins that stimulate appetite, even if the dose is not excessive.

*"It has long been known that B vitamins at doses below their toxicity threshold **strongly promote body fat gain**. Studies have demonstrated that formulas, which have very high levels of vitamins, **significantly promote infant weight gain, especially fat mass gain**, a known risk factor for children developing obesity."*
(Zhou, 2014).[914]

There is also a matter of the regulation of supplements by the FDA. Supplements are not as closely regulated and are not as rigorously tested as prescription medication.[915]

Therefore, if you do require supplements, make certain that you diligently do your homework. It is important to figure out which brand has "Vitamin-looking-stuff" in an attractive packaging, and which brand really delivers the necessary potency. The Internet is the best place to evaluate ratings. Just make certain that the web site is reputable so you get the best information possible. Look at several web sites to evaluate and compare if the information is relevant.

By now you're probably thinking that I'm against supplements. Absolutely not!!! In fact, **Vitamins have the ability to combat a multitude of <u>specific ailments</u> if taken in mega doses**[916] **in <u>certain</u> situations**. What I'm saying is that supplements have their rightful place, but only when necessary. Let's look at the best place for obtaining real Vitamins and minerals.

ALL-INCLUSIVE VITAMIN AND MINERAL BUFFET

So, besides in the form of a pill, where do these life-saving substances come from? You get most of them from food! It is imperative that food is used as your all-inclusive Vitamin and mineral buffet. Why am I saying most? Well, because when you're out in the sun, you get Vitamin D-boosting benefits, which we'll talk about later. For now, let's concentrate on food:

"Most individuals can obtain all the Vitamins and minerals needed to meet the recommended dietary allowances and adequate intakes by eating a variety of foods"
(Bellows, Moore, & Gross, 2013) [917]

Your body cannot produce calcium; some of the richest sources of calcium are leafy green vegetables, broccoli, and fish.[918] Even canned salmon, mackerel, and sardines are loaded with calcium. [919] There is also calcium in dairy products, but you have already been through that section.

As you will read in the "**WHAT TO EAT**" chapter later, the Living Wonderfully vegetable base or "LW-base" will include most of the Vitamins and minerals that your body needs. The rest you will get from other foods. That does not mean that you may not be deficient in certain Vitamins and minerals. Everyone is different, and your absorption of Vitamins may be different from someone else's. You may require the infusion of additional Vitamins from other food sources. On the other hand, you may have to remove some foods or beverages that may impede your Vitamin absorption. Don't fret; everything will be explained shortly.

The next logical question is, how do I know what Vitamins and mineral deficiency I might have? I'm glad that you asked this question, because I have a great answer for you.

FIGURING OUT YOUR VITAMIN DEFICIENCY

I was puzzled at the reasoning behind my former doctors' willingness to feed me liver-toxic prescription medications[920] [921] [922] rather than discussing the benefits of Vitamins and minerals that were critically lacking in my "Western-dead-food" diet. Why didn't my doctors discuss the benefits of Vitamins, especially those which I was extremely deficient? After all, information that I'm providing in this chapter was readily available in every possible scientific and government publication. Yet my doctors, who should have been aware of such fundamental benefits, did not concentrate on this easily obtainable material. Perhaps it was their training? **The truth of the matter is that <u>I was seeing the wrong doctors all along</u>.**

Once again, I have my wife to thank, as she located a Medical doctor who combines the best of conventional and non-conventional medicine. This doctor became our family's primary care physician. Wow, what a change!

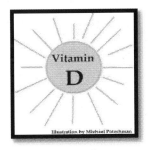

He immediately took all of the necessary conventional blood tests and a full Vitamin and mineral panel. Although my evaluation was almost perfect, I was deficient in **Vitamin D**, as a lot of people are. After I learned of my deficiency, I exposed myself to more sun. Also, as the sun is not as strong in the winter, I take supplements in addition to eating fish regularly. My Vitamin D deficiency is now a thing of the past.

Although my wife and I were eating incredibly potent foods, her Vitamin and mineral evaluation revealed iron deficiency. It was difficult to comprehend why my wife would be iron deficient or have mild anemia. Although our eating structure was evolving at the time, we were consuming most, if not all of the foods that are listed in the "**WHAT TO EAT**" chapter. We also couldn't understand why she was feeling tired. So why iron deficiency?

We knew that we got more than enough Vitamins and iron from our food. Even though my iron level was textbook-perfect, we had to narrow down foods that were robbing my wife of iron. A quick search of archives of the U.S. National Library of Medicine revealed a study with an interesting title: "*Effect of tea and other dietary factors on iron absorption.*"[923] "TEA?" Was the first word that came out of our mouths! We were indeed drinking tea consistently with every meal.

Drinking **tea or coffee** during meals can reduce the amount of iron your body can absorb from food, even if you're taking supplements. [924] [925] [926]

Another study revealed a scary outcome. Only <u>one cup of tea</u> decreased iron absorption from a hamburger meal by a whopping 64%.[927]

The components in tea such as phytates and polyphenols can inhibit the absorption of iron.[928] The study suggested not to drink tea during meals, but between meals in order to prevent tea's effect on iron absorption.[929]

My wife immediately began taking **iron supplements** in order to re-build her iron level and stopped drinking tea or coffee until her iron level normalized. After she rebuilt her iron, and got a glowing report from our new awesome doctor, she stopped taking supplements and re-started drinking small amounts of tea between meals. Most of the time, she substituted tea with hot water and a wedge of lemon or lime. The subsequent tests did not register any other Vitamin or mineral deficiencies! Yippee! ☺

The next mineral that we had to fit into our <u>daily</u> routine was an **Iodine** supplement in order to support the thyroid gland, as we discussed in the "**ALCOHOL**" and "**DETOX**" chapters. Keeping in mind that the thyroid gland controls many bodily functions including metabolism, thyroid gland requires iodine in order to convert iodine that's found in different foods into thyroid hormones which are called T3 and T4.[930]

The names of hormones are unimportant. What is important is that we weren't getting iodine in Himalayan (pink salt) that we were/are using. Although regular table salt does contain added iodine, in many cases, it also has additional "stuff" added to it, i.e., dextrose (corn sugar,) as well as, anticaking agent - calcium silicate, which are the prime examples of what we would not put into our bodies.

You can also get Iodine through Iodine-rich foods such as sea kelp, different types of sea vegetables, fish, and different types of seafood, among others. But are you getting enough? Although my family and I consume these foods consistently, we continue to supplement. Our tests show that our Iodine level is textbook perfect. Keep in mind that you should not over-supplement, as hyperthyroidism (overactive thyroid) caused by excess Iodine causes slew of problems. Thus, Iodine blood test is essential.

The final supplement that we added to our daily routine is **Magnesium**. Although we get Magnesium through our wonderful vegetables, there may not be enough of it in the soil where even organic greens grow.

"Magnesium is one of the most depleted minerals, yet one of the most important."
(Dean, 2017)[931]

As such, we supplement regularly with this life sustaining mineral. You may ask why one needs Magnesium. The answer is simple. Not only does this vital mineral support thyroid function, but is important for most bodily functions, and is regarded as liver detoxifier and blood cleanser. [932] [933] [934]

Numerous studies show that there is a link between **Magnesium deficiency and aging**.[935] Furthermore, Magnesium deficiency may contribute to heart failure, heart disease, insomnia, high blood pressure (hypertension,) neurological problems, osteoporosis, fatigue, cramps, and even bowl disease, among many, many other illnesses and diseases. [936] [937] [938] [939] [940]

"As magnesium deficiency worsens, numbness, tingling, muscle contractions, cramps, seizures, sudden changes in behavior caused by excessive electrical activity in the brain, personality changes, abnormal heart beat and coronary spasms might occur."
(Jahnen-Dechent & Ketteler, 2012)[941]

As you can see by the examples above, we supplemented only with Vitamins and minerals that were necessary and not what the health gurus or industry were dictating. Keep in mind that even though we were eating the same food, our Vitamin/mineral deficiencies were completely different. The most exciting news is that we are now getting the majority of these Vitamins and minerals from our "LW-Base" and toppings as will be outlined in the "**WHAT TO EAT**" chapter.

So, go and find a medical professional with the knowledge of not only how to prescribe liver-toxic medicine, but one who can evaluate you from a holistic perspective.

ESSENTIAL VITAMINS

What type of Vitamins do you really need? Even though my family and I are getting almost all of our Vitamins from food, it is important to understand which Vitamins make our bodies operate at their peak. There are a number of essential Vitamins, 13 to be exact, that your body needs to function properly.[942] These Vitamins are divided into two categories: fat and water soluble.

- **Fat Soluble**

  Vitamins A, D, E, and K are fat soluble, which means that they dissolve in fat and then are stored in adipose (fat) tissue in your body and in your liver. Because they're stored in fat, they can build up to toxic levels.[943] [944] That's why I go nuts when companies and some doctors advocate to blindly take supplements without knowing whether or not you're deficient.

- **Water Soluble**

  Vitamins B1(thiamine,) B2(riboflavin,) B3(niacin,) B6(Pyridoxine,) B12, C, Biotin, Folate (folic acid), and Pantothenic acid are water soluble.[945] Water soluble means that the body must use Vitamins as soon as possible because they dissolve in water and can be excreted through urination.[946] The only anomaly out of these eight is Vitamin B12 as it can be stored in the liver for prolonged periods.[947] Don't think that if you take water soluble Vitamins you can "pee them all out." Not true! You can still get intoxicated by these Vitamins if taken in large quantities.

Each Vitamin that's addressed above performs a special function in your body and is found in certain types of foods or the environment. The chart of functions of these Vitamins and the type of foods that contain these necessary substances is located in **Appendix I**, at the end of the book.

ESSENTIAL MINERALS

Besides Vitamins, there are essential minerals that we must consume in order to stay healthy. The following are some examples of these vital minerals and foods in which they are found:

Name	Function	Food Sources
Zinc	"…helps the immune system fight off invading bacteria and viruses. The body also needs zinc to make proteins and DNA, the genetic material in all cells. During pregnancy, infancy, and childhood, the body needs zinc to grow and develop properly. Zinc also helps wounds heal and is important for proper senses of taste and smell."[948] **Should you come down with a common cold, which is less likely when following the Living Wonderfully lifestyle, this wonder mineral will help fight off this pesky bug. If taken within 24 hours of symptom onset, it has the power to reduce the duration of cold symptoms in healthy people.[949]** [950]**As with everything, check with your doctor first, as some people may experience side effects.**	"•Oysters (best source of zinc) •Red meat, poultry, seafood such as crab and lobsters, and fortified breakfast cereals. •Beans, nuts, whole grains, and dairy products, which provide some zinc."[951]

Magnesium	"Magnesium is important for many processes in the body, including regulating muscle and nerve function, blood sugar levels, and blood pressure and making protein, bone, and DNA."[952]	"•Legumes, nuts, seeds, whole grains, and green leafy vegetables (such as spinach) •Fortified breakfast cereals and other fortified foods •Milk, yogurt, and some other milk products" [953]
Iodine	"The body needs iodine to make Thyroid hormones. These hormones control the body's metabolism and many other important functions. The body also needs Thyroid hormones for proper bone and brain development during pregnancy and infancy."[954]	"•Fish (such as cod and tuna), seaweed, shrimp, and other seafood. •Dairy products (such as milk, yogurt, and cheese) and products made from grains (like breads and cereals). •Fruits and vegetables, which contain iodine, although the amount depends on the iodine in the soil where they grew and in any fertilizer that was used. •Iodized salt. Processed foods such as canned soups, almost never contain iodized salt."[955]
Chromium	Essential mineral Chromium is not made by the body. Chromium is vital to storage and metabolism of fat, carbohydrate, and even protein. It also helps regulate Insulin, among other important functions.[956]	•Broccoli •Beef •Eggs •Bananas •Chicken •Turkey •Oysters[957]
Copper	"…works with iron to help the body form red blood cells. It also helps keep the blood vessels, nerves, immune system, and bones healthy."[958]	•Dark leafy greens •Oysters and other shellfish •Organ meats (kidneys, liver) •Cocoa •Beans •Nuts •Potatoes •Prunes •Black pepper •Yeast •Whole grains[959]

Manganese	Used to reduce premenstrual syndrome(PMS) symptoms. Used to keep bone and cartilage healthy. A study showed that diabetics with higher levels of manganese in their blood were better protected from bad cholesterol (LDL).[960]	•Leafy green vegetables •Legumes •Nuts •Seeds •Pineapple •Whole grains[961]
Iron	"The human body needs iron to make the oxygen-carrying proteins hemoglobin and myoglobin. Hemoglobin is found in red blood cells and myoglobin is found in muscles. Iron also makes up part of many proteins in the body."[962]	•Red meat •Turkey or chicken giblets •Oysters, clams, scallops, and other shellfish •Liver •Egg yolks •Dark, leafy greens (spinach, collards) •Prunes •Raisins •Iron-enriched cereals and grains (check the labels) •Beans, lentils, chick peas and soybeans •Artichokes[963]
Potassium	"•Builds proteins •Breaks down and uses carbohydrates •Builds muscle •Maintains normal body growth •Controls the electrical activity of the heart •Controls the acid-base balance"[964]	•Broccoli •Potatoes (especially their skins) •Peas •Lima beans •Tomatoes •Sweet potatoes •Winter squash[965] •Bananas
Selenium	"Selenium helps the body with: •Making special proteins, called antioxidant enzymes, which play a role in preventing cell damage •Helping your body protect you after a vaccination Some medical studies suggest that selenium may help with the following conditions, but more studies are needed: •Prevent certain cancers •Prevent cardiovascular disease •Help protect the body from the poisonous effects of heavy metals and other harmful substances"[966]	•Fish •Shellfish •Shrimp •Red meat •Liver •Grains •Eggs •Chicken •Turkey •Liver •Garlic •Spinach •Lentils [967] [968]

Sulfur	Important for joint health, connective tissue such as ligaments and tendons.[969]	• Meats • Fish • Poultry • Nuts • Legumes [970] • Cruciferous vegetables

As you will read later in the "WHAT TO EAT" chapter, almost all of the foods that possess these minerals are included as part of our "LW-Base" and respective toppings.

JOINT HEALTH AND VITAMINS

As I worked on this chapter, I shared my knowledge with some of the members at my local gym. Everyone kept asking if I would include joint health as part of the Vitamin section. The fact is, joints are critical in everything we do when it comes to movement and strength.

The mechanism that allows us to move are the joints that connect one bone to another and permit us to be flexible. Bones are attached by ligaments. Tendons attach bone to muscle. Cartilage is located between the joints in order to cushion the movement, otherwise our bones would be grinding together; not a good thing. Because we perform countless movements daily, joint health is just as important as every other aspect of our health. So, let's keep our joints healthy with the following awesome Vitamins and minerals.

We already looked at **sulfur** which is important for the health of connective tissue such as ligaments and tendons.[971] Just to remind you, sulfur can be found in meat, fish, poultry, cruciferous vegetables, nuts, and legumes.

Calcium and **Vitamin D** are essential to bone health. Vitamin D helps with the absorption of calcium. Besides exposure to the sun, Vitamin D is found in fatty fish such as tuna, salmon, and mackerel, as well as in small amounts in egg yolks, beef liver, and cheese.[972]

Excellent sources of calcium include leafy green vegetables, broccoli, and fish.[973]

Omega-3 fatty acids cannot be made by the body, so we have to get them from food or supplements. As we discussed earlier, Omega-3 fatty acids can be found in fatty fish, such as salmon, halibut, tuna, and even algae, nuts, and different plants such as chia and flex seeds, etc. Studies have shown that Omega-3 reduces joint stiffness and pain.[974]

Exercise coupled with great food that contains calcium, as we will be discussing in later chapters, also leads to healthy weight maintenance. It is a very simple formula; the more weight you carry the more stress you put on your joints, especially your knees and ankles.

Regular exercise helps to improve your joint flexibility and muscle strength, as well as bone density.[975] Strength training, yoga, swimming, and even dancing are good for your joints.[976] Make certain that your exercise routine is as "low-impact" as possible. Perhaps, instead of the treadmill, choose an elliptical trainer. In other words, exercise caution when exercising.

IS GLUCOSAMINE SUPPLEMENT AN ANSWER TO JOINT PROBLEMS?

Glucosamine is produced by our bodies in order to build cartilage.[977] Unfortunately there are very few food sources for glucosamine, but there are supplements. Glucosamine supplements are generally made out of the outer shell of lobster, shrimp, or crabs.[978]

Keep in mind that there is no conclusive evidence that glucosamine repairs or grows cartilage. Furthermore, Consumer Reports evaluated multiple studies that show that Glucosamine and Chondroitin may not be the answer, but actually pose risks as it can react negatively with other medicines.[979]

I have not taken this supplement myself, but I've spoken to many people who swear by it. So, talk to your doctor and see if Glucosamine may help you with your joints.

WATER: CAN IT GET ANY SIMPLER?

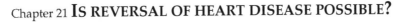

As simple as it sounds, water is essential. Water lubricates and cushions joints.[980] Sometimes you may experience joint pain which comes from dehydration.[981] Thus, always stay hydrated not only for the sake of your joints but for your overall health. Most experts recommend six to eight 8-ounce glasses of water per day for an adult.[982] Keeping this figure in mind, you need to account for exercise that may require additional hydration. Although this is not an exact science, you have the framework to give you an approximation of how much water you need to drink. I, for example, drink over a liter of water per day. On the days when I exercise, I may even drink close to two liters. One thing to consider, the six to eight glasses per day figure does not account for your size. Also, keep in mind that you get at least 20 percent of water from food, whether it comes in a form of kale or a piece of fish. Therefore, if you overhydrate, you may be peeing important electrolytes out of your system.

Now that you have your "prescriptions" so to speak, and you're well versed in bad foods and dieting conundrums, let's examine what else can be done to improve, and in some cases, reverse the ailments that you may be experiencing.

Chapter 21 IS REVERSAL OF HEART DISEASE POSSIBLE?

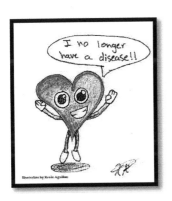

As I mentioned at the beginning of the book in the "SICK AND SICKER" chapter, during my visit to a cardiologist after a cardiac catheterization procedure, I received disturbing and demoralizing news. My doctor informed me that I had progressive heart disease, and considering my family history, I had to stay on prescription medications for the rest of my life.

This particular news had devastated me the most, and actually sunk me even deeper into the mindset of hopelessness. Because of this grim prognosis, I was thinking that I didn't have much longer to live, and that I would follow in the footsteps of my mother, who passed away from heart disease at the age of 58.

What my cardiologist failed to mention is that there are studies and tangible scientific evidence that heart disease can be stopped from progressing and even reversed![983]

Even in the most severe cases, heart disease can be partially reversed, all **without cholesterol lowering drugs or coronary bypass surgery**.[984]

My case wasn't the most severe, yet the picture that my doctor painted was quite chilling. Perhaps my doctor hadn't read such research. Perhaps he did not want to lose a patient who would be in need of prescription medications for the rest of his life, and therefore provide a steady cash flow to his business. Perhaps my doctor was benefitting from pharmaceutical companies.[985] I will give my doctor the benefit of the doubt because we'll never know what his motivation was. Perhaps he genuinely didn't know that **coronary disease reversal programs existed.**

Dr. Dean Ornish, MD., founder of Preventive Medicine Research Institute and Clinical Professor of Medicine at the University of California, San Francisco, has published numerous books on the subject of reversing heart disease. In one of his books, "The Spectrum", he describes patients with severe heart disease who were on the waiting list for heart transplantation. The most impressive phenomenon was that some of the patients who enrolled in Dr. Ornish's program, while awaiting heart transplants, have improved to the point that they no longer needed this procedure.[986] The simplicity of Dr. Ornish's program incorporates **proper foods, exercise, and stress reduction techniques**.[987] That is it!

Another 20-year study was conducted by Dr. Caldwell Esselstyn, Jr., an internationally renowned surgeon.[988] He headed the section of Thyroid and ParaThyroid Surgery and was the president of staff and a chairman of the Cleveland Clinic Breast Cancer Task Force. In 1991 he organized the first national conference on Elimination of Coronary Artery Disease.[989]

In his book, "Prevent and Reverse Heart Disease", Dr. Esselstyn describes a group of patients with conditions so severe that they were told by their cardiologists that they had one year left to live.[990] After following his **plant based whole food diet**, their condition began to improve within months. What's even more mind-blowing is that __20 years later their symptoms have not returned__.[991] As a side note, Dr. Esselstyn's study showed even more radical improvement after he **eliminated dairy products** from his patients' diet. I'm certain that you already suspected that after reading the "DAIRY" section of "WHAT NOT TO EAT" chapter earlier.

Numerous studies on the subject of the reversal of heart disease were published decades before I saw my cardiologist. Despite this information being publicly available, I was put on a regimen of liver-toxic medications and fat-free or low-fat foods that exacerbated my already fragile condition.

Now that we know that the reversal of heart disease is clearly **possible**, how does your body fight this ailment that's considered by some industry professionals as irreversible?

RIDDING THE BODY OF HEART DISEASE

The human body has the capacity to heal itself, as long as one provides favorable conditions for such healing to take place. A good example would be a simple finger cut. If we keep the cut clean, use antibacterial ointment and a bandage, most cuts will heal swiftly. We have essentially created favorable conditions for the body to heal itself.

Therefore, if there is damage to the heart, arteries, or other organs, the body is constantly crying out for help so it can heal itself. All that's required is favorable condition where healing is possible, just like in the finger cut example. Here's how it works.

The lining of our arteries and veins consists of endothelial cells which produce nitric oxide gas in order to protect vessels [992] and help to eliminate inflammation. These cells facilitate dilation of blood vessels to **keep our blood flowing freely without sticking, thus inhibiting the formation of plaque.**[993] As we continue to eat processed or "almost foods", simple carbs, or typical foods associated with "Western diet", we damage the endothelial cells to the point that they are no longer efficient at protecting arteries from forming plaque. [994]

Studies reveal that after we begin eating plant based whole foods, we not only stop the damage but we instigate the reversal of the artery disease by rebuilding the endothelial cells.[995]

THE ELUSIVE VITAMIN K2 FOR HEALTHY ARTERIES

Why is this Vitamin so elusive? Well, it's because none of the doctors, including cardiologists that I saw in the past, recommended or even mentioned that I should tackle my progressing heart disease with this seemingly simple substance.

In order to understand how this Vitamin works, one needs to understand how heart disease is created. Although you already got a glimpse of this artery saving Vitamin in the "**FATS**" chapter, we will get a little more involved in this section, because it's that important!

The clogging of the arteries begins with a lesion, tear, and/or inflammation in the walls of the arteries, and/or damage to the endothelial cells as we discussed above.[996] [997]   Just like when you have a finger cut and cover it with a bandage, so is your body covering a cut or a tear, and/or inflammation inside the damaged artery with its own version of a bandage – plaque.

As we continue to eat foods that are described in "**WHAT NOT TO EAT**" section, we continue to keep our body inflamed and cause more damage to the endothelial function, so plaque continues to build. [998] Overtime, the plaque hardens, arteries become narrow, and blood flow that is oxygen rich doesn't get to the heart as it used to. [999]   What I just described is called atherosclerosis. [1000] As scary as this all sounds, there is a way to reverse it.

Besides what you read earlier about saying a big NO to processed foods and a loud YES to organic plant based diet, there is something equally as potent that has the ability to clear plaque out of the arteries, and works in conjunction with LIVING WONDERFULLY lifestyle and foods that will be described in Section 6 later in the book.

VITAMIN K2 TO THE RESCUE

In order to understand how this incredible Vitamin can offer its assistance in unclogging of the arteries, one has to know what artery clogging plaque consist of.

Plaque that's covering the arterial damage is made up of fat, cholesterol, calcium, among other substances that are present in blood.[1001]

Vitamin K2 works with Vitamin D3, and is responsible for taking calcium out of the arteries or soft tissue where it does not belong, and distributing it into the bones and teeth[1002] **where it does belong**.

To illustrate this, imagine a Vitamin K2 cargo ship sailing through your blood stream inside your arteries. It comes upon plaque. It stops, and gets loaded with calcium and continues sailing. It sails on with its calcium cargo until its next stop, where Vitamin D3 crane helps to unload the ship or to absorb calcium into your bones and teeth as illustrated in the drawing below.

What this means is that Vitamin K2 promotes cardiovascular and bone health while lowering the chances of heart disease, arthritis, and osteoporosis. [1003] [1004]

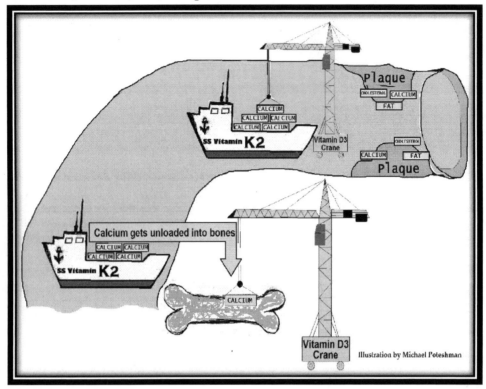

Without Vitamin K2, you may end up with calcium plaguing in the arteries. I'm certain that you've noticed some older people who are quite stiff and have difficult time moving. Chances are they may be deficient in Vitamin K2, and their soft tissue is calcified. **Vitamin K2 also increases elasticity and flexibility of your arteries,**[1005] **which means that you may see improvements in your high <u>blood pressure numbers</u>**.

As we discussed in the "FATS" chapter, you already know that the best sources for Vitamin K2 are <u>grass fed (**not grain fed**) organic beef, organic chicken, organic egg yolks, organic organ meats</u>, [1006] among other foods that my doctors prohibited. These foods are high, and in some cases, very high in saturated fat and cholesterol. Although I consume them daily, my cholesterol numbers are perfect!

As a vegan, you can find this vitamin in natto, [1007] a fermented soy product. Check with credible nutritionist if natto will provide sufficient amount of Vitamin K2 for your dietary needs. Also, vegans can enjoy fermented vegetables such as sauerkraut that contain Vitamin K2, but not in the same quantity as in natto or animal products.

Although the entire Living Wonderfully puzzle has not been revealed, as we're more than half way through the book, I believe that you now have an idea of how I went from Living Dead to living a dream of health at the age of 53! I'm actually reversing what used to be a progressive heart disease!

Now that we know that we can reverse heart disease, let's concentrate on an equally important subject: your second brain.

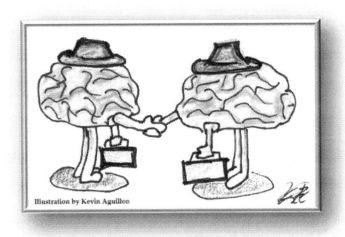

Illustration by Kevin Aguillon

When I embarked on the subject of gut health, I began to understand multiple reasons behind my declining health of the not so distant past. The constant feeling of unhappiness, and even despair, had a lot to do with my gut.

Would you have ever thought that you had two brains? When I pose this question, most of the time I hear; "The second brain is in my tongue, as sometimes it has a mind of its own". Funny, but not the correct answer. Many doctors and scientists refer to the gut as the second brain. The reason behind this phenomenon is that your "second brain", or gut, uses the same neurotransmitters and neurons that are found in your central nervous system.[1008] [1009]

"The gut contains 100 million neurons - more than the spinal cord. Major neurotransmitters like serotonin, dopamine, glutamate, norephinephrine and nitric oxide are in the gut. Also two dozen small brain proteins, called neuropeptides are there along with the major cells of the immune system"
(King, 2013).[1010]

As we grow and transform in our mother's womb, there are two nervous systems that are formed: the actual brain with the attached spinal cord or central nervous system, and something that is called "enteric nervous system" which is located within the lining of the stomach, small intestine, esophagus, and colon. [1011] [1012] [1013] In order to communicate, both the central nervous system and the enteric nervous system are connected via the vagus nerve. [1014] [1015] An interesting fact is when the nerve is severed, both continue to operate independently,[1016] hence the nickname, "second brain."

To illustrate the connection between the main and the "secondary brain", I recall my teenage years when I would have "butterflies in my stomach" when I wanted to ask a particular girl out on a date. I'm certain that I'm not the only one that had this type of experience.

It was especially noticeable when nerves were kicking in about a new job or a speech I had to give. For some reason I felt queasy and had indigestion. Let's explore why people have "butterflies" or feel queasy in stressful situations.

ONE BRAIN AFFECTS THE OTHER

If you are experiencing problems in your gut, your brain may suffer as a result. [1017]

"The gut's brain is reported to play a major role in human happiness and misery"
(King, 2013). [1018]

This means that whatever happens in the brain may affect your gut, and whatever happens in the gut may affect your brain.

There is a simple explanation for these brain-gut connections.

Ninety five percent of all of the serotonin in your body is located in your gut and not your brain.[1019]

Serotonin is the neurotransmitter which relays messages from one part of the brain to another, and influences the majority of brain cells.[1020] [1021] The impact on our behavior through serotonin is immense as it influences brain cells associated with **sleep, mood, appetite, sex drive and performance, learning abilities, memory, cardiovascular system, muscles, temperature regulation, and even social behavior!** [1022] [1023]

If your gut is out of balance, any of the functions listed above can be affected in a very negative way. For example, the post mortem examination of **Alzheimer's** patients revealed serotonin deficiency. [1024] [1025] Such deficiency may manifest into Attention Deficit Hyperactivity Disorder (ADHD,) as interaction between dopamine and serotonin in the brain is believed to affect the attention span.[1026]

"Ailments like anxiety, depression, irritable bowel syndrome, ulcers and Parkinson's disease manifest symptoms at the brain and the gut level"
(Brown, 2005).[1027]

One study showed a connection between gut bacteria and **childhood autism**.[1028] [1029] When compared to non-autistic children, it was evident that autistic children suffered from low level of gut bacteria.[1030]

We know that when the second brain is out of balance it causes harm to the entire system. So, how do we bring our gut into balance? For that we have to become gardeners, but not what you think. We have to grow and cultivate a very special kind of garden.

THE GARDEN INSIDE YOUR GUT

Figuratively speaking, the garden that resides inside your gut is home to different bacteria, fungi, and yeasts, collectively known as "intestinal flora." According to a large study, our intestinal flora consists of more than 35,000 species.[1031]

As with any garden there are plants that are beneficial and there are weeds that may cause damage to your entire crop. It is the same with intestinal flora. There are numerous microorganisms or "good bacteria" which play a huge role in the development of the immune system. These bacteria are necessary for digestion, killing of destructive pathogens in your intestines, and production of Vitamins, among other important functions.[1032] [1033]These good microorganisms are generally referred to as **probiotics**, which we will be discussing shortly.

WEEDS IN THE GARDEN

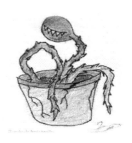

Just as you have weeds in every garden, there is also "bad flora" or yeasts and bacteria that develop in the gut. There are different species of bacteria, parasitic worms, or microorganisms that may be acquired when traveling overseas or domestically. How many times have you heard of food related illnesses that originate from sick employees or mishandling of food at restaurants?

"A 2002–03 study of foodborne illness outbreaks in restaurants found that food handling by an infected employee was a contributing factor in two-thirds of the outbreaks."
(FDA, 2013)[1034]

How about this sobering estimate?

"The CDC estimates of 3,000 deaths, 128,000 hospitalizations and 48 million illnesses associated annually with foodborne pathogens…"
(Taylor, 2012)[1035]

Besides bad flora, **improper diet is the cause of overall declining health in most people**.[1036] [1037] Most of the bad flora, especially in the Western diet is a result of ingesting foods that literally demolish your internal garden. For example, non-beneficial yeasts or fungi such as "candida albicans" feed on **sugars** supplied in abundance by processed, sugary and starchy foods, even those foods that contain **simple and complex carbohydrates**.[1038] These are the type of "almost foods" discussed in "**WHAT NOT TO EAT**" section.

If you decide to indulge in white bread, cake, pasta, white rice, pizza, or anything with refined grain, sugar, sugary drinks, and even fruit juices, understand that you are taking your body's chemistry out of balance.

Although "almost food" is detrimental to your gut health, there are other offenders. Taking certain antibiotics, for example, may not only destroy the good flora,[1039] but cause major damage to the liver.

"The most common drugs leading to Drug Induced Liver Damage in the United States are antibiotics, central nervous system agents, herbal/dietary supplements, and immunomodulatory agents."
(Ghabril, Chalasani & Björnsson, 2010)[1040]

Although antibiotics may provide relief for different ailments, they often don't discriminate between good and bad bacteria in your gut. According to Michigan State University, **the cause of most vaginal yeast infections in American women may be attributed to antibiotic use**.[1041]

How could this happen you may be asking? We all learned that antibiotics don't create infection, they clear up infections, but this is not true in all cases. For example, a woman may be prescribed an antibiotic to clear up a certain infection. The antibiotic not only kills the infection but the beneficial bacteria, which throws off the balance in "vaginal ecosystem." [1042]

Besides antibiotics, other drugs such as pain killers, acid blockers that I took for decades, and drugs that we know and love such as Tylenol (acetaminophen), may contribute to disrupting or disturbing the good flora or damaging your digestive tract. [1043] [1044]

Food chemicals such as **Aspartame, monosodium glutamate, preservatives, additives, sweeteners, and artificial sweeteners among many other chemicals, may irritate the intestines, reduce good bacteria, and throw off the pH balance in the gut**. [1045] [1046] [1047]

Homogenized and pasteurized dairy products, through "subtle allergic reactions", may damage the intestinal tract and its flora. [1048] [1049] [1050] Not only that, but as you recall from the "Dairy" chapter, the homogenization process breaks up fat molecules into very small particles so fat becomes suspended in milk and no longer rises to the top.[1051] These particles or proteins that are usually digested in the stomach can bypass digestion and travel through the bloodstream.[1052] [1053] Once in the bloodstream, they can cause damage to the arterial walls, and as time progresses, may cause heart disease. [1054] [1055] Only imagine what the homogenization process may do to your gut if homogenized particles have the ability to pass through your digestive system.

There is also a matter of alcohol that we discussed as part of the **ALCOHOL** chapter earlier. Please recall our discussion about ethanol that gets converted to Acetaldehyde, a known carcinogen that wreaks havoc on a person's gut and liver. We also discussed that ethanol, through conversion into Acetaldehyde in the liver, **has the ability to produce holes in the gut (permeation of the intestines)**[1056] **to become big enough for the molecules of bacterial toxins (endotoxins) to fit through**. [1057]

The permeations (holes) in your intestines allow the proteins that haven't been fully processed, toxic bacteria as discussed earlier, as well as some waste product, among other undesirable "garbage" to leak out into your blood stream and cause undesirable side effects. [1058] [1059] [1060] [1061] Adverse conditions of the permeated intestines may include irritable bowel syndrome, inflammatory bowel diseases, inflammatory joint disease, food allergy, celiac disease, metabolic diseases, and obesity, among others.[1062] [1063] [1064] Another serious condition that's worth mentioning is the autoimmune response, where your immune system begins to attack healthy cells and/or organs in your body.[1065] [1066]

There are "almost foods" and beverages that we discussed earlier, and there are some that we haven't discussed. There are also environmental chemicals that have the ability to wreak havoc on your precious internal garden. Now you know what to watch out for. But before we leave this section, let's discuss the role of antibiotics, and what they have to do with weight gain and your gut.

ANTIBIOTICS, GUT, AND WEIGHT GAIN

As we discussed earlier, antibiotics don't discriminate between killing the good or the bad bacteria in your gut. So, what does it all have to do with gaining weight? Everything!

In the, "living-dead" past I always knew that antibiotics found in food weren't exactly good for you. But I never suspected that they could actually make you gain weight. As I began to study the side effects, read articles and studies, the following headings began to pop up:

- From Berkeley Wellness – *"Are Antibiotics Making Us Fat?"*[1067]
- From CBS News – *"Chemicals in Food Can Make You Fat"*[1068]
- From Fox News – *"6 foods that can damage your metabolism the moment you eat them"*[1069]
- From The Dr. Oz Show – *"The Fat Drug: How Antibiotics Make You Gain Weight"*[1070]

It's beyond simple of how antibiotics may cause weight gain. While your body is attempting to keep its gut bacteria in perfect balance, antibiotics kill off some of the flora, thus disturb the precious balance in the gut.[1071] These changes may be triggered by antibiotics and/or other antimicrobial agents.[1072]

A study entitled, *"Obesity in the United States – Dysbiosis from Exposure to Low-Dose Antibiotics?"* suggests that weight epidemic may be attributed to being exposed to the **low-residue antibiotics from food supply**.[1073] By the way, the word dysbiosis means the imbalance of bacteria. Here's how it works.

"If you have an imbalance of bacteria—too much of the type that breaks food down into energy—you may be absorbing more calories from the same amount of food you eat than you would otherwise."
-University of California, Berkeley Wellness-[1074]

Here's an excerpt of the conclusion of yet another study entitled, *"Risk Assessment of Growth Hormones and Antimicrobial Residues in Meat"*. I believe that it will drive the message home:

"The induction of resistant bacteria and the disruption of normal human intestinal flora are major concerns of human health for antimicrobial growth promoters."
- Toxicological Research -[1075]

As you can see, the common denominator is the disruption of gut flora and consequences that follow. So, next time you go to a restaurant, ask if the chicken or steak that you're about to order is organic? If not organic, I believe that you are already aware of the risks that we discussed here as well as in Chapter 12, "ANTIBIOTICS IN MEAT, CHICKEN, SEAFOOD... AND THE CONSEQUENCES THAT FOLLOW".

"…organic growers are not allowed to use any antibiotics on chickens from hatching to slaughter."
(Hotcamp, 2011)[1076]

RE-PLANTING YOUR GARDEN WITH GOOD FLORA

Perhaps you are thinking that you've ingested too many bad flora items and that it may be too late because the damage is done. I used to have similar concerns not so long ago, and thought that nothing would help. Although results may vary from person to person, in my case I began to see incredible results within three months. When I switched to the "Living Wonderfully" routine, which includes eating foods that are rich in probiotics, I stopped getting frequent colds, my lifetime allergies went away, and my bathroom visits became "fast and delightful."

The biggest change took place when I was finally able to see the world from the perspective of a contented person rather than a guy who was constantly questioning his existence. As we discussed at the beginning of this chapter, your "second brain" affects your central nervous system and as a result of your renewed gut health, the world just seems brighter.

Replanting your garden is much easier than you think. We do this with the aid of probiotics. **All you have to do is eat**.

> *"Probiotics are the 'friendly' bacteria that reportedly help improve or maintain health. Generally speaking, non-harmful bacteria are formed during the fermentation process"*
> (Hackert, 2013).[1077]

Keeping in mind that pasteurization or heat treatment destroys "valuable" live bacteria or cultures,[1078] it is important to look for foods that have not been subjected to these processes. The following <u>raw</u> and <u>raw fermented</u> foods contain probiotics:

- Sauerkraut – not only loaded with "good" live bacteria, but contains Vitamins A, B, C, and K.[1079] According to the study "DNA Fingerprinting of Lactic Acid Bacteria in Sauerkraut Fermentations" published by the American Society for Microbiology, raw shredded sauerkraut was so potent that it contained more species of bacteria than was previously thought.[1080] You will find my easy family recipe for sauerkraut in the "LIVING WONDERFULLY RECIPES" section at the end of the book.

- Kimchi – almost the same as sauerkraut but made with Napa or Bok Choi cabbage, hot pepper and other ingredients. It can also be made with different vegetables such as radishes and even cucumbers. Besides the healthy bacteria found in yogurt, similar to sauerkraut, kimchi contains Vitamins A, B, and C, as well as an abundance of minerals. [1081] [1082] People in Korea eat this food at practically every meal including breakfast. Health magazine published an article that was titled "World's Healthiest Foods: Kimchi (Korea)."[1083] *"Koreans eat so much of this super-spicy condiment (40 pounds of it per person each year) that natives say 'kimchi' instead of 'cheese' when getting their pictures taken"*(Raymond, 2008). [1084] A very simple kimchi recipe is located in the recipes section at the end of this book.

- Pickles – brine cured without added vinegar.[1085] That also includes pickled carrots, cauliflower, ginger, string beans, mushrooms, tomatoes, etc. Talking about simplicity; check out the recipe section.

- Miso – fermented soybean that originated in Japan. According to WebMD, miso contains over 160 strains of different bacteria.[1086] In addition, it contains "protective antioxidants" and B Vitamins.[1087] Japanese people eat this food for breakfast.

- Tempeh – fermented soybeans that originated Indonesia. It contains B12 Vitamins that are derived from bacteria during fermentation,[1088] a category of natural antibiotics to fight particular bacteria, as well as probiotics.[1089] [1090]

- Spirulina – considered a superfood. It is a spiral shaped algae, hence its name. According to the University of Maryland Medical Center, spirulina contains nutrients including manganese, beta-carotene, gamma linolenic acid (an important fatty acid), copper, Vitamin E, B complex Vitamins, zinc, iron, and selenium.[1091] In addition, this superfood is very high in protein, provides immune support, and may boost the growth of good bacteria. [1092] In a placebo-control study, it was shown that spirulina reduced pre-cancer growth lesions in people who chewed tobacco. [1093]

- Chlorella – considered a superfood. It is a fresh water algae that is generally grown in Taiwan or Japan. Chlorella has "good bacteria" that helps treat Crohn's disease, colitis, ulcers, among other diseases, and is used as medicine for prevention or protection against certain diseases and even side effects after certain medical procedures. [1094]

- Non-dairy yogurts and kefirs are available with added live probiotic cultures, as long as these products contain live bacteria, or live and active cultures. Watch out for products with <u>added sugars and chemicals</u> as they will feed the bad bacteria or destroy good bacteria in your gut, thus counteract the effects of live bacteria.
- Dairy yogurts including Greek yogurt, among other dairy concoctions including cheeses, contain different forms of good bacteria, but only non-pasteurized or not heat-treated kinds. So, why did I place yogurt and cheese at the end of this list even though they contain an abundance of probiotics? For that information, you have to refer to the earlier "DAIRY" section. But for the sake of full disclosure, I have to list these foods for their probiotic content.

According to Probiotic Factsheet published on Dr. Oz's website, non-pasteurized or non-heat treated yogurts and certain cheeses contain good bacteria such as Lactobacillus bulgaricus, Streptococcus thermophilus, Lactobacillus acidophilus, Lactobacillus casei, and Bifidobacteria.[1095] Taking a second look at **raw sauerkraut**, an interesting picture will emerge. According to the study published in the "Applied and Environmental Microbiology" publication, raw sauerkraut contains incredible number of good bacteria. Although difficult to pronounce, here are some examples: Pediococcus pentosaceus, Lactobacillus brevis, Leuconostoc citreum, Leuconostoc argentinum, Lactobacillus coryniformis, Lactobacillus paraplantarum, Leuconostoc mesenteroides, Weissella sp, Leuconostoc fallax, Lactobacillus plantarum, among others.[1096] Why wasn't my doctor discussing the tremendous benefits of this seemingly simple probiotic-boasting food? Perhaps because it does not require a prescription? Let's give him the benefit of doubt as it was for lack of nutritional knowledge.

- There is another form of probiotic, and I couldn't bring it to you at the beginning of this section because you may have closed the book. So here it is. How about consuming a little bit of dirt? I don't mean to go out in your garden and shove a spoonful of garden soil into your mouth. What I'm saying, don't peel the carrot or radishes; just wash them, for as long as they were grown in the organic soil. Those little brown elements in the crevices of the vegetable skin contain probiotics. And yes, they look like dirt, because they are.

Studies show that consumption of beneficial bacteria that are in the dirt, have the power to assist in fighting allergic diseases through stimulation of the immune system.[1097] [1098] How's that for eating dirt?

There are other foods with probiotics and antioxidants such as raw cacao beans;[1099] that's what real chocolate is made out of. Also, probiotic supplements are available in health food stores everywhere. Be aware of the source because not all supplements are created equal. In my opinion, there is nothing better than live bacteria that are derived from food, which may keep your "second brain" humming like a well-oiled machine!

PRE-BIOTICS: THE FERTILIZER FOR GOOD FLORA

There is another important part to the gut health that is called pre-biotic. This is not to be confused with pro-biotics.

Pre-biotics can be regarded as food or fertilizer for probiotics (good bacteria) that I listed above. The main function of pre-biotics is to keep the beneficial bacteria healthy.[1100] [1101]

My family and I consume this great stuff daily as part of our every meal. You find pre-biotics in foods like raw onion and garlic, beans, chicory root, bananas, some whole grains, kale, lentils, and seaweed, among others.[1102] [1103] [1104] Be mindful of the grain you use, as grains have the ability to raise your Insulin level. So, nurse your probiotics with these seemingly simple foods and your "second brain" will pay dividends.

ESTABLISHING GUT FLORA FROM THE BEGINNING OF LIFE

It is a well-known fact that human breast milk can be regarded as "liquid gold" as it contains hormones, cells, and antibodies that help infants fight diseases and illnesses.[1105]

According to the U.S. Department of Health and Human Services Office on Women's Health, breast fed children are at a lower risk of developing asthma, obesity, type 2 diabetes, lower respiratory infections, and even gastrointestinal tract disease that affects preterm infants.[1106]

One of the reasons behind this phenomenon is that breast milk contains large quantities of pre-biotics that help develop and optimize the good bacteria in a baby's gut.[1107] If breast milk is unavailable, consult your pediatrician for other sources of pre and pro-biotics for your baby as it's "that important" for the rest of your baby's life.

OPTIMIZING YOUR GUT FLORA

As with any garden, drought will cause damage and destruction, but over-watering will kill or damage it as well. It is the same with your internal garden or gut flora.

When you drink water or any type of liquids with your meal, you flood your digestive enzymes, and only partial digestion may take place.[1108] Dr. Gillian McKeith recommends not drinking water or other liquids during the meal, but 30 minutes before or after you eat.[1109]

Although I understand that not drinking water during meals is important, sometimes I get thirsty while eating. Thus, I take a few sips rather than gulping water like I used to for years. Most of the time, I drink 30 minutes before and after a meal, and I can truly see the difference in my digestion.

Chewing slowly is another important factor in optimizing your gut flora.[1110] When saliva comes in contact with food, the digestive process begins.[1111] Once the chewed food hits your digestive system, the maximum amount of nutrients is extracted from food instead of partially passing through your system undigested.[1112]

Drinking a glass of warm water and juice of half or a whole lemon first thing in the morning not only cleans mucus out of your system from the day before, but stimulates your digestive system, which helps your body to better absorb nutrients.[1113] [1114] It also makes it easier to flush toxins out of your liver.[1115] Dr. Oz took it one step further and added hot sauce to this concoction as it contains capsaicin that increases particular enzymes as well as blood flow for liver detoxification.[1116]

Now that your second brain is in check, let's look at a chapter that may bring you one HUGE step closer to Living Wonderfully.

Chapter 23 SLEEP, WEIGHT GAIN OR WEIGHT LOSS

*"In epidemiologic studies, shorter sleep has been correlated with incidence of **obesity**, hypertension, and other metabolic disorders."*
(Spivey, 2010).[1117]

Sleep is an ancient phenomenon that on the surface may not require explanation, but it really does, especially in my case. I never thought that not sleeping enough hours, or having disjointed sleep, could lead to certain ailments that I experienced in the past. Some of these ailments stemmed from weight gain. But how did I get to the point of "Living Dead" besides making bad food choices? **Bad food choices led to a vicious cycle of disjointed sleep and weight gain. Disjointed sleep led to additional weight gain. Weight gain led to more health problems, which led to even shorter sleep duration, which resulted in additional weight gain.**

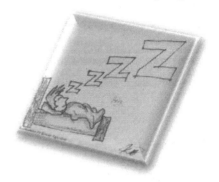

At the beginning of the book I described that in my state of "Living Dead", I sometimes slept in 15 to 30 minute intervals, which is unacceptable in "Living Wonderfully" land! Not having sound sleep, even if you are in bed for seven or eight hours, is just as bad as having short sleep duration.

*"...studies link short or disrupted sleep to elements of one of the major health problems linked to **obesity**: metabolic syndrome, which includes a variety of symptoms that can lead to **heart disease, stroke, or diabetes, including high triglycerides and cholesterol, hypertension, Insulin resistance, and glucose intolerance**."*
(Spivey, 2010).[1118]

I'm certain that you noticed the word "obesity" besides all the other problems that stem from the disrupted sleep. Why do we gain weight when we don't get restful sleep or we sleep for shorter duration?

A large Wisconsin study of 1,024 volunteers explored the association between sleep and weight gain. *"Short Sleep Duration Is Associated with Reduced Leptin, Elevated Ghrelin, and Increased Body Mass Index"*[1119] is the title of the study that I will interpret next.

We already discussed Leptin from the MSG chapter earlier. Just to remind you, Leptin is a hormone that tells your brain to stop eating. Ghrelin, is a hormone that is secreted from your stomach and tells your brain when to eat.[1120] The way Ghrelin does its job is by making high calorie foods look more appetizing. The more Ghrelin produced, the more you want to eat high calorie and/or foods rich in fat, as high levels of this hormone simulate a fasting condition.[1121] [1122] [1123] I'm certain that you're familiar with sayings: "hungry like a wolf", or "I could eat a horse." That's Ghrelin at work as it's regarded in scientific circles as the "hunger hormone".[1124]

Let's return to the Wisconsin study which noted a direct correlation between short sleep duration and weight gain. *"Participants with short sleep had reduced Leptin and elevated Ghrelin"* (Taheri, Lin, Austin, Young & Mignot, 2004).[1125] In other words, when a person does not get enough sleep, the levels of Leptin go down, in essence telling the brain **to continue eating**. Furthermore, short sleep duration or deprivation causes your body to produce more Ghrelin which tells your body that you **need to eat more**. So we eat because our body forces us to, and the result is weight gain and its associated problems.

SLEEP AND INSULIN SENSITIVITY

I often hear people say that they control their appetite and try not to succumb to coercion of uncontrollable hunger because they eat by the clock. They believe that because they eat during certain times of the day, not getting enough sleep is not a big deal. Here's the problem with this thinking:

*"When you're sleep deprived, your body almost immediately develops a condition that resembles **Insulin resistance of diabetes***"
(Shaw, 2012). [1126]

Studies show that people who are sleep deprived exhibit weakened glucose tolerance and Insulin sensitivity.[1127] As you've learned from the "Sugar" section earlier, having too much Insulin coursing through your system leads to additional fat storage.

Even though you decide to eat by the clock, your body will still remain out of balance if you don't get enough sleep.

If you don't gain additional weight due to Insulin resistance caused by sleep deprivation there are still consequences. Your out of balance body may take its vengeance by being constantly tired, sluggish, and having brain fog. Unfortunately the infusion of caffeine through energy drinks or coffee may put an additional toll on your already exhausted system. **The only true remedy that you have at your disposal is sleep!**

When I get through my explanation about sleep, people usually realize that they're not doing themselves any favors by not sleeping. As a result, I get the same two questions every single time I discuss this subject:

1. "I can no longer sleep normally; my sleep pattern is already wrecked. How do I normalize my sleep and how much sleep is enough?"
2. "I know some people who sleep only 6 hours a day and function absolutely normally. So why are you saying that we need more hours than that?"

Let's take a look at the answers.

HOW MUCH SLEEP IS ENOUGH?

Although most of us are probably aware of how much sleep is necessary, the National Institutes of Health (NIH) came up with general recommendations per age group:[1128]

Recommended Amount of Sleep Per Age Group

Age	Recommended Amount of Sleep
Newborns	16–18 hours a day
Preschool-aged children	11–12 hours a day
School-aged children	At least 10 hours a day
Teens	9–10 hours a day
Adults (including the elderly)	7–8 hours a day

Obtained from:
http://www.nhlbi.nih.gov/health/health-topics/topics/sdd/how much.html

The amount of sleep may vary from person to person. The chart above should give you an idea of how many hours you should be sleeping.

SIX HOURS OF SLEEP: IS THIS ENOUGH?

Sleeping six hours per night and functioning in a normal way is indeed possible but not for the predominant majority of **the human population**. Over twenty years ago I knew one lucky co-worker who slept five hours per night and always functioned at his peak. He was the only person that I met with this type of sleep pattern over the years. Perhaps there will be others, but highly unlikely. There is a reason behind being able to function normally at five or six hours of sleep per night. According to a study conducted by the University of California in San Francisco, researchers identified a specific mutation of the gene "DEC2" that allows people to sleep only six hours per night.[1129] [1130] That's the good news. The bad news is that this gene is so rare that it's found in **less than 3% of the human population**.[1131] If you happen to be one of those fortunate people in the "less than 3% club", who can exist on six hours of sleep, congratulations! For the rest of us, we need to adjust and normalize our sleeping patterns or circadian rhythms to be at the top of our game. Let's examine remedies that will enable us to achieve a full night's sleep.

THE WRONG REMEDY

So how do we go about getting some true restful sleep? When I ask this question, there's always someone who says with a grin, "You take sleeping pills." Then everyone laughs. After I finish my discussion about sleeping pills, not a single person remains laughing or even smiling. Instead, they're all thinking about the harm that they may have caused to their own health by taking sleep aids. Taking sleeping pills is a risky business. Here's why:

You don't normalize your sleep by taking sleeping pills, as most of the time they cover up the symptoms and don't address the actual cause of sleeplessness. Like a lot of the prescription drugs, sleep aids are not without side effects, which are probably even riskier than you ever thought. **Sleeping pills are linked to an increased risk of death and cancer.**[1132]

"Most alarmingly, a large study of 30,000 people published in the February 2012 issue of the British Medical Journal found a 300% increase in death in people who took fewer than 18 sleeping pills a year"
(LoGiudice & Bongiorno, 2012).[1133]

A 300% increase in death due to sleeping pills is enormous. When taken in higher doses, the risk increases to a whopping 500%! [1134] Besides increased mortality risks, 35% of people who took sleeping pills were at an increased risk of developing major cancer, excluding melanoma.[1135]

"The top third of sleeping-pill users had a 5.3-fold higher death risk. They also had a 35% higher risk of cancer, the study found"
(DeNoon, 2012).[1136]

Some of the sleeping pills mentioned by their generic name in the study were identical to what my doctor prescribed to me or my family members in the past such as Ambien or Lunesta. [1137] Luckily, I was always opposed to sleep aids as I felt that they were toxic and addictive. Thus, I wasn't in a habit of taking sleeping pills even when my sleep pattern was completely shattered. I guess I was proven right.

As far as I'm concerned, there has to be a truly extenuating circumstance to use these drugs.

"…according to Dr. Lee Green, a professor in the department of family medicine at the University of Michigan, the risks outweigh the benefits. 'We tend to think that a sleeping pill once in a while is harmless, but there's no such thing as a medication free of risk'"
(Salahi, 2012).[1138]

Before you consider taking a sleep aid, consider some remedies that will help you combat sleep deprivation.

THE RIGHT REMEDIES OR NORMALIZING THE CIRCADIAN RHYTHM

Circadian rhythm can be regarded as an **internal body clock** that regulates approximate 24-hour sleep/wake cycles.[1139] The different psychological and biological processes including cell-regeneration and hormone production, are related to circadian rhythm. [1140] It can be affected by sun light and temperature.

Because circadian rhythm is one of the most important factors in determining your sleep patterns, having it "out of whack" causes a multitude of problems and disorders related to sleeping, eating, neurological, and many ailments we discussed earlier.

Perhaps it takes you forever to fall asleep. You wake up in the middle of the night, and you don't feel rested even after you've spent more than eight hours in bed. If you have experienced these symptoms, you're not alone. After 10 years of fragmented sleep, this is how I fixed it in five easy steps:

1.   **NORMALIZING THE INTERNAL CLOCK**

We begin by normalizing our internal clock or circadian rhythm. **It is absolutely non-negotiable to be in bed at the same time every night!**[1141] For example, if you start work at eight o'clock in the morning, you should be in bed by 10:00 PM. That way you will have 15 minutes to read a book before falling asleep, sleep for 8 hours, and have remaining 1 hour and 45 minutes to take a shower, get dressed, and travel to your destination. If you don't need that much time in the morning, adjust your time accordingly. **It is imperative to plan your day around your sleep.**

The key is to go to bed at the same time and allow yourself eight or more hours of sleep every single night!

If you're working the night shift, adjust your schedule to allow for eight or more hours of sleep. It's just a matter of shifting your schedule to a different time frame. Your days off should follow the same sleeping schedule as the rest of the week. The reason is that <u>it's extremely easy to affect your circadian rhythm negatively by just sleeping **90 minutes longer than usual**</u>.[1142]

DAY/NIGHT IDENTITY

The next non-negotiable item is day/night identity. Just like any clock that displays AM/PM, your body has to differentiate between day and night patterns. If at all possible, schedule your wake up time to correspond with sunlight. As soon as you wake up, try to expose yourself to outdoor light[1143] for 20 minutes or longer, even if it's cloudy. If it's impossible to go outside after you have awakened, try to spend at least 20 minutes outdoors in the mid-morning or early afternoon.

Another remedy is to purchase a therapy lamp that simulates daylight. It's available on-line and in stores.

Belos is the photo of the daylight lamp called "Happy Light." It gets a lot of use in our home, especially during winter months.

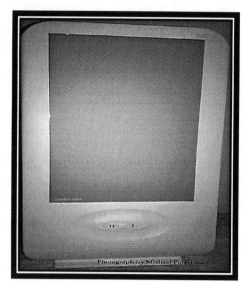

Photograph by Michael Potashnick

ROOM DARKENING

Just as vital as exposure to daylight when you wake up, room darkening plays a huge role in your quality of sleep. Get room-darkening blinds which will almost completely shield the light from the windows. The problem with just installing blinds is that sides and corners may allow light to seep in. For that, use "blackout" curtains made out of heavy fabric.

NO DEPLETION OF MELATONIN BEFORE BED TIME

I've always regarded myself as a night owl, as I regularly worked on my computer before going to bed. Unfortunately, I didn't know that light from the computer or tablet screen actually decreases the level of melatonin. Recall that melatonin is a hormone secreted by your brain in order to control sleep/wake cycles. A study published in the *Applied Ergonomics Journal* showed that if you use a computer tablet for only two hours prior to going to bed, you will decrease your melatonin level by a whopping 22%! [1144]

There are two ways to combat this problem:

1. Limiting or stopping the use of your computer before bed time would be ideal.[1145] In our modern age that may not be possible due to work load. Fortunately, there is another method.
2. If you have no other alternative but to work on your computer when it gets dark, the blue light that emanates from your screen must be blocked. The University of Toledo study showed that using amber lenses to block blue light not only significantly improved the quality of sleep, but elevated the mood of the test subjects.[1146] Thus, if you have to work at night as I do, purchase a good pair of glasses with amber lenses. I'm aware that I don't look trendy or sophisticated when I wear these glasses, but take my word for it, they really do the job! I'm not wearing this piece of "equipment" to look stylish, but to preserve my

precious night's sleep. I love my ugly glasses! They're worth every penny of the $14.99 that I spent on them.

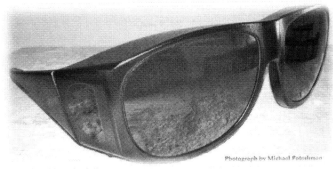

Photograph by Michael Poteshman

Finally, in order to prevent disruption to melatonin, replace your regular light bulb with amber light bulbs in your night lamp. That way, while reading a book before bed, the blue light will be adequately filtered out. If you decide not to purchase amber light bulbs, you can also use your glasses with amber lenses while reading a book before going to sleep.

ALARM CLOCK AND SLEEP

In the past I paid no attention to color and brightness of the digits on my alarm clock, and what it had to do with the quality of my sleep. I discovered that incorrect light color that emanated from the digits of my alarm clock was robbing me of melatonin. Regrettably, it was practically the same "blue" discussed in the section earlier, except that the clock was pointing at my face throughout the night. So, I purchased an alarm clock with amber digits which block out the blue light.

If it's not in your budget to purchase a digital amber alarm clock, make use of the dimmer settings to dim the digits, and turn the clock away from your face. Another alternative is to use the alarm clock function on your cellular smart phone, as it lights up when it's time to get up.

A gentleman once explained that he took a piece of amber tape and pasted it over the digits on his alarm clock. He said that he was extremely happy with the outcome, as he believed that it improved his quality of sleep. Although I never tried this method, it may be a viable alternative to spending additional money for a new alarm clock.

2.   EATING AND DRINKING BEFORE BED

When I was younger, I used to favor eating before going to bed. I preferred it because it made me fall asleep much faster. Even though I fell asleep faster, I never had restful sleep as I kept waking up to go to the bathroom or just wasn't able to fall back asleep. The reason this happens is that the digestion of food is an intense process that requires energy.

Every last fragment of food you consume must be processed and broken down into amino acids, glucose, and fatty acids.[1147] The process of digestion is intense, and takes hours.

It takes from **six to eight hours** for food to be processed by the stomach and passed to the small intestine.[1148] Therefore, **if you eat before bedtime, you're almost guaranteed not to have a quality night's sleep**.

There is also a very important matter of temperature regulation, specifically the increase in body temperature after eating. According to a Columbia University, as it gets darker, your internal clock begins to adjust by slowing down your metabolism, which results in a slight reduction in body temperature.[1149] [1150] But when you eat before going to bed, your temperature rises, which throws off your internal clock.[1151] If you thought it was difficult, and in some cases impossible to maintain sound sleep, escalating temperature has a lot to do with it.

ACID REFLUX

Another issue is acid reflux or heart burn, where the acid backs up into your esophagus. When you are resting in a horizontal position, food that you just consumed can press against the valve or lower esophageal sphincter that keeps acid from going into your esophagus.[1152] If the valve remains partially open or is opening frequently, acid can seep into your esophagus, causing heartburn, and eventually may manifest into acid reflux disease.[1153] Gravity is to blame. When we remain upright after a meal, food stays where it belongs, in the stomach. **If one goes to bed on a full stomach, it's almost impossible for the body to be in a restful state; hence sleeplessness**.

OVERCOMING FOOD RELATED SLEEPLESSNESS

To overcome sleeplessness associated with eating before bedtime, the Minnesota State University suggests that if you have no other alternative but to eat late, have a light dinner two hours prior to going to bed.[1154] As I've been my own guinea pig during my transformation into "Living Wonderfully", my last meal takes place four to five hours prior to "hitting the sack".

If for some reason you get seriously hungry because you missed your meal, as outlined in the "EATING TO LIVE" chapter later, have a handful of in-shell pumpkin or sunflower seeds, almonds, or any type of nuts, [1155] but only a handful! If that isn't available, eat an egg, or a <u>tiny amount</u> of boiled or baked beans that you prepare yourself with no sugar or chemicals added.[1156] Other options include a small piece of organic roasted turkey, or a piece of fish, or a couple of pieces of shrimp.[1157] But as a rule, definitely **no food within three to four hours before bed time**, <u>even if it's a very small amount</u>! Do not, under any circumstances, eat fruit before going to bed, as you will be raising your blood sugar level.

Just keep in mind that your body has to do a lot of work in order to metabolize even a small amount of food, let along fructose. That means that your sleep will be negatively affected.

The reason for eating nuts, beans, egg, turkey, tuna, or seafood, is that they contain the natural amino acid L-tryptophan, which triggers the production of serotonin, a chemical which naturally helps with sleep cycles.[1158] If you're wondering why not milk or yogurt as they also contains L-tryptophan, please refer back to the "DAIRY" section of the "WHAT NOT TO EAT" chapter.

USE CAUTION BEFORE GOING TO BED

SPICY AND ACIDIC FOODS

Even if you eat two hours before going to bed, stay away from anything spicy or acidic such as tomatoes or any type of hot peppers or pepper sauces. Also, fatty foods put an additional burden on your system, preventing you from staying asleep. Keep in mind that if you eat four to five hours prior to bed time, you can try to introduce spicy and acidic foods in small amounts in order to assess your tolerance level. I, for example, have no problem digesting food that contains spicy and acidic ingredients as long as I eat between four and five hours prior to bedtime.

SUGARY OR SIMPLE CARB FOODS

Here's this "S" word again, as if we didn't spend enough time on it in the "SUGAR" section. Unfortunately, sugary or simple carb foods that convert rapidly into glucose have a lot to do with sleeplessness.

"Eating a diet high in sugar and refined carbohydrate and eating irregularly can cause a reaction in the body that triggers the "fight or flight" part of the nervous system, causing wakefulness"
(Murray, 2006). [1159]

Perhaps you decided to eat a seemingly innocent piece of bread, a small bowl of ice cream, or a tiny bowl of pasta before bed. Although you fall asleep, you keep waking up and tossing and turning. The reason that you can't sleep when you eat these foods is that simple sugars break down rapidly in your body and cause a quick burst of energy. Your pancreas releases Insulin or it spikes, and tries to quickly lower your blood sugar level, thus you experience a crash. Hypoglycemia or low blood sugar is one of the causes of sleeplessness.

Your body's natural defense mechanism is to recognize when sugar drops to a certain level, thus stimulating the brain to be awakened. [1160]

If that wasn't bad enough, additional research shows that although the taste of sugary foods before bed may seem to have calming effect, it actually causes nightmares. [1161]

CAFFEINE

Any foods or beverages containing caffeine should not be consumed prior to going to bed. That means no coffee, espresso, or caffeinated teas. Something as benign as green tea may be loaded with caffeine, unless labeled "caffeine-free." Also, check the labels on foods, as they may contain caffeine, i.e. chocolate and even chewing gum.

Even a lot of **headache and pain pills contain caffeine** for faster and better absorption. [1162] [1163] [1164] In fact, the added caffeine makes these drugs 40% more effective. [1165]

A study published in the *Journal of Clinical Sleep Medicine* concluded that ingesting caffeine **even 6 hours before going to bed could decrease sleep by one hour**.[1166] [1167] Prior to the study, the effects of caffeine were not only underestimated by the public, but by doctors.[1168]

If you're going to bed around 10:00 PM, discontinue consuming products containing caffeine at around 3:00 PM or 7 hours before sleep.

Since I occasionally enjoy black tea and coffee, I tried different time frames closer to bed time, only to learn that the study, especially in my case, was proven correct.

As far as limiting of caffeine consumption, *"Health Canada recommends no more than 400 milligrams of caffeine per day — about three 8 ounce cups (237 ml) of brewed coffee — with a lower limit for women who are pregnant, breastfeeding or planning to become pregnant."* (CBC News, 2013)[1169]

ALCOHOL

When it comes to alcoholic beverages, there shouldn't be any alcoholic consumption at least 4 to 6 hours prior to going to bed.[1170] In a not so distant past, I always thought that alcohol helps you sleep. This is only partially true.

> *"While alcohol does help people fall into light sleep, it also robs them of REM and the deeper, more restorative stages of sleep. Instead, it keeps them in the lighter stages of sleep…"*
> (Perricone, N., MD., 2008).[1171]

So, when you wake up in the morning after having a couple of drinks, you feel tired, groggy, or remain sleepy. This is partially because you have not entered deep sleep, although you believed that you "slept like a baby."

3.   EXERCISE

Although I'm a committed proponent of exercise, there are mixed opinions that exercising before sleep may actually keep you awake instead of letting you rest. The reasoning behind this is that your pulse and body temperature increase, resulting in being more awake and alert.[1172] This is certainly true for me, although some studies point out that a number of people don't experience sleeplessness immediately after exercise.[1173] [1174]

According to the University of Maryland Medical Center, exercising in the afternoon can actually improve sleep. On the other hand, your ability to fall asleep may be reduced by exercising even two hours before going to bed.[1175] I usually work out in the morning or late afternoon. If I exercise even two hours before bed, I have restless sleep.

4.   COMFORTABLE SLEEPING ATMOSPHERE

DROWN OUT NOISE

Before I discuss sleeping atmosphere, I have to reveal another secret of sleeping soundly. Since my early childhood I've had an unfortunate ability to wake up at the faintest sound. I tried ear plugs, but after a while I realized that they hurt my ears. To solve this problem I tried different remedies such as a white noise generator or desktop fan. The best solution that I found was a motorized air cleaner that makes a consistent "whooshing" sound. The benefit of this gadget besides cleaning the air, it drowns out the majority of noises that may occur at night: air conditioning cycles, wind, creaks in the attic or floors, etc.

There are different white noise generators available. Some emulate sounds of the rain forest, ocean surf, or chirping birds. As long as it works for you, it's a winner!

ROOM TEMPERATURE

Temperature in the room is one of the most important sleep-related factors. As discussed earlier, when your body is getting ready to fall asleep, your temperature drops slightly. In order to easily achieve this decrease in temperature, H. Craig Heller, PhD, professor of biology at Stanford University, suggests that the temperature of your bedroom should be cool instead of warm.[1176] [1177] It is important because the temperature affects your deepest sleep cycle or REM sleep, which is the stage of sleep where you dream.[1178]

Ideally, the room should not be hot or cold, but comfortably cool at around 60°F to 67°F or 15.5°C to 19.4°C.[1179] If these temperatures are uncomfortable, keep experimenting until you find the sweet spot where your sleep is the most restful. In our family, for example, we prefer sleeping under warm blankets at temperatures below 65°F or 18.3°C.

5.   CAT NAPS

A lot of people are worried that if they sleep during the day, they won't be able to sleep well at night. They are only partially correct. In the past, I've had some of those sleepless nights when I napped during the day, as I had no other alternative.

I did it all wrong! "Cat Nap" signifies exactly what it is, a sleep that is short in duration. According to Harvard Medical School, a daytime nap should be kept short; approximately 20 to a **maximum** of 30 minutes in duration.[1180] Furthermore, a Harvard Health Letter states that sleeping for a short duration, even for a couple of minutes, is beneficial.[1181] If this model of "Cat Napping" is followed, there shouldn't be any interference with sleeping through the night.[1182]

Normalizing sleep actually plays a huge role in the next chapter, which offers limitless health possibilities! How about prolonging your life?

If you only take away one thing from this book, this chapter would be "It!" Everything that you've read and learned up until this point has prepared you to put it all together. This chapter is the universality for the entire book.

Let's look at the big picture. Do you want to live a longer, healthier, happier, and more productive life, or have a sick, sad, and unsatisfied existence? The answer should be obvious, but before I began to live "Wonderfully", I really didn't care one way or the other because of my progressing health problems. But that was in the past!

The bottom line is that you only have one life, and then that's it. The power that you now possess by reading this book is that **you may not only live a happier life, but be able to prolong it!** Yes, I know what you might be thinking, as I didn't believe it either. By the time you finish this chapter, I hope that a smile on your face will emerge as you recognize that your health problems can be overcome quite effectively!

It all comes down to one single factor: **"Insulin!"** I mentioned the word Insulin and Insulin resistance several times throughout the "**WHAT NOT TO EAT**" and other chapters. Recall the "**NITRATES**" section where halting Insulin production in the brain was linked to Alzheimer's and Parkinson's diseases. [1183] [1184] As you can see, most of the discussions lead back to Insulin. Now we know that this life-sustaining or "life-destroying" substance that our body produces has an even greater purpose!

Although people with Type 1 diabetes cannot produce Insulin, they may also benefit from the information in this chapter.

TO 100 AND BEYOND… OR AS LONG AS YOUR GENES CAN POSSIBLY ALLOW

"We know now that the variability in life span is regulated by Insulin"
(Rosedale, 2008).[1185]

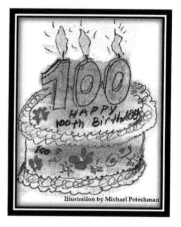

How powerful is that? The way your body regulates Insulin may determine not only your longevity but the degree of health throughout your lifetime.

When we think about cardiovascular diseases, certain forms of cancer, or the common cold, all can be attributed to some form of **Insulin involvement**. [1186] Ever since I began to eat as outlined in the "**WHAT TO EAT**" chapter that's coming up later in the book, my constant colds have gone away. Before this change, it didn't matter whether it was winter or summer, as I was getting colds regularly. This doesn't mean that I may not catch a virus in the future. What I'm trying to impart is that my semimonthly colds and perpetual allergies have disappeared. What does that have to do with Insulin or life extension? Read on…

Illustration by Michael Poteshman

People who live to 100 years of age or beyond, have one thing in common. No matter what their lifestyle is or was throughout their lifetime, the blood sugar "relative to their age", triglycerides, and Insulin were in check.[1187]

Until I was controlling my Insulin production by eating foods that kept my body on an even keel or without Insulin spikes, I couldn't lose weight or feel contented with my life. Unfortunately, I didn't know that **Insulin production or Insulin resistance was at the center of my entire existence,** and that it could be easily controlled. As a result, I paid the price as described in previous chapters.

A study published in *The Journal of Applied Research* found a **direct correlation between aging and elevated Insulin levels**.[1188]

Extending your lifespan by controlling Insulin production and Insulin resistance through <u>what you put in your mouth</u> is much easier to achieve than you think.

The hormone Insulin determines whether you are storing fat or burning fat.[1189] By controlling Insulin on the "Living Wonderfully" routine, I feel younger, stronger, and more vibrant in my early fifties than when I was in my thirties. Having potency as if I were in my twenties is another powerful indicator that the body is rebuilding itself. How's that for life extending strategy? My blood pressure, blood test results, and overall wellbeing are confirming this, as I'm living without any prescribed or over the counter medications! In the past, when people were having seasonal allergies twice a year, I had them practically year-round for over 20 years. **I have no allergies now!** How's that for life prolonging strategy?

I'm now a believer as I'm living this dream of health and vitality. **By regulating Insulin, we can get rid of or reduce diseases, prolong our lives, and have absolutely awesome outcomes and experiences!**

"…the actual rate of aging itself can be modulated by Insulin. We should be living to be 130, 140 years old routinely"
(Rosedale, 2008).[1190]

That's right, by controlling Insulin we could be living to 100 and beyond!!! How cool is that? My family and I have already signed up. Now it's time to get you in the club of "Living Wonderfully" until the ripe age of over 100 or the maximum age that your telomeres may allow.

TELOMERES OR NATURAL AGING

Although "Telomeres" may sound like something that's on TV, they have nothing to do with television. Telomeres represent another factor that regulates our longevity, and involves our natural genetic predisposition. Telomeres are pieces of DNA protective structure located at the end of chromosomes. This DNA structure protects our genetic information that involves aging, division of cells, etc.[1191]

Imagine a shoe lace with a plastic piece at the end that keeps your shoe lace from fraying. Using this example, think of telomeres as "plastic pieces" that keep chromosomes from fraying. Chromosome fraying essentially muddles or jumbles the genetic data and thereby may result in cancer or even death.[1192] Every time your cells divide, the telomeres get shorter, and eventually they get too short. This phenomenon is associated with aging, different types of cancer, and death. [1193]

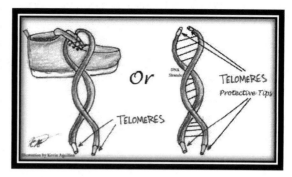

We all have telomeres. Some are longer, which represents longer life. Some are shorter, which may dictate that life expectancy of an individual will not be as lengthy. There is even a telomere blood test to predict your biological age. I will not be undergoing this blood test because I don't want to have mental susceptibility that would dictate my demise.

Let's take one step at a time and extend our lives for as long as possible so we don't expire prior to the expiration of our telomeres. You never know, you and I may have telomeres that last to 100 and beyond! I know that mine have a much better chance now that I'm "Living Wonderfully." By having a healthy lifestyle, you don't accelerate telomeres reduction, which may just extend your life.

"Recent evidence suggests that a high quality and balanced multiVitamin will also help maintain telomere length. Specifically, studies have linked longer telomeres with levels of Vitamin E, Vitamin C, Vitamin D, omega-3 fatty acids and the antioxidant resveratrol"
(SpectraCell Laboratories, 2014).[1194]

"Telomeres are known to respond well to a healthy lifestyle. A person who maintains a good diet, exercises regularly, and is free from constant heavy stress, is not likely to endure accelerated telomere shortening"
(Telomeretesting.net, 2013). [1195]

In order to get you into this "longevity club", we will begin by briefly recapping why Insulin is produced and overproduced. Next, we will assess what happens when you develop Insulin resistance. Finally, we'll move on to an "even keel" or leveled Insulin production strategy. There will be no ambiguity as to why I've been eating monstrous portions and have lost an incredible amount of weight, got rid of constant colds and allergies, and improved my overall health. Let's begin.

INSULIN PRODUCTION AND RESISTANCE

When I was on my many doctor-directed low fat diets, trying to desperately lose weight, I was inadvertently spiking my Insulin with these diet foods. I had no idea that **my obesity was due to excessive Insulin or Insulin resistance**.[1196]

Your body uses Insulin as a key in order to unlock your cells to absorb glucose, the food source that cells require in order to exist.

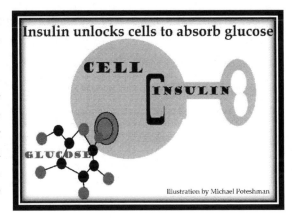

Unlike complex carbohydrates or fibrous foods, when you eat foods that are quickly converted to glucose such as cake, pasta, bread, pretzels, potato chips, white rice, bagels, candy, doughnuts, cookies, etc., your pancreas releases Insulin or it produces Insulin spikes in order to combat the onslaught of sugar on your system. In other words, your body is desperately trying to stabilize your glucose level.

Here's how it works. Your body first stores glucose in cells for immediate energy use. Next, your body stores glucose in the form of glycogen for later use.[1197] Glycogen is a product of glucose stored primarily in the **liver and muscles**. The purpose of glycogen is once your body determines that blood sugar is low during the periods when you don't eat, some of the stored glycogen is sent back into the blood stream to be used as energy. Unlike fat, there is only a limited amount of glycogen that can be stored in the liver and muscles.[1198]

Once your body has filled up its cells and glycogen stores, the excess, if any, has to go somewhere. You guessed it; **it is stored as fat**, specifically visceral fat, as we will discuss in the next section.

Keep in mind that **if glucose is not utilized as energy, your body converts it to fat**.

The more simple carbohydrates and sugar you ingest, the more Insulin will be produced. Thus, when Insulin levels remain high, or your pancreas produces continuous Insulin spikes in order to regulate glucose, your body develops Insulin resistance. The cells that Insulin is supposed to unlock for glucose absorption can no longer appropriately respond to the actions of Insulin. Sort of like you're yelling at your kids, and after a while they ignore you. You try to get their attention by yelling at them louder. In the case of Insulin resistance, your pancreas produces more Insulin in order to combat cells "not hearing" or not appropriately responding to Insulin.

Because of additional Insulin production, your body struggles to effectively use fat reserves, resulting in **more fat being stored**.

This downward spiral leads to heart disease, obesity, diabetes, high blood pressure, and strokes, among other serious ailments, some of which will be discussed in the next section. [1199] [1200]

Don't think that Insulin is a bad thing. In fact, it is wonderful for your body in normal or **low amounts**. After all, if it weren't for this "wonder hormone" we would not only die of glucose intoxication, but also our muscles, our organs, and especially our brain would have nothing to feed on. [1201] [1202]

Once again, too much Insulin "spiking" for too long, and your organs begin to develop Insulin resistance. Because of Insulin resistance, your body struggles to use Insulin properly, and as a result, multitude of problems begin to manifest.[1203]

"Insulin resistance is the basis of all of the chronic diseases of aging."
(Rosedale, 2008).[1204]

The result of Insulin spikes or consistent increase of blood sugar level is that **your body is directed by the Insulin hormone to use carbs for energy instead of fat**.[1205]

In addition, your body is directed by this hormone to <u>store fat and not to release fat</u>. "*...Insulin converts almost half of your dietary carbohydrate to fat for storage*" (Mercola, 2006).[1206] Essentially, the residual sugars and carbs don't just contribute to your weight gain, but **you become "resistant to weight loss"**.[1207]

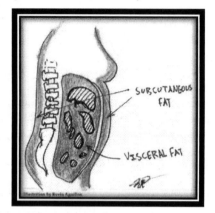

As you continue to create Insulin spikes by eating foods that rapidly turn into glucose, you begin to develop a unique kind of fat known as, "Visceral fat." [1208] This is fat growing inside the abdominal area;[1209] sometimes referred to as "beer gut" or belly fat. Visceral fat is not subcutaneous or located underneath the skin and abdominal wall as indicated by the illustration.

Instead, visceral fat resides a lot deeper in your belly, as it surrounds <u>your inner vital organs</u>. It may be in the pancreas, or you may have a condition known as fatty liver, enlarged intestines, enlarged spleen, fatty kidneys, or all of the above.[1210] [1211] [1212] [1213]

You don't have to be obese or overweight to have accumulated visceral fat. Even a person with normal weight who's sporting a protruding belly has already "stockpiled" visceral fat. I'm certain that some of you have heard the term TOFI, not to be confused with tofu. TOFI stands for "Thin on the Outside, Fat on the Inside." What that means is that even though you are skinny on the outside, your organs may be incrusted with fat.[1214] It also means that you're just as susceptible to heart disease or diabetes as an overweight person. [1215]

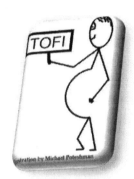

"Visceral fat literally encrusts the vital organs: the kidneys, liver, stomach, and others"
(Hartley, 2009)[1216]

Why is this fat so "unique?" It is unique for one very disturbing reason. **Visceral fat is a hormone producing organ that is "<u>metabolically active</u>."**[1217]

In essence, this "home grown" organ wreaks havoc on your entire body. An example is that visceral fat produces an enzyme called "aromatase." **Aromatase converts the male hormone - Testosterone into the female hormone - Estrogen**.[1218] [1219]

"Visceral fat produces so much aromatase that it's literally feminizing men, by robbing them of Testosterone"
(BodyMeasure, 2013).[1220]

Males are growing female breasts, which is one of the prime examples of Testosterone being converted into Estrogen.[1221] Perhaps you've witnessed the man-boobs or "moobs" phenomenon. According to American Society of Plastic Surgeons, male breast reduction surgery is one of the fastest growing cosmetic procedures for men, which accounts for over 40% of all breast reduction surgeries across the United States.[1222]

As production of Testosterone declines, males not only gain more body fat, but lose strength and muscle mass, and suffer from a diminished sex drive.[1223] [1224] Thus, the vicious downward spiral gains momentum. As more weight is gained, more aromatase is produced, more Testosterone gets converted into Estrogen, and more weight is gained in the mid-section. The more Testosterone that is lost, the more muscle mass is lost, and so on.[1225]

Although men begin collecting visceral fat earlier in life than women, neither gender is exempt from visceral fat's damaging effects. According to Harvard Medical School, **visceral fat in women is related to cancer and the need for gallbladder surgery where gallbladder is removed**.[1226]

This "home grown wonder" **produces substances that cause inflammation**, which is the foundation for additional devastating health problems:

According to the research, heart disease, type 2 diabetes, strokes, colorectal cancer, increase of LDL or bad cholesterol, and decrease of HDL or good cholesterol, blood vessel constriction which causes high blood pressure, among other diseases, **are triggered by visceral fat**. [1227] [1228] [1229]

I will leave you with something that made me think twice before I even had an inkling of putting a piece of Insulin-spiking "almost food" or "simple-carb and/or sugary junk" in my mouth. Let's reflect on the possibility of dying before your time.

"Research also has associated belly fat with an increased risk of premature death — regardless of overall weight."
(Mayo Clinic, 2013)[1230]

Several studies found that men with large mid-section and surplus of belly fat are at risk from what is called **all-cause mortality or premature death from any cause**.[1231] [1232]

Scary? You bet! But as long as we're alive there's good news. That means we can do something about it, and it's coming up next.

"EVEN KEEL" OR LOW INSULIN PRODUCTION STRATEGY AND REVERSING OF DISEASES

When I discuss the subject of regulating Insulin production and improving quality of life, I always hear, "I'm too far gone", or "I have type 2 diabetes, so it makes no sense to go through the motions as I'm already taking Insulin." In the past I gave myself an out by saying, "My blood pressure is through the roof because my doctor told me that my arteries are partially blocked, hardened and constricted. Let me enjoy the years that I have left in peace." These excuses were perfectly reasonable when I had no clue that anything could be done about these diseases and my overall health.

The awesome news is that even if you are pre-diabetic or suffer from type 2 diabetes, in a lot of cases it can be reversed!!![1233] [1234] [1235]

As you read earlier, even if you have hardened and/or partially blocked arteries, the scientific evidence clearly shows that heart disease can be reversed.[1236] This incredible news of coronary disease and type 2 diabetes reversal were not only music to my ears, but a turning point in my beliefs and judgment about the future.

I'm the prime example of this phenomenon. After only **three months** of "Living Wonderfully", my blood and urine samples were not only normal, but in most cases, better than the recommended levels. After six months, my blood pressure normalized. This tells you that your body wants to heal itself. **The reversal of a 15-year miserable and sick existence on prescription medications, suffering, and "Living Dead" was put on its head in <u>six months!</u>** The primary factor was getting my Insulin to normal or low secretion levels, something that I call an "even keel" strategy. This is much easier to achieve than you think.

There are four components to achieving the even keel Insulin production which will inadvertently improve or reverse your heart disease, type 2 diabetes, and overall health:

1. Reducing Stress
2. Meal frequency and eating "Real-anti-inflammatory" food
3. Physical activity
4. Sleep

1. REDUCING STRESS

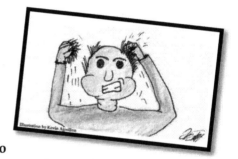

Why is stress reduction the number one item on the list for regulating Insulin? It's because when you're stressed, you produce a steroid hormone known as **"Cortisol" which over time raises blood sugar level**, [1237] [1238] and thereby gets your Insulin out of balance. As Cortisol is secreted, your body is "flooded" with glucose/blood sugar.[1239] [1240] What happens then is overtime, due to consistently raised cortisol, **you begin to store fat**. When you're constantly stressed, your other body processes also get disrupted. For example:

- Weight gain; specifically through **relocating triglycerides to visceral fat cells.**[1241] [1242] Just to remind you, visceral fat resides deeper in your belly, as it surrounds <u>your inner vital organs.</u>
- Cardiovascular disease [1243]
- Depression[1244] [1245]
- Insomnia[1246]
- Digestive disorders [1247] [1248]
- Problems concentrating, especially in cases of cortisol induced insomnia[1249]

Another reason that stress reduction is the first item on the list is that it's one of the most difficult conditions to overcome and control. As you will learn in the "YOUR STATE OF MIND" chapter later in the book, "THE FIVE-MINUTE MIND CLEANSE" technique worked wonders for me and for my family. For now,

I'm hoping that the rest of this "Stress reduction" section helps you reset your mind in order to deal with anything that life throws at you.

"With every rising of the sun, Think of your life as just begun"
-Ella Wheeler Wilcox-

Isn't that beautiful? Ella Wheeler Wilcox truly captured the meaning of "Living Wonderfully" in this one simple sentence. Indeed, <u>every day is the beginning of the rest of your life</u>. Therefore, it is imperative to always stay happy and positive. N**o matter how tough your day is going, don't let this new day become ruined.**

"Happiness is one of the most important treasures. It is within your soul. All you have to do is dig it out and enjoy it."
-Remez Sasson-[1250]

The following few activities are rudimentary, but truly life-changing.

BREAKING OUT OF THE SELF-IMPOSED PRISON OF MISERY

When I began to break-out of the "Living Dead" existence, I came to a realization that *"We are all creatures of habit who continuously build self-imposed prisons of misery!"* Just like millions of others, I built mental prison borders that prevented me from enjoying my past accomplishments.

The question that I'm often asked is how do you smile if there is no reason for it? Think about something pleasant in your life, something enjoyable such as past memories or new pleasant achievements that you want to come to fruition.

We can go even further in order to induce a bigger smile. Although you may be thinking that a problem is really tough, inject some humor into it. Make it somewhat comical. Pretend that this "thing" that bothers you is buzzing around your head like an annoying fly and you're trying to swat it. You will eventually swat this pesky "fly-problem." You know that you have done so in the past, and you will do it again, but this time with a huge smile on your face. So smile; it's not the end of the world! Just remember that this new day is only the beginning of the rest of your life!

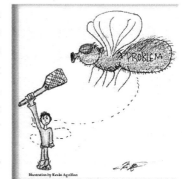

Illustration by Kevin Aguillon

An article in *Psychology Today* by Ronald E. Riggio, Ph.D., Professor of Organizational Psychology, affirms that smiling and laughing produces positive changes in your brain:

"…the serotonin release brought on by your smile serves as an anti-depressant/mood lifter"
(Stevenson, 2012).[1251]

In addition, when dopamine, endorphins, and serotonin are released into your system, the body goes into resting or relaxing state, and blood pressure may be reduced as a result.[1252] So, smile and laugh from sun up to sun down and beyond, as it's really good for you! The great news is that there are no bad side effects, only excellent results that contribute to an even keel Insulin production.

BE GRATEFUL FOR THINGS YOU HAVE

Be grateful for what you already have and what you have accomplished. A lot of people are never satisfied with what they have. Thus, the quest for more becomes a very unhappy place where you always feel dissatisfied. Instead, look around you and take inventory. Whether it's your family, friends, or material things that you own, be grateful. Your lifestyle may be better than someone else's. Who cares if the "Joneses" have a bigger TV or better car! Make a list of what you're grateful for and recite it at the beginning of each day. This activity will distract you from the unhappy "I don't have" thoughts. Therefore, if you're happy with what you have, and still want more, it will give you a baseline from which to start. Once you complete your inventory, you'll realize that no matter how much or how little you have, you are wealthy. Whether the wealth is financial, family, or health related, you've achieved it!

MAKE A RESOLUTION TO STAY UPBEAT

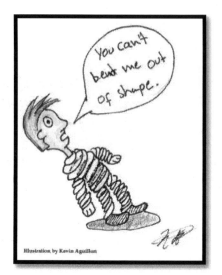

Illustration by Kevin Aguillon

You might say, "How can I be happy when this person that I work with is such an a*%@#*e?" Perhaps you're too tired to be happy because your boss is so demanding. While excuses are made, life is passing you by. So when will you be happy? When you retire?

Happiness is a state of mind. Use my favorite phrase that helped many of the managers that I trained throughout my career: **"You are flexible enough not to be bent out of shape!"**

This means that even if you're working next to an "a**@%e", that person will not be able to destroy your joyfulness. Keep in mind, **when you're getting upset over someone's actions, this person wins!** Instead, by keeping upbeat, you will always be the winner! Instead of leaving work in a miserable state of mind, you will be in high spirits and full of life.

Remember, time waits for no one. **The time to be happy is NOW and every single day thereafter, for the rest of your life!**

2. EATING REAL-ANTI-INFLAMMATORY FOOD – YOUR BODY IS NOT A GARBAGE CAN

<u>**The hormone Insulin determines whether you are storing fat or burning fat.**</u>[1253] If you abstain from high carbohydrate, sugary or processed, as well as other Insulin spiking "almost-foods" that we discussed in "WHAT NOT TO EAT" chapter, your Insulin remains low. **As a result of very low or no Insulin production, <u>your body uses stored fat for energy instead of glucose</u>.** [1254] This is where the stored fat that you've been trying to get rid of throughout your lifetime begins to vanish, almost magically.

Although exercise is one of the four most important methods to achieving the even keel Insulin production, it is ineffective without the crucial component of food. You can exercise until you're blue in the face, and you may achieve some positive results as I have in the past. But if you're treating your body like a garbage can by eating simple carbs sugar, processed foods with added chemicals, or what I call "garbage", it will be very difficult, and in some cases, impossible to normalize Insulin. As I mentioned earlier, when I was in my teens, twenties, and early thirties, I had no problem metabolizing "almost food" items. Therefore, I continued to treat my body like a garbage can. The sad reality is that over the years it caught up with me with a vengeance, as the effects are cumulative. For those readers who are in their teens or twenties, don't think that you're invincible. Unless you are one lucky

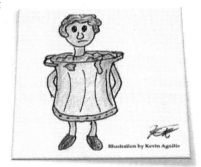

Illustration by Kevin Aguilis

centenarian who naturally has normal blood sugar level, low triglycerides, and normal Insulin, you are not exempt. Unfortunately most of us aren't, thus **we have to do things that will turn us into centenarians**.

You've already read about the destructive foods in the "WHAT NOT TO EAT" chapter. These types of simple carbohydrates and processed foods are responsible for a multitude of illnesses, elevation of blood sugar, different types of cancer, and are the prime cause of blockages in the arteries

I replaced "almost foods" with absolutely delicious and astounding combinations of different foods that possess anti-cancer, anti-inflammatory, and anti-aging properties. All was done without the need for dieting or some sort of special routine as you will read in the "WHAT TO EAT" section later. The most wonderful news is that <u>you stop being resistant to weight loss</u>, and begin to heal from the inside out!

The best part of this new way of eating is that all types of cravings unexpectedly disappear, your mind begins to clear up, and you are feeling like you're "on the top of the world!"

As to the meal frequency, all will be explained in the "HALF BREAKFAST" section later in the book. For now, it's important to keep in mind that there is **no snacking** in the Living Wonderfully land, as we want to keep our insulin production down to a minimum, while utilizing glycogen and stored fat respectively. Once again **as a result of very low or no Insulin production, <u>your body uses stored fat for energy instead of glucose</u>**.[1255]

Suddenly your skin begins to glow, chronic aches begin to ease, and your mood begins to lighten. Now for the third part of the even keel strategy.

3. PHYSICAL TRAINING

"One of the key health benefits of exercise is that it helps normalize your glucose, Insulin, and Leptin levels by optimizing Insulin/Leptin receptor sensitivity"
(Mercola, 2013)[1256]

When you exercise and build muscle, your body begins to respond better to Insulin. According to a study, exercise training facilitates the normalization of **glucose metabolism**.[1257]

In order to melt your visceral fat and normalize your Insulin production, your body must be put in motion. The cold and sobering reality is that we must move in order to maintain good health.

Although it's dreaded by many, unfortunately I have to use the word "exercise." When I speak about exercise I hear the same excuses that I used in the past: "I don't have time" or "I'm too tired."

You can start by walking 20 to 30 minutes per day around your neighborhood. If you don't feel like it, whenever you are at work, take your lunch break outside, and walk around instead of sitting at your desk or in a restaurant. If you don't have 30 minutes, try to do something physical for at least 15 minutes. If you have time to watch TV for 15 minutes, it means that your time can be spent preserving your health and extending your life by walking or doing sit-ups!

As you build your stamina by walking briskly or doing other physical activity such as walking up and down stairs, you can begin to add more vigorous exercises. For example, I lift moderate weights three to four times per week, do sit-ups, and use an elliptical machine; all without resting between exercises as will be explained in the next section. During the other three/four days I either walk briskly around the neighborhood or use a low impact elliptical machine at home. Elliptical trainer machines are available on line or your favorite big box store, starting around $130.00 for the basic model.

STEPS FOR CONDITIONING YOUR BODY FOR GREAT REWARDS

"…for every extra 1lb of muscle you have, your body uses around an extra 50 calories a day! This means an extra 10lb of muscle will burn roughly an extra 500 calories a day without you doing anything - and that's a sufficient amount to lose 1lb in a week"
(Kellow, 2004)[1258]

1. Walking, climbing stairs, or anything that puts your body in motion is the first step to the rest of your life as it may help you with reversal of diabetes and/or heart disease. Take it easy, as Rome wasn't built in one day; don't overexert yourself. This is only the beginning to the rest of your life!
2. Once your body is ready for more moderate exercise, your next step is 25-30 minutes of continuous elevation of heart rate three times per week.
3. The final step is to get your body to the point where you will be able to endure 30 minutes of vigorous exercise such as aerobic training about every other day or 4 days per week. Even vigorous exercise on a low impact elliptical trainer will do the job. As I read extensive research papers and by experimenting on myself, I learned that high-intensity circuit training gets rid of fat faster than anything I ever tried.[1259] [1260] Circuit training means keeping your heart rate up throughout your workout routine as you move from exercise to exercise with little to no rest. For example, I lift weights, do sit-ups, and use a low impact elliptical machine in between exercises, all without stopping to rest.

I have every confidence that you will be able to condition your body to get to this point, but first we must walk before we can run. Start slowly and work your way up to the point of getting rid of this

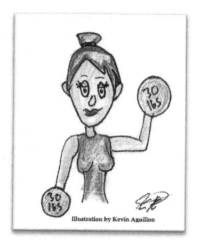
Illustration by Kevin Aguillon

horrible "home grown" visceral fat. Check with your doctor first before embarking on an exercise program.

Don't give yourself an out by saying "I only have 10 minutes to exercise, and those 10 minutes don't count." Not true at all. Any physical activity, even 10 minutes of moving, is better than 10 minutes of sedentary existence. Your body will respond accordingly by being less sluggish, more alert and vigorous.

Before you begin any exercise routine, keep one very important thing in mind. Do not over-exert yourself by over-exercising, as you will be generating cortisol.[1261] That's the _stress hormone_ that we discussed earlier. Please recall, when cortisol is secreted, your body is "flooded" with glucose/blood sugar.[1262] [1263] Overtime, **Cortisol will prevent you from burning fat until it's out of your system**. Therefore, instead of losing weight, you will continue to store fat. That's the reason I advocate baby steps when starting any exercise routine. _Begin with a low intensity exercise, and build up to a more strenuous routine_ **without stressing out your system**.

Don't think of exercise as boring. Get your MP3 player and load it up with audio books, your favorite music, or different audio classes.

4. SLEEP

You are already aware of the benefits of sleep from the previous chapter. Keep in mind that productive sleep plays a huge role in achieving an even keel strategy.

Although this concludes the "Insulin" chapter, the rest of the book will provide crucial information on keeping your Insulin levels in check.

Chapter 25 **EATING TO LIVE**

"Eat to live, don't live to eat."
-Benjamin Franklin-

I believe that I'm speaking for a lot of people when I say that I depended on food to make me feel happy, or to pleasantly occupy my time. As a result, I was eating when I wasn't really hungry. I planned my entire schedule and majority of activities around food.

When my family and I went on vacation, the number one priority was to find facilities that served a variety of food around the clock. Consequently, we went on cruises, or as I called them "food-cruises", where food was in abundance 24 hours per day. Even around midnight, when I wasn't hungry, I regularly paid visits to the pizza kitchen. Although I had dinner just a few hours earlier, it was really pleasurable to eat fresh pizza on the deck of the ship. The end result was more headaches, brain fog, higher blood pressure, higher cholesterol, exacerbated acid reflux, and sadness.

Although I understood that what I was doing was wrong, eating while not hungry made me feel really good. Later, it caught up with me with a vengeance. It's almost like an addict snorting cocaine to feel good for a short time, only to return to the misery of craving the drug.

There are a number of reasons why we eat when we're not hungry, and sometimes overeat, and why our lives revolve around food. The food additives, as described in previous chapters, have a lot to do with eating uncontrollably. Recall earlier discussion of Leptin insensitivity. There are other reasons why we eat the way we eat. Once I understood those reasons and was **brutally honest with myself**, I was able to stop the insanity. I began to listen to my body as an indicator for food, which we will discuss at the end of this chapter. Now that my life is not revolving around food and eating, I focus on the present and bright future because my outlook on life has changed. The following are some examples of how the majority of us "Live to Eat", and how some of us have gotten to this rotten place of "Living Dead".

FOUR DOUBLE CHEESEBURGERS FOR FOUR DOLLARS: HOW AWESOME IS THAT?

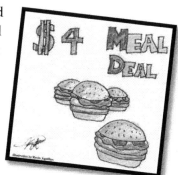

I was especially guilty of this offense! I used to love to visit fast food restaurants and feast to my heart's content on cheap foods that were devoid of nutrients. I used to eat three double cheeseburgers and then made a point to stop at a convenience store to get a huge diet soda, and my favorite, chocolate candies. How is that for blocked arteries in the making? I'm certain that I was full after eating only two double cheeseburgers or even one, but I kept eating because it was delicious, cheap and plentiful, and I was used to it. "The more the merrier" was my motto. How stupid was that?

What about all-you-can-eat restaurants? You consume one plate of food and it usually fills you up. But you end up overeating because it's all-you-can-eat and it's all paid for. "Let's get our money's worth!" In essence, you end up eating when you are completely full.

How about those membership food megastores where they give you free samples of food? I used to make a point to drive by those stores to try different food samples, even though I wasn't hungry. After all, what would these small samples really do to you? That was a completely wrong mentality and I was paying for it with my health.

WELL-INTENTIONED FOOD PURVEYORS; BET YOU KNOW ONE

One day my wife and I were enjoying ourselves at a party at my friends' house. In walked another good friend with an absolutely gorgeous cheesecake. He said, "Michael, why don't you try this?" I apologetically told him that I no longer ate this stuff because of the refined sugar and dairy. His response was swift, "You have to try it because I made it! I had to get up early this morning to make it fresh for everyone to enjoy!" I felt defeated as there was no arguing with a person who was on the edge of getting offended over non-appreciation of his hard work. At the end I had no other alternative but to eat a very small piece of cake that **I did not need, enjoy**, or want, in order to avoid hurting his feelings.

I'm certain that you have "food purveyors" in your circle of friends and family. Although my excuse didn't work on my friend in that particular situation, I always have a number of excuses handy. You can say that you just ate and can't eat another bite. Alternatively you can say that you're on a strict diet. For the sake of your health, you can even lie and say that your doctor prohibits you from having a particular food that your friend or family member is pushing on you. After all, people love you and don't want you to go against your doctor's advice. When they hear the "doctor excuse," most of the time, they will back off.

EMOTIONAL HABITS ARE A KILLER; LITERALLY!

Your day is going really badly. Everything you touch turns into a disaster. You end up turning to food to calm your nerves and relieve stress. But does it make you feel better? Indeed it does while you're eating, and even an hour or less after the meal. Then there is a crash, and you're worse off than when you started.

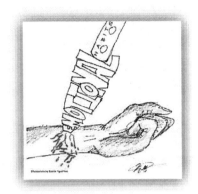

Being stuffed after a meal may redirect your attention from the bad day that you're having, but it gets even more miserable later. As the old European saying goes, "Misery breeds misery".

The very next day, everything is going great. There is a reason to celebrate, so you go out and you eat, usually more than you need. After all, this is a celebration! What's the best way to celebrate but to stuff your face?

It is crucial that you keep track of your emotional eating habits as they will eventually turn into unneeded pounds, and undoubtedly cause a decline in health.

CLEAN PLATE SYNDROME

"You can't leave the table until you clean your plate!" Have you heard this before? This was the story of my life. Growing up, my parents told me that many children around the world were starving and I was fortunate to have food on my plate. Therefore, I had to leave my plate completely clean. Consequently, I developed a habit of eating everything on my plate even when I was completely full.

As I've changed my life and habits, here's what I do now. I eat until I'm full, and if there are leftovers on the plate, I put them in the refrigerator. This also applies to restaurants where you can ask for a carryout containers or a doggie bag. Most of the time, the food can be reheated. On rare occasions, reheating may not be advantageous, so the food has to be thrown out or given to a pet. Ponder on this:

Even though you may throw out two or three dollars' worth of food, you will save <u>thousands</u>, if not **tens of thousands of dollars in medical expenses**.

I believe that this logical math speaks for itself as you will not only be saving money but your own life along the way.

For those of you who do not like to throw any food away, all you have to do is switch to a smaller plate. If you believe that you're still hungry, add a little more food to that small plate. That way there will be no leftovers, nothing to reheat, and nothing to throw away.

Most of us have eaten out of boredom. You open your refrigerator and stare inside even though you're not hungry. You find a morsel or two, and you put it in your mouth. Because this morsel is so delicious, you go back and get more. All of a sudden, it's all gone. Two hours later you're eating your dinner on a full or semi-full stomach. Sound familiar? Here's how to combat this habit of eating out of boredom.

As soon as you head to your refrigerator, or to any food source, check if you're truly hungry. If you're not hungry, how about going for a walk instead? Perhaps go to the gym, play a video game or watch a movie. Almost <u>any activity is better than eating on a full stomach</u>.

Use this "Eating out of boredom" as a trigger to do something else which is fun and makes you happy. That way, you will turn this debilitating habit into something that's life infusing, and something that you may have a lot of fun doing.

I SEE FOOD, I EAT IT: THE "SEE FOOD" DIET

When I first made a commitment to my wife that I would not be eating processed foods for at least one month, I asked her to remove all of the sweets, cereals, bad carbohydrates, especially my favorites, cookies and chocolate, from the house. As a result, I wasn't tempted to practice my "see food diet" at home. I also made changes at the office where "junk" was readily available everywhere and on the work desk of every colleague.

When you go to your office tomorrow, the first order of the day should be to move that bowl of candy, pretzels, or sugary snacks from your desk into a trashcan. If you have a cookie jar filled with cookies, it should follow the same path. Instead, fill a jar with in-shell nuts of your choice. This will be something to hold you over until your next "real" meal. Before you contemplate eating even one nut on a full or semi-full stomach, **check your hunger levels**, as will be discussed next.

IT'S TIME TO EAT, BUT IS IT REALLY?

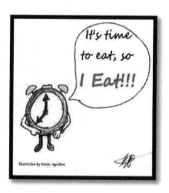

I believe that the majority of us are guilty of this flawed thinking. You check your clock, and it says noon, which means that it's time for lunch. But is it really? Not really! There are no rules stating that you have to eat at a particular time. It's just what we are programmed and conditioned to do. It's imperative to check your **hunger levels**. You get hungry for a reason. This indicator has been forged into our bodies for millennia. Cavemen did not have clocks to tell them they were hungry. They ate when their hunger indicated that it was time to eat. With all the progress in the world, as far as food consumption is concerned, it is essential that we revert to a caveman mentality, and here's how:

25-180

Cavemen did it right. How can we, seemingly an advanced civilization, behave like cavemen? We begin by listening to our bodies.

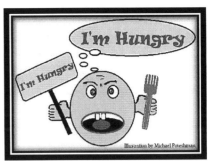

Because no one ever showed me or explained what hunger levels were, I was following my learned habits of eating incorrectly for decades. As I delved into getting myself out of the "Living Dead" nightmare, I realized that simplicity is what it takes to overcome such habits.

Different nutritionists and researchers define hunger in 10 or more levels, steps, and sub-steps.[1264] [1265] [1266] [1267] I distilled this process into three simple levels:

1. **Slightly hungry**: You pay a visit to your kitchen, and see that you have food left over from prior meals, but you really don't feel like eating it. Instead, just to pass the time, you decide to munch on chips and other "almost food" items that have no nutritional value. I know this pattern well, because I did this over and over again in the past. All I had to show for it was a big gut, ridiculously high blood pressure, and a slew of medications. Thus you should not eat at this level. **Not even a snack!**

2. **Moderately hungry:** You pay a visit to your kitchen again, and leftovers look a bit more enticing, but you just want something different. What does that mean to you? It means that you should not eat, as your system may not have fully processed foods from the previous meal. So, if you eat when you're moderately hungry you are not fully engaging your metabolism. **No snacks** at that stage either.

3. **Hungry**: You open your refrigerator door with determination, and everything, including your two-day old casserole, looks tempting. The food looks so good that you want to eat everything as soon as possible.[1268] What your body is telling you is that it's time to refuel. It's also telling you that your metabolism is engaged, and the food from the previous meal has been processed. This is a perfect time to eat, not because the clock strikes noon, but because you're hungry. At this level you can actually control the amount of food you will be consuming without overeating.

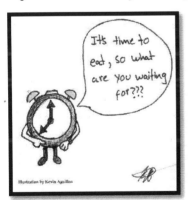

Although hunger occurs on average about two to three times per day, it varies in different people. Some get hungry twice a day, while others only once. Play it by ear, as you are unique! Remember, you are engaging your metabolism at this level. Eating when hungry constitutes yet another piece of the puzzle of "Living Wonderfully."

Please keep in mind that the only time to **have a small snack** is when you know that you will not be eating a full meal for a while, and you're already at the third level - **Hungry**. If this is the situation that you found yourself in, you should eat a small handful of nuts or a snack that does not cause your Insulin to spike. This is done for the sole purpose to hold yourself over until the next "real" nutrient dense meal.

Even if you're eating good quality foods that are high in nutrition when you're not hungry, you begin to accumulate pounds. It happens because your metabolism is not engaging properly.

Embrace your hunger, as it's there for a reason. It will keep you balanced. Eat when your body tells you to eat by checking your hunger levels, but never wait until extreme hunger kicks in; have a snack or a full meal.

The preceding hunger levels only hold true unless you are intentionally fasting, thus, these rules will only partially apply. For example, if you're fasting through breakfast, there is absolutely no snacking before lunch; only water is allowed. The same scenario applies if you're fasting through both, breakfast and lunch.

"Eating to Live" will not only make you feel like a champ, but play a huge role in every aspect of "Living Wonderfully."

SECTION 5. DETOX – WHY AND HOW?

Chapter 26 FORMAL INTRODUCTIONS BEFORE DETOX

Let me introduce you to "You", specifically to your body; the ancient, most elaborate, most complex and intricate piece of machinery that hasn't changed from the inception of humanity!

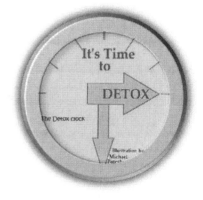

Some scientists believe that humans evolved to their present form approximately 2,000,000 years ago.[1269] Some researchers believe that we evolved 6,000,000 years ago.[1270] According to various religions, our bodies have been operating in the same manner between 2,000 to 5,000 years. The consensus in the scientific and religious communities are quite uncomplicated; the human body structure as well as its inner workings are not just ancient, but prehistoric, and remains <u>unchanged</u>. Since our bodies haven't changed in millennia, and we are digesting and metabolizing food in the same "ancient" way, what has really changed? **Everything has changed,** with the exception of our inner-workings!

Less than 150 years ago we breathed air without air pollutants such as car exhaust, industrial fumes, plastics vapor, and recycled air. There were no refrigerators, with the exception of crude ice boxes. Therefore, food had to be eaten fresh because there were **no chemical food preservatives, artificial flavors, or flavor enhancers.**

Although our bodies and their functions have remained the same for millions of years, the food and the environment have changed drastically in a little over a century.

Please meet your liver; the biggest organ inside your body and the most important detoxifier.[1271] Besides filtering blood, the liver performs many vital tasks such as regulating blood clotting, regulating different chemical levels in blood, storing Vitamins and iron, and other important functions.[1272] This organ gets the brunt of the aforementioned pollutants, and tries to deal with them the best way it can.

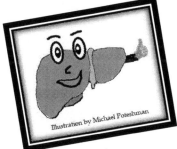

Illustration by Michael Poteshman

From the inception of the human race until now, your liver has not been exposed to the chemicals, liver-toxic medications, and "almost foods" discussed in earlier chapters. So, how do we expect this organ to deal with the current chemical assault?

It really tries its best, to do its job in order to protect our bodies from the toxic elements in food, water, and indoor and outdoor pollution. Unfortunately, as we consume by swallowing, inhaling, or absorbing immense amounts of toxic substances through the skin, the capacity of the liver diminishes.

Because the liver cannot metabolize all or even the majority of foreign toxins that it receives, it stores them.[1273]

I was truly astonished when I learned about the enormous number of chemicals stored inside our liver. The data from the National Health and Nutrition Examination (NHANES) survey revealed that out of 200 pollutants such as lead, organochlorine pesticides, and mercury, among many that were studied, *"...111 chemical pollutants which were commonly found in at least 60% of NHANES subjects"* (Doheny, 2009). [1274] Can stored "garbage" in the liver have anything to do with the shocking statistic below?

According to the study "Environmental Toxins & Liver Disease: A Link", Matthew Cave, MD, assistant professor of medicine at the University of Louisville explains, *"'More than **one in three** U.S. adults has liver disease...'"* (Doheny, 2009).[1275] This unfortunate statistic tells us that some of us may have liver damage without even knowing it.

Even if the damage has not been diagnosed, the overloaded liver that isn't functioning to its full capacity presents a slew of problems. Think of the liver as a filter that you would use in your air conditioner unit at home. As the filter clogs up, and you fail to change or clean it, free flow of air becomes restricted. Eventually, the air ducts will clog with dust, and ultimately burn out your air conditioning unit. As you continue to accumulate toxins, the overloaded liver will wreak havoc on your immune system. As with your A/C filter at home, instead of changing it every month, your liver releases bile that carries toxins or other undesirable waste products for elimination through the rectum.[1276] "Bile is a liquid released by the liver. It contains cholesterol, bile salts, and waste products such as bilirubin" (NIH, 2013).[1277] Since it can only work within limited capacity or is fully obstructed, different types of illnesses and even chronic diseases begin to rear their ugly heads. For example, if you have an obstruction of bile ducts you may even have jaundice, which causes yellowing of the skin.[1278]

Without additional explanation of liver functions or liver diseases, it's abundantly clear that the environment that we live in possesses a high degree of risk to our health. Although we can, for the most part, avoid foods, alcoholic beverages, and even medications (acetaminophen among others) that are treated with different types of chemicals, it's quite difficult to avoid the surrounding environment. Furthermore, seemingly benign items that we're accustomed to using daily may be contributing to liver intoxication.

THE INTOXICATING ROUTINE

Most of us begin intoxicating our bodies automatically -- from the time we get up to the time we go to sleep. Sometimes we don't even know that we're doing such a huge disservice to our entire system. Let's look at a couple of examples of automatic intoxication:

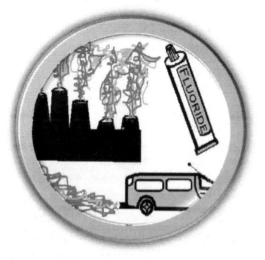

You wake up in the morning and the first thing you do is you stick a toothbrush with toothpaste in your mouth. You probably think that I'm crazy because everyone does it several times per day. The fact is that your ordinary toothpaste is loaded with different types of chemicals including **fluoride**. These chemicals either get absorbed into your system through your mouth, or you inadvertently swallow them. Here's what happens:

When fluoride enters your stomach, it mixes with the hydrochloric acid that your stomach produces.[1279] As a result, fluoride changes to hydrofluoric acid or **hydrogen fluoride**.[1280] Hydrofluoric acid has a tendency to penetrate stomach tissue and cause inflammation, irritation, and corrosion.[1281] *"Hydrogen fluoride goes easily and quickly through the skin and into the tissues in the body. There it damages the cells and causes them to not work properly."* (CDC, 2013).[1282] Consider some more examples:

"...according to a 500-page scientific review, fluoride is an endocrine disruptor that can affect your bones, brain, thyroid gland, pineal gland and even your blood sugar levels"
(Mercola, 2013)[1283]

An article in the Harvard School of Public Health publication entitled "Impact of fluoride on neurological development in children" truly shocked me. In a study entitled *"Developmental Fluoride Neurotoxicity: A Systematic Review and Meta-Analysis"*, researchers from Harvard School of Public Health along with China Medical University have combined 27 studies on fluoride.[1284][1285] After analyzing 8,000 school age children, it was concluded that ingestion of fluoride may impact cognitive development of children in a negative way.[1286] What this suggests is that **IQ in children who were exposed to fluoride was lower than those who weren't exposed**.

"The average loss in IQ was reported as a standardized weighted mean difference of 0.45, which would be approximately equivalent to seven IQ points for commonly used IQ scores.[1287][1288] **Some studies suggested that even slightly increased fluoride exposure could be toxic to the brain"** (Dwyer, 2012).[1289]

Although fluoride can affect many organs in your body, one organ is worth mentioning specifically. Besides brain as we discussed above, studies show that fluoride is also toxic to the **Thyroid gland,** as it worsens hypothyroidism or lowers production of thyroid hormones.[1290] It does this by binding to iodine and by obstructing the thyroid hormones. [1291]

We always hear that fluoride forms a protective layer on tooth enamel that prevents cavities. Indeed it does, but the layer is so thin that scientists are questioning if this protective layer can really act as a defense against cavities.[1292]

All hype aside, the layer of fluoride is only 6 nanometers thick. [1293] [1294] If you were to compare it to the thickness of human hair, it would take approximately 10,000 of these 6-nanometer layers to span the thickness of a single human hair. [1295] What that means is that as soon as you begin to chew, this thin layer quickly disintegrates.[1296] Since it does not do much to protect our teeth, what does it really do to our bodies?

If you're still using fluoride toothpaste, make sure that you don't swallow while you're brushing your teeth. Also make certain that you thoroughly rinse any residue that remains in your mouth after brushing. Ensure that you gargle with water to prevent any ingestion of fluoride, or just purchase a **non-fluorinated toothpaste**, which is what we used at home not so long ago. Currently we make our own toothpaste with all natural ingredients, and without chemicals, additives, or preservatives. You will find the easy toothpaste recipe in the LIVING WONDERFULLY RECIPES chapter at the end of the book.

Besides fluoride in toothpaste, processed foods, and fluorinated water,[1297] your intoxicating daily routine continues with other toxic chemicals that seem benign. But there is nothing benign about them:

- You step into the shower and begin to use shampoo and soap, among other chemical bathing products. They are absorbed through the skin while you are lathering up. There are, however, soap products available that are completely natural. We also began making our own soap and shampoo at home with food grade ingredients.
- Both men and women shave. We lather up our body parts with shaving cream. The chemicals in different shaving creams get absorbed through the skin into our system. Consider using shaving and after shave creams that are 100% natural.
- You get into your car to go to work or to go shopping. You inadvertently breathe exhaust fumes from your car's exhaust system, as well as from passing cars that are coming in and out of the parking lot where you park.
- You get to work and immediately begin to breathe recycled air which contains a slew of airborne pollutants. According to the Department of Health, here are some examples of the pollutants we ingest through breathing while in the office:
  - "…cleaning or deodorizing products
  - mold growth from damp or wet porous areas such as carpeting, ceiling panels, and sheetrock or from poorly maintained HVAC (heating, ventilating and air conditioning) systems
  - chemical leakage from the coolant in water coolers or fuel oil containers
  - contamination from nearby renovation or construction within the work area or office setting
  - vapors and gases such as ozone or VOCs (volatile organic compounds)
  - particulates such as airborne fiberglass, carpet and partition fibers
  - combustion pollutants such as carbon monoxide and nitrogen dioxide

- Chemicals found in some office or personal care products are also potential indoor air pollutants"

(Vermont Department of Health, 2013).[1298]

You can't even escape the air pollutants in your own home or when you go to your local gym. As most gyms and homes have carpeted floors, the vapor from synthetic carpet fibers and adhesives, especially when they're new, cause indoor chemical pollution.[1299]

So, how do we get rid of these horrible substances that made their way into our bodies? First, we go to see a doctor to make certain that there is nothing serious, and then we detoxify!

WITH JUST A LITTLE HELP FROM US

Over the years I've seen many elaborate television commercials claiming that a particular "body cleanser" will detoxify your system. The problem is that I have absolutely no idea what is in those pills or liquids, who manufactures them, what ingredients are not included on the label, and what is actually included. The reason behind this distrust is that the **majority of these so-called remedies are not government regulated**.

Before I came to this realization, I tried different types of "snake oil" detox solutions in response to ads on television or the radio. I was younger, my system was able to metabolize the majority of the "snake oil detox solutions", but in reality, I spent my money without noticeable results.

"Living Wonderfully" doesn't just involve eating proper foods, detoxifying with "real" food ingredients, exercising, and mind cleansing. It also involves internal cleansing, which it is a big part of this entire puzzle.

As you've read earlier, I'm a big proponent of letting our bodies do most of the work. Your body knows what to do, and it really wants to get itself back on the right track. You just need to create a favorable atmosphere. Although pharmaceuticals may be necessary in some situations, it is important that the body use its own faculties to detoxify, with only a little help from us:

Chapter 27 SAUNA – WHAT'S THE BIG DEAL?

You've heard the phrase, "Today is so hot and sticky; it feels like a sauna." In the summer months, most of us routinely seek shelter from the hot and sticky atmosphere. We accomplish this by rushing into an air-conditioned environment, whether in your home, office, or car. Why would someone intentionally sit in a hot room for more than 15 minutes just to sweat and feel uncomfortable? It is done for a very important health related reason, which we only recently began to understand. Here's a little history for those of you who are not very familiar with the sauna concept or have never experienced it.

A sauna is an insulated room inside a building - an independent free-standing structure. Cedar wood is traditionally used for construction due to its natural aromatic and long lasting qualities. Cedar is also resistant to rot, fungus, and bacteria. It's nearly free of resins that other woods possess.

There are two types of saunas: traditional and infrared. The traditional sauna uses electric, gas, or a wood heater/stove to heat up rocks located on top of the unit. These rocks keep the sauna warm. Depending on the stove and user preference, the temperature of the traditional sauna ranges between 160°F and 220°F (71°C and 104°C).

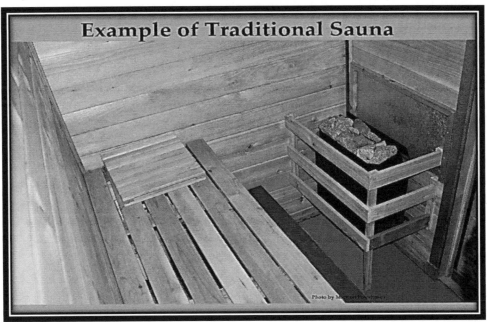

The infrared sauna uses several infrared electric heaters that are hung on the wall. Thus, instead of heating up the room from a single source as in the traditional sauna, infrared heaters radiate heat directly upon the user. The temperature of the infrared sauna ranges between 120°F and 140°F (43°C and 60°C); depending on user preference. Some units may generate even higher heat.

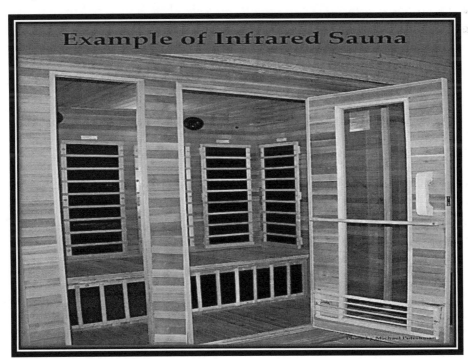

Traditional and the infrared saunas have similar applications. But because of the heat distribution and lower temperature, the infrared sauna can be enjoyed for longer periods of time. Instead of 15-20 minutes, the infrared sauna may be utilized for 30 minutes or longer with similar results. It all depends on your comfort level. You sweat just as much in the infrared unit as in the traditional sauna. The infrared sauna is tolerated better than the traditional sauna by patients with serious medical conditions such as congestive heart failure; more on that later.

It is estimated that the sauna was invented by Finns over 1,000 years ago, give or take 200 years. The sauna is not a novel concept and is enjoyed all over the world. Initially it was used for relaxing and unwinding, bathing, healing the sick, relaxing muscles after a long day of work, and even for giving births.

Okay, enough history. It's time to unravel the sauna's enormous benefits from a modern perspective. There is no shortage of books, studies, or documentation about the benefits of a sauna, with broad consensus. I will dispose of minutiae, and share some of the most important benefits of this particular form of detoxification:

TOXINS - BE GONE!

"Saunas do more than just help you relax; they help clear toxins out of your body. It's done not only through the predictable means—the sweat—but because the forced constriction and dilation of blood vessels that happens when you go into and out of the heat releases the chemical nitric oxide."
(Oz & Roizen, 2007)[1300]

According to the book "Never Be Sick Again" by Raymond Francis, M.SC and Kester Cotton (2002),[1301] the sauna detoxification process consists of melting fat and oils located beneath the skin, which transport the dissolved toxins to the surface of the skin through sweat.

"Heat from the sauna increases skin temperature, causing those fats and oils to 'melt' and ooze out of the skin's oil glands."
(Francis & Cotton, 2002) [1302]

The more your skin is exposed to heat, the more water and oil soluble chemicals will be released.

On my **LIVING WONDERFULLY** journey, I began to use sauna consistently after workouts, approximately three times per week, for 15 to 20 minutes per session. The first couple of times after I used the sauna, I experienced an uncomfortable tingling sensation on my skin. As soon as I took a shower and washed off the sweat with soap and water, the tingling stopped. I thought to myself, "Could this be the chemicals that were coming to the surface of my skin through the pores?" Indeed they were!

"As sweat and oil are secreted, the toxins dissolved in them are secreted as well. By excreting these toxins and then washing them off your body, your toxic load is lowered and cellular health improves"
(Francis & Cotton, 2002).[1303]

Incidentally, I only experienced tingling sensation during the first two sauna sessions, then it completely ceased.

It is imperative that after you finish using sauna, you immediately take a shower with soap and water to wash off the excreted chemicals and salts from the surface of your skin. Otherwise, the chemicals will get partially reabsorbed into your skin, which would defeat the purpose of this entire exercise.

Keep a couple of things in mind.

1. Make certain that you are thoroughly hydrated by taking a **stainless steel or glass bottle of water into the sauna** with you. Unfortunately, polycarbonate drinking bottles can release BPA's or bisphenol A or Phthalates that are used to make PVC plastics. The ugly truth is that these chemicals can have neurotoxic estrogenic effects[1304] (toxic to the nerve tissue or nerves,) among other problems. The release of these toxins is further amplified when heated, [1305] or in the hot environment, such as sauna. Even BPA free plastics are in question. Here's an exerpt from a study:

"Almost all commercially available plastic products we sampled—independent of the type of resin, product, or retail source—leached chemicals having reliably detectable EA (estrogenic activity,) ***including those advertised as BPA free.***"
(Yang, Yaniger, Jordan, Klein, & Bittner, 2011)[1306]

2. Wear a sauna hat in order to protect your brain from overheating. There is approximately 1" or 2.5 cm. of bone separating your brain from the heat of the sauna.

   It is very easy to overheat the brain, and the resulting heat stroke would put an unnecessary burden on your body. Below is the picture of my younger son wearing a traditional sauna hat. Sometimes these hats look a bit ridiculous, but the hat with the superman logo just adds to the fun of using sauna.

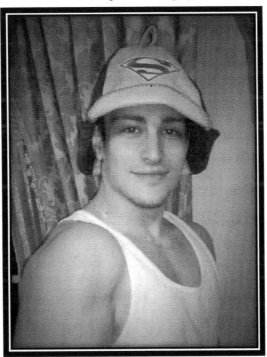

If you feel remotely dizzy or somewhat uncomfortable, exit the sauna immediately. Before using a sauna, check with your doctor to assess if you're physically fit for such an activity. Have your doctor recommend the maximum duration that you're allowed to remain in the sauna, as well as your tolerance level to heat.

Perhaps you're still wondering why you need to go through all this trouble of purchasing an ugly sauna hat, sitting in an uncomfortable hot room, and wasting 30 minutes of your life. I promise that by the time you finish this chapter you will be convinced.

HEALTHIER SKIN

The next phenomenon that took place as a result of using sauna is that my skin began to look healthier. I really thought that sauna would dehydrate my skin because of the dry heat, but the complete opposite occurred. Once again, my research confirmed this observation.

In his book, "Ageless: Living Younger Longer", Ben H. Douglas, Ph.D., explains that when you sweat, the infusion of liquid to the skin immerses skin cells in nutrients, and enhances the removal of metabolic waste products. [1307]

"As blood flows through the capillaries, fluid containing vitamins, minerals, and nutrients filters out and flows to the sweat glands, bathing all the structures in the skin."
(Douglas, 1990)[1308]

Furthermore, a study showed that "constant exposure" to FAR Infrared sauna or specialty devices that emit FIR radiation <u>increase collagen content of the skin</u>.[1309]

Therefore, when you sweat during your regular sauna sessions, you are practically **cleaning your pores from the inside out**, which may reduce acne. Recollect from the "SUGAR" chapter where collagen happens to be the main structural protein which makes the skin "plump and springy". [1310] I believe, we can safely regard **sugar as an Anti-Collagen destructive force, and Sauna as Pro-Collagen.** That does not mean that you should go and load up on sugar or simple carbs. The sad reality is that <u>sugar always wins</u>!

Without going into deep details, a study conducted at the Department of Dermatology at Friedrich Schiller University in Germany concluded that **regular use of the sauna causes protective effects on skin**.[1311]

Let's summarize. The increased blood circulation and sweating during sauna sessions increases the amount of nutrients that are transported to the skin, which promotes healthier and younger looking skin.

After using a sauna, your pores will be open, therefore an immediate shower will essentially exfoliate your skin without the need to take expensive trips to a beauty salon.

THE BEAUTY IS NOT ONLY SKIN DEEP – IT'S FROM THE INSIDE OUT

When I began my research into detoxification, I was only thinking of getting rid of chemicals that accumulated in my system over decades. What I wasn't thinking about, is something that occurred as an incredible side effect, confirmed by yet another study.

For approximately one month, as I was getting used to the sauna, I began to vary my routine. Thus, instead of sitting in a sauna for 15 to 20 minutes for one session, I would sweat for 12 to 15 minutes and then take a cold shower. When my heart rate fully normalized, I immediately got back in for another 12 to 15 minutes of heat. It was a fascinating phenomenon, as every time that I used sauna for an extended period I experienced a feeling of ease. It was almost like something heavy was lifting off my shoulders.

One day I came home after a workout and sauna routine and decided to measure my blood pressure, just to see if anything had changed. To my surprise, my blood pressure dropped by over 10 points, both systolic and diastolic. I realized that the feeling of ease was simply the reduction of constant throbbing in the back of my head caused by high blood pressure. Over the years, whenever that throbbing would increase, I instantly knew that my blood pressure was high. Those were the days when I would double up on my blood pressure medication, but no more!

One among many studies pertains directly to the phenomenon of blood pressure reduction. Published in the 2009 issue of the *Journal of Human Kinetics*, the study was named "The Effects of Finish Sauna on Hemodynamics of the Circulatory System in Men and Women."[1312] The word "Hemodynamics", means the study of blood flow or circulation. This research was administered by studying 74 men and 127 women with the average age of 22.[1313]

Here are the parameters of the study:
"Each sauna session consisted of three phases:
Phase one: direct overheating: air temperature in the sauna room – 115°C (239°F), humidity–35%, time spent in the sauna room – 12 minutes.
Phase two: cooling by submerging the whole body three times under water of 10°C (50°F),
Phase three: passive relaxation for 24 minutes"
(Prystupa, Wołyńska, Ślężyński, 2009). [1314]

Although the time I spent in the sauna was identical to the study, the temperature during my sessions was not as hot as 115°C or 239°F, as the sauna at my local gym maxed out at 85°C or 185°F. In addition, the cold shower that I took was warmer than the study's 10°C or 50°F. Despite the variances in temperature, my results echoed those of the study.

Scientists have concluded that when sauna is used consistently, the positive effects on blood flow, blood pressure, respiratory system, endocrine glands, and immunological system, were evident. [1315]

"It can be concluded that a bath in a Finnish sauna positively influences the hemodynamics of blood pressure and pulse. A series of sessions in the Finnish sauna leads to a considerable decrease of the systolic and diastolic pressure and an increase of pulse among male and female volunteers"
(Prystupa, Wołyńska, Ślężyński, 2009). [1316]

To clarify, I began to see positive results after varying my routine: 12 to 15 minutes in the sauna, and then an immediate cold shower. The study specifically addressed this phenomenon.

"The systolic blood pressure in the examined men decreased considerably from the statistical point of view under the influence of alternating hot and cold effects of the sauna sessions"
(Prystupa, Wołyńska, Ślężyński, 2009). [1317]

IMMUNE SYSTEM ON "STEROIDS"

As I continued to eat healthy and use sauna, I noticed something different. Throughout the first winter of my "Living Wonderfully" routine, <u>I did not get a cold or even a runny nose</u>. In comparison, throughout my "earlier" life, I got sick quite often. Some may say that my consumption of proper foods was the main factor in strengthening my immune system. I completely agree with that notion as you are definitely what you eat. Although change in food was crucial, there were other contributing factors emerging as I researched the benefits of sauna.

A six month study revealed that people who used sauna had roughly **half the incidences of common cold** as compared to the control group who did not use sauna.[1318]

The removal of toxins allows our immune system to operate more efficiently and deal with the remaining contaminants. Although I understood the connection, I didn't fully understand how and why I felt better and stopped having colds. Well, that's how:

> *"Give me the power to create a fever, and I shall cure any disease"* [1319] [1320]
> (Hippocrates, 460 BC – 370 BC)

The father of medicine, Hippocrates, was definitely onto something over 2,000 years ago.

As I continued my research, one area truly surprised me. When one uses the sauna for prolonged intervals, it simulates fever. That's right, you read it correctly; I did say "fever." This phenomenon is regarded as "Artificial Fever."[1321] When a person gets a severe cold or flu, for example, the body's natural defense is to raise its temperature in order to slow down the progress of infection, or in some cases stop the disease altogether. Artificial fever works in a similar way. By artificially elevating the body's temperature, your body is able to deflect some of the infectious bacterial organisms. **That means that consistent use of sauna has the power to stop cold or flu before they take root and become full blown**!

I was extremely excited when I read this research for the first time. Now you are also armed with this information, and you will soon be ready to beat your winter cold, but only after you complete this entire book. There is more to "Living Wonderfully" than meets the eye!

SAUNA AND WEIGHT LOSS

As seen in my before and after weight-loss photos, I can say with certainty that sauna, to some extent, is responsible for my 60+ pounds or 27 kilogram drop in weight. You may wonder, how sitting in a hot room and doing literally nothing would contribute to weight loss.

As I continued to read articles and studies, there were different claims to weight loss or calories burned.[1322] A name of one particular study was truly as unambiguous as its results:

> *"Sauna-Induced Body Mass Loss in Young Sedentary Women and Men"*
> (Podstawski, Boraczyński, Choszcz, Mańkowski, & Markowski, 2014)[1323]

Some articles and studies claimed that depending on your metabolic rate, using sauna may help you burn 300 calories in a single session. "A person weighing around 160 lbs. will burn about 300 calories during a 30-minute session in the sauna" (Stellner, 2011).[1324] Others did not specify the weight loss or calorie burned figures. The author for the Mayo Clinic, Brent A. Bauer, MD., inferred that *"The appeal of saunas in general is that they cause reactions, such as vigorous sweating and increased heart rate, similar to those elicited by moderate exercise"* (Bauer, 2011).[1325]

Whether the figures were precise or imprecise, there was one common and undeniable denominator:

Using sauna aids in burning calories through the increase in metabolic rate, hence it is responsible to some degree for weight loss.

There is another very pleasurable and satisfying side-effect…

FEELING HAPPY AND DON'T KNOW WHY?

I often hear comments from people at the gym: "I don't know why, but when I use the sauna, I feel really good and it puts me in a good mood." I jokingly reply, "You're probably happy to get out of this scorching hot room, and that's what makes you happy." All joking aside, sauna does have a calming effect, as most physicians agree.

"One of the most important benefits of a sauna that hasn't changed much over time is how it can help relax your mind and body … how it can provide an exhilarating feeling of well-being"
(Mercola, 2014).[1326]

As to why after using the sauna, people generally are in a good mood. The answer is quite simple:

Using the sauna simulates exercise. Thus, by increasing body temperature and escalating your heart rate, endorphins are released into your system.[1327]

Endorphins are neurotransmitters inside your brain that are responsible for feel-good sensations. [1328] "Endorphin: A hormonal compound that is made by the body in response to pain or extreme physical exertion. Endorphins are similar in structure and effect to opiate drugs" (MedicineNet.com, 2011).[1329]

Although using the sauna simulates exercise, I don't believe in substituting sauna for exercise. With a sauna you're not using your muscles to raise your heart rate. It's done purely through heat. Thus, your muscles will weaken over time. Physical exercise is essential, especially with the added benefit of sauna. Using the sauna is a huge contributing factor towards good mood and feeling happy.

You now have enough tangible evidence and knowledge to use sauna to detoxify, heal, or just plain feel good. Before we conclude this chapter, there is something that is equally as important: excuses and misconceptions about using sauna.

NO EXCUSES!

In talking to some of my friends, acquaintances, and family members, I've heard excuse after excuse why they would not use sauna for therapeutic purposes. The number one excuse: "It's way too hot, and I don't tolerate heat that well." Another excuse was, "My heart is too weak to sit in a hot room for prolonged periods of time." The excuse that really took the cake was, "I'm too old and sick for the sauna. In my condition I have to be in an air conditioned environment instead of putting so much stress on my body with extreme heat."

For all the doubters, skeptics, cynics, and excuse makers, I say, "Hogwash!"

I will provide undisputed evidence to debunk the arguments of all of the "Doubting Thomases." This debunking begins with study that I found in the files of the US National Library of Medicine, National Institutes of Health - Clinical Cardiology Review, titled, *"Beneficial effects of sauna bathing for heart failure patients."*[1330] Congestive Heart Failure or CHF is the condition where the heart does not adequately pump blood in order to fully satisfy the demand of the body.

As you can tell by the title of the study, arguments such as, "I'm too old" or "My heart is too weak", do not hold water. The following conclusion affirms that sauna is *"...well tolerated and improved hemodynamics has been shown in patients with chronic heart failure after a single exposure and after a four-week period of sauna bathing (five days per week)."* (Blum N., PhD. & Blum A., PhD., 2007).[1331]

As you can see, people with <u>severe</u> cases of Congestive Heart Falure (CHF) were not only able to tolerate the heat of the sauna "five days per week", but showed improvement in blood circulation. How wonderful is that? Can you imagine the possibilities of improving your health if you haven't suffered such health predicaments?

Keep in mind that this study was conducted with the use of far infrared sauna operating at 60°C or 140°F, [1332] which is not as hot as the traditional sauna. Thus, if you have low tolerance to heat or have a medical condition that prevents you from using the traditional sauna, the infrared unit may be the answer.

People often ask me where to purchase an Infrared Sauna. There are number of websites that you can find by entering the name "Far Infrared Sauna" in the search bar of your favorite search engine. At the time of this writing, one-person units were as low as $500 and went up from there. The sauna usually arrives disassembled for shipping purposes. Assembly is not that difficult as you don't need any special tools. The sauna that I have at my home came with a video which was extremely easy to follow. You don't need any special electrical connections, as usually the sauna just plugs into a standard electrical outlet. It is only when you get into multiple person units that you may have to worry about the additional electrical load.

LET'S SUM IT UP FROM THE PERSPECTIVE OF A TV DOCTOR

On the 2009 Oprah Winfrey show, "Extreme Life Extension",[1333] Dr. Mehmet Oz gave a perfect summary when it came to the overall benefits of using a sauna:

"...the high temperature helps lower blood pressure and increase blood circulation. It gets your heart to beat faster, and it burns calories. It raises your metabolism a little bit, and also when you sweat, you sweat out toxins through the skin"
(Oz, 2009). [1334]

Please keep one thing in mind: "Living Wonderfully" is not a "one trick pony" proposition. Although sauna helped me with detoxification, reduction of my blood pressure, among other wonderful things, it was coupled with another crucial form of detox...

Chapter 28 FOOD DETOX AND RESULTING WEIGHT LOSS

You are already familiar with detoxification that involved the use of a sauna. This chapter shows you not only one of the major reasons **why your body retains fat**, but how to rid your system of detrimental toxic substances through eating in order to release this fat.

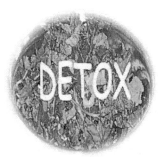

Because we don't live in a vacuum, from time to time toxins may slip in, but as you continue your daily food detox, your body will be better prepared to face adversity. You won't have to do anything difficult or time consuming in order to fight toxins. I promise you that it will be much easier than you ever thought possible. In fact you do not have to do anything different than what's outlined in the "**WHAT TO EAT**" chapter later in the book.

TOXINS AND WEIGHT RETENTION

A recurring question that I'm asked is, "Even though I'm in the gym four times per week and I'm on a low calorie diet, why do I still have these love handles and this gut that I can't get rid of?" Here's why:

"A person who has too many toxins to process will make new fat cells and store those toxins along with fat in them" (Richards, 2012). [1335]

Many toxins are lipophilic or attracted to fat.[1336] As a result, toxins are absorbed through the fat cells. [1337] [1338] **Your smart body protects itself by keeping those toxins out of the way of your major organs by storing them in your fat**. [1339] [1340]

If you're trying to lose accumulated fat, your body doesn't easily give this up, as toxins may get released into your system and pollute your major organs including your brain.

Your smart body continues to protect itself by holding on to this fat, and in many cases, **generates even more fat where these toxins can be confined**. [1341] [1342]

So, here is the story that I come across regularly. Even though you're going to the gym for an exhaustive workout, and use sauna to sweat some of these toxins off, for some reason, your body is resisting by holding on to fat. Consequently, you try to force the fat loss by doing more cardio, more weight lifting, and cutting calories. To your delight, eventually, some of this stubborn fat comes off. All true, but right after the gym you decide to eat processed foods that contain toxic substances that you read about in "**WHAT NOT TO EAT**" section. Bottom line, if you're consuming more toxins than you're eliminating by sweating them off in the gym or sauna, <u>your body will continue to resist weight loss, and more importantly, fat loss</u>.

Because your smart body requires protection against these poisons, <u>it protects itself by retaining or generating more fat so it can store those toxic substances</u>.

There is an additional problem with this scenario in the long term. Even though we want to believe that these chemicals and pollutants are confined within the fat cells, they can't stay there forever. As these poisons are festering inside your body, they are slowly released from the fat cells into the blood stream. [1343] The saddest part is these toxic substances are released into the blood stream at an accelerated rate <u>during weight loss</u>. [1344]

Your body, being an incredibly efficient machine, wants to rid itself of these poisons. All you have to do is help it by:

1. Not eating processed foods and drinking beverages that contain toxins, and
2. Eating foods that detoxify the body. Luckily, in "Living Wonderfully" land you're not only getting incredible Vitamins and minerals, but every time you eat, you effortlessly detoxify with food! Most of the detoxification you require is located in the "LW Base" which is coming up later in the section titled "THE BASE IS KEY."

Some of the most incredible detoxifiers already in your "Base" are cruciferous vegetables such as kale, collard greens, cabbage, broccoli, cauliflower, and rutabaga. Brussels sprouts also belong to the cruciferous family. Incidentally, there is a very simple and delicious roasted Brussels sprouts recipe provided in the recipe section at the end of the book. All these vegetables are jam-packed with Vitamins, minerals, and most importantly, natural dietary fiber which helps with elimination of waste products from your system.

As you will see in the vegetables shopping list later, it is imperative that your "LW BASE" contain cilantro, parsley, dill, and spinach. Here's why.

Cilantro detoxifies by binding to the heavy metals in your system such as mercury[1345] that you find in a lot of fish. Parsley, dill, and spinach, due to their high concentration of <u>chlorophyll</u> reduce inflammation[1346] and cleanse your blood, as well as liver.[1347] [1348] Just make certain that the vegetables as well as animal products are organic!

There are other potent detoxifiers such as chia seeds that are soaked in water, seaweed,[1349] and Aloe Vera[1350] that removes heavy metals and other toxins using its gelatinous delivery system. [1351] If you feel adventurous, as Aloe Vera is quite bitter, slice it in your "Base", as we will be discussing later. That's exactly what I do. Believe it or not, because of the variety of delicious ingredients in my meal, I can't even taste the bitterness of this super plant!

FOODS INSTEAD OF DRUGS

When I talk to people about my present health condition, they find it difficult to believe that I no longer suffer from frequent colds and allergies, anxiety, blood pressure, and acid reflux. How can this happen without any medication? Well, it's easy. My family and I use food instead of drugs.

The majority of the ingredients that promote healing and staying healthy are **already** a part of our "Base" or greenery mix, LW Smoothies, as well as toppings that you will read about in the next chapter. The following are the healing properties of seemingly simple foods; all you have to do is eat:

- Common cold – By eating fresh raw sauerkraut, kimchi, tempeh, miso, and other foods high in probiotics at every meal, will promote gut health, which strengthens the immune system.[1352] [1353]
- Anxiety or minor depression – Foods such as dark leafy green vegetables, cabbage, mackerel, sardines, beans, nuts, salmon, and olive oil, can help lower the risk of depression.[1354]
- High blood pressure – Foods such as collard greens, kale, broccoli, carrots, beet greens, tomatoes, spinach, squash, bananas, and other foods high in potassium, magnesium, and fiber may help control blood pressure.[1355] [1356] In addition, one study clearly showed that purple potatoes (not the ones that just have purple skin, but the potatoes that are purple all the way through) lowered systolic blood pressure.[1357]
- Acid reflux – Anti-inflammatory foods such as turmeric, aloe vera, green leafy vegetables, parsley, celery, broccoli, asparagus, wild-caught fish, and ginger, may help you fight acid reflux. [1358] While on the ginger subject, how about prevention and treatment of gastrointestinal cancer? *"Ginger has been found to be effective against various GI cancers such as gastric cancer, pancreatic cancer, liver cancer, colorectal cancer, and cholangiocarcinoma."* (Prasad & Tyagi, 2015). [1359]
- Heart disease – Blueberries, salmon, spinach, turmeric, mackerel, sardines, walnuts, chickpeas, kidney beans, bananas, and other foods high in magnesium and potassium, are your heart disease fighting allies. [1360] [1361] [1362] [1363] [1364]

The foods I described above help your body function the way it was intended to function in order to ward off disease or illness. For example, my decades of allergies were obliterated after only two months of eating foods that I just described. Even the unrelenting colds that I suffered from "have left the station!" I suppose that it is possible to catch a cold, but for now, I've been cold-free for over three years.

And now for the final form of cleansing and healing, perhaps the toughest one yet…

Chapter 29 YOUR STATE OF MIND OR ANOTHER FORM OF DETOX

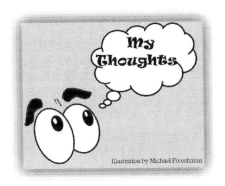

Illustration by Michael Poteshman

"Thoughts have power; thoughts are energy. And you can make your world or break it by your own thinking."
-Susan L. Taylor-

Approximately 70,000 thoughts go through the average person's mind in a day.[1365] Your brain is constantly working as thoughts keep streaming into your mind at a high rate of speed. After all, that's what the brain is for, isn't it?

Most of us concentrate on negative thoughts more than we do on positive ones. In most cases, negative thoughts are easier to reflect upon than the positive ones. These types of thoughts seem very real and come to fruition easily.

Positive thoughts are more difficult to imagine and bring to realization. As human beings, we tend to process negative information more thoroughly than positive,[1366] hence the habit of dwelling on negativity.

Let's look at how to control every thought that comes into the mind, and how to rid yourself of the unnecessary negative "mind babble."

"Dwelling on the negative simply contributes to its power."
- Shirley MacLaine -[1367]

What type of thoughts come into your mind? Are they positive or negative? Don't feel bad if the thoughts are mostly negative. This is absolutely normal. There is nothing wrong with you; you are not evil or crazy. Everyone maintains negativism as part of their thinking.

Make an effort to be aware of your thoughts from the time you get up to the time you go to sleep. To help me with this task, I put a small Post-it note on the mirror in my bathroom with the phrase "track your thoughts." In my office I taped a small piece of paper on my computer monitor. Using clear tape I placed the same phrase onto my watch band as an additional reminder.

Within three weeks into this exercise, I no longer needed prompts, and I'm now completely aware of my thoughts. As soon as a negative thought comes in, I process it by immediately redirecting negative into positive, solving it, or completely discarding it. **As you will be performing this exercise, you will realize that a lot of the negative thoughts are to be <u>discarded</u> because they're simply inconsequential.**

The way I usually correct my thinking is by mentally saying "Stop!" I used to say it out loud when I could, but within three days, the word "stop" became purely mental.

Don't get upset if you're only being partially successful at the beginning of this process. As you continue to practice, all of a sudden you will begin to form a habit of thinking wonderful thoughts.

PAY SPECIFIC ATTENTION TO UNRELENTING THOUGHTS – USE HUMOR

"If you realized how powerful your thoughts are, you would never think a negative thought."
- Peace Pilgrim -

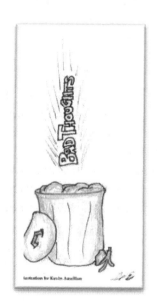

As you begin practicing being aware, you will very quickly find thoughts that just keep spinning in your head. Indeed, I had my share of those and they were polluting my existence. Once I got rid of unrelenting thoughts, my outlook on the future completely changed. Just imagine an insistent thought spinning in your head. Now imagine that same thought spinning and spiraling into a garbage can.

When I teach people how to stop unrelenting thoughts, I ask them to imagine a cartoon elephant wearing a little hat. Then I ask them to imagine that insistent thought lying on the ground, and the elephant stomping all over it and demolishing it.

Illustration by Kevin Aguillon

Sometimes I even imagine a bad thought crashing against a concrete wall with a thud. I try to make it comical, as it puts a smile on my face. You can come up with unique scenarios if you use imagination.

And now for the final and the most important remedy.

THE FIVE-MINUTE MIND CLEANSE

"A negative mind will never get you a positive life."
- Dale Partridge -

Some call it meditation, some call it achievement of inner peace, and I call it a simple five-minute mind detox to prime your positive thoughts. You don't need to sit for hours in a room, humming a single note or muttering something under your breath just to be able to let go of your thoughts. Although I don't see any harm in prolonged meditation, you will just spend a lot of time doing it.

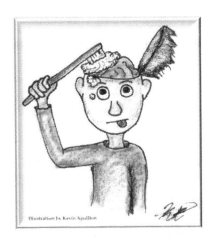

Earlier we discussed how to cleanse your body. The following simple technique is used to cleanse your mind. I use this method every other day after I finish my workout at the gym. Because of how little time it takes, some people practice it twice a day or even more. My former colleague uses this technique every time he goes to the bathroom. He justifies his venue by saying that no one bothers him while he's on the commode, and he couples "pleasant with necessary." It's completely up to you where and when you want to detox your mind, as long as you follow few simple parameters. Just make certain that if you perform this technique on the commode as in the example above, you limit your time, otherwise you may get hemorrhoids.

You can perform this technique at any time, especially after a difficult workday. I recommend using this technique after you've interacted with people or dealt with a circumstance that has unraveled your emotions. The good thing is that you don't need to purchase any special equipment, join a group, or spend any money to be successful. **The only thing required is that you're able to breathe**. Let's begin.

1. First, try to find a very quiet room with a door. I prefer a darker room. It does not have to be completely dark, just a room with little light. Remember, this only takes five minutes, so your family or roommates will understand that you need complete quiet for a brief five-minute duration. You can even follow my colleague's advice and use your bathroom; it's your choice.
2. Find a dining room chair, bar stool, or any chair that doesn't have soft cushions. Sit upright in the chair with your back straight. The reason for this type of chair and for sitting in the upright position is so you don't fall asleep when performing this exercise. Your mind must be relaxed but not drowsy.
3. You can close your eyes completely or leave them partially open. Begin to breathe through your nose. If you can't breathe through the nose, the mouth will suffice. There is no special way you have to breathe, whether fast or slow. Just breathe normally.
4. As you breathe, begin to listen and concentrate your attention only on your breathing. Remember, your entire universe for these five minutes revolves around listening to your breathing **only**. Nothing more. Breathe in, breathe out. Just listen and do nothing else.

5. As thoughts begin to come in, whether good or bad, tune them out by continuously listening to your breathing. At first it will seem like your "mind babble" intensifies. What your mind is really telling you is how it's being bombarded relentlessly with all kinds of thoughts and scenarios. This is the perfect time to tune these thoughts out and continue to concentrate on your breathing.

6. As you continue to breathe, you may find that you stray away from listening to your breathing by following one of the thoughts. As you recognize that you have strayed away, return your mind to concentrating on your breathing immediately.

Don't be discouraged if your mind wanders as it will. In the span of five minutes you may have to bring your mind back to listening to your breathing more than a few times.

Keep in mind that Rome wasn't built in one day. Your first couple of attempts will be a little more difficult because your mind and body are getting adjusted to this new experience. Never fear. With a bit of effort, tuning out thoughts will become a breeze and actually quite enjoyable. Keep bringing your mind back until all you hear and think about is your breathing, nothing else.

If in the middle of the workday you are faced with a stressful situation, don't wait until you finish work. Find a quiet room for five minutes, or step out to your car, excuse yourself and enjoy a mind cleanse.

So, what is the point of this entire exercise besides getting rid of bad thoughts, feelings, and emotions? I will speak from experience. Every time I perform this exercise, my mind feels incredibly clean and lucid, hence the name, "five-minute mind cleanse." This mind detox creates a feeling of cleanliness, contentment, and euphoria, which opens up your mind to better problem solving. The reason is that you've gotten rid of a barrage of unnecessary minutia without outside distractions or interference.

Once you learn to control your thoughts, your daily toils will become a lot easier to handle. Difficult people that you've dealt with in the past will seem to be not as difficult. Your complicated problems will not seem as complicated. Perhaps your new, improved, and contented mind found a way to deal with such difficulties. The most interesting thing is that you will begin to smile more often, and will begin to live "Wonderfully." I will conclude this chapter with the words from an ancient philosopher:

"Watch your thoughts; they become words. Watch your words; they become actions. Watch your actions; they become habit. Watch your habits; they become character. Watch your character; it becomes your destiny"
- Lao Tzu --

At the beginning and throughout the book I mentioned that I was completely off all medications for the illnesses that I suffered from in the past. Perhaps by now you can easily speculate how this was accomplished. Let's explore the **final piece of the puzzle to Living Wonderfully – Food!**

Chapter 30 LIVE FOOD VERSUS DEAD FOOD

I'm constantly asked how my wife and I are so effortlessly maintaining the weight that we lost three years ago. Besides everything that you've already read about "almost foods", gut health, exercise, Insulin, and detox of the mind and body, one significant item remains: FOOD! I'm shouting this word from the rooftop because in the past I had no clue how life could get turned around just by eating!

The concept of "**dead food**" raises a lot of eyebrows and causes controversy. I completely understand this sentiment, as my family and I have been indulged in dead food throughout our lifetimes. When I talk about this subject, some people get very upset because I impose on them a new concept that is often at odds with their traditions and customs. How can you argue with what your parents and grandparents taught you? I now can! So, here goes:

Live food = Raw food
Dead food= Processed and most cooked foods

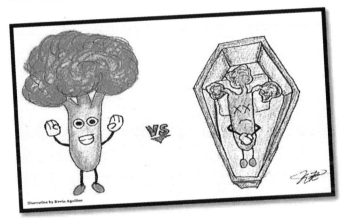

Immediately after I outline these definitions, I often hear: "Why do you call foods that are cooked, dead? This is ridiculous! I've been cooking food all my life, and nobody died or got sick from it!" I always ask for a little patience until I get a chance to explain. After I finish, the skeptics still remain somewhat upset, but the concept begins to sink in, and eventually I hear: "Michael, you were absolutely right!"

The truth is that there is no profound voodoo science in answering this question, as the answer is very simple.

When most vegetables are cooked, or even lightly steamed, depending on the temperature and cooking time, heat may kill most, if not <u>all</u> of the digestive enzymes and even Vitamins. Furthermore, some cooking methods may cause foods to form dangerous and even carcinogenic substances.[1368]

As you've read in the "GUT HEALTH" chapter earlier, digestive enzymes are extremely important for digesting foods and nourishing your "gut flora."

"The idea is that heating food destroys its nutrients and natural enzymes, which is bad because enzymes boost digestion and fight chronic disease. In short: **When you cook it, you kill it***"*
(WebMD, 2013).[1369]

Let's take a step back. By no means am I advocating only eating raw food! There are definitely some positives when it comes to several forms of cooked foods. Although vegetables lose enzymes when heated, some have their nutritional value amplified through heat application.

For example, beets, broccoli, onion, and red bell pepper among others, should be consumed raw because they lose too much nutritional content when cooked. [1370] [1371] On the other hand, when cooked, carrots release more beta-carotene,[1372] tomatoes release more lycopene; you absorb more magnesium, calcium, and iron when eating cooked spinach; cooking mushrooms releases potassium; steamed asparagus has substances to help fight cancer. [1373] [1374] That does not mean that you should be eating these vegetables in only cooked form. They need to be consumed in both raw and cooked state as will be explained in the "60/40 RULE" section later in this chapter.

For now we must delve into the mechanics of the body in order to understand why it reacts the way it does to live versus dead foods. Only then you will appreciate the significance of the fine balance, which is the key to "Eating Wonderfully." It is this balance that will deliver benefits for the rest of your life that you never thought possible!

YOUR BODY, YOUR PROTECTOR, YOUR INDICATOR

"Whenever a germ or infection enters the body, the white blood cells snap to attention and race toward the scene of the crime"
– World Health Organization – [1375]

This concept is incredibly important for the reader to understand because "Eating Wonderfully" centers on the balance between live and selectively cooked foods.

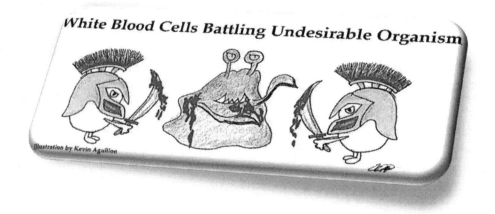

The white blood cells in your body essentially act as an army of soldiers. As soon as they sense anything dangerous, they deploy numerous weapons to protect your entire system. Their strategy may vary, as they may surround the undesirable organisms and just devour them, or release special enzymes that kill the "unwelcome" germ.[1376] What does white cell deployment have to do with food? **Everything!!!**

What I'm about to tell you may seem foreign or even preposterous, but research says otherwise. When you eat only cooked foods, your body generates a condition known as "digestive leukocytosis" or above normal count of white cells in the blood. [1377] [1378] [1379]

What that means is your body reacts in the same manner towards cooked foods as it would react towards infection or a toxin that it has to protect itself against. [1380]

That's one of the reasons for the deployment of these "white blood cell soldiers." "Leukocytosis is significant because it is often just one indicator of an inflammatory response" (Mihalik, 2012).[1381] There are other reasons for white cell deployment such as parasitic infections, bacterial infections, tumors, and emotional stress,[1382] but these may not be directly related to digestion.

So, how can we nourish our bodies without deploying our "soldiers?" For that we have a "51/49% MODEL".

THE 51/49 MODEL[1383]

In the First International Congress of Microbiology that took place in Paris in 1930, a doctor from Switzerland, Paul Kouchakoff, M.D., demonstrated that when a person's food intake consists of more cooked food than raw, the body reacts defensively, almost as if it were invaded by foreign organisms.[1384] [1385] On the flip side, when a person consumes more natural raw food, the "leukocytosis" or white cell release is **not** triggered.[1386] [1387] According to Dr. Kouchakoff's research, the raw food "neutralized" the effects of cooked or heated foods. [1388] His study also affirmed that manufactured/processed foods increased the white blood cell count.[1389] This research was confirmed in the present day by the study conducted at the Logan Chiropractic College where the participants were given processed chili, crackers, cheese, and water in order to emulate the modern Western diet.[1390] The study showed that Dr. Kouchakoff's research remains relevant today.

When you eat a meal that consists exclusively of cooked food, your immune system becomes burdened, and in some cases, overstrained with constant release of white blood cells. If your diet consists of more organic raw food, your immune system will not be weighed down with unnecessary work.[1391] Instead it will stand guard with vigor to fight "real" diseases and toxins that may enter its domain as opposed to responding to the "false alarm"[1392] of cooked and processed food.

As I studied this seemingly simple concept, I began to understand that my former sniffles, allergies, aches and pains were associated with my overburdened immune system. Thus, my family and I began to experiment with eating more raw foods with every meal. The most interesting phenomenon occurred when we began to increase the amount of live food from 51% to 60%.

As my family and I embraced the 51% raw food concept with open arms, we learned very quickly that additional raw foods yielded greater results.

When I began to substitute part of the meal with raw foods or "greenery", as my wife and I now call it, my body began to change. The change became so radical that my thought process began to evolve and life began to take on a new meaning. Suddenly there was light at the end of the tunnel where I precipitously looked out the window and smiled at the brightness of the day, something that I hadn't done in a long time. The fog had lifted, and suddenly my thoughts became razor sharp, just like 20 years ago.

As I added more "greenery" to my meals, my body began to respond with accelerated weight loss and a mind-blowing increase in energy and vigor that was reminiscent of an 18-year-old.

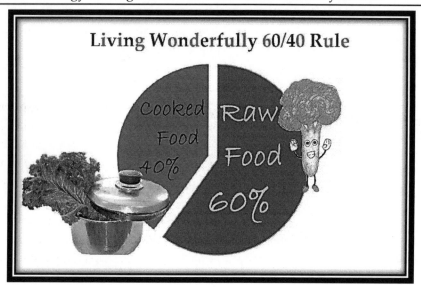

In addition, when I switched to 60% "greenery", I not only stopped being drowsy in the afternoon, but became invigorated and full of life after lunch.

So, why not 70% or 80% of raw food vs. cooked? It was simply a matter of taste, although more "greenery" may have been even more beneficial. Let's be honest, if food doesn't taste great, we won't eat it or eat it for a short time and then revert back to the old way. **The ability to sustain this new way of eating for a <u>lifetime</u> is of vital importance!** Therefore, the new rule of a minimum of 60% live food had to be the new norm or the new 60/40 rule. What's even more important is what we eat that makes our way of life incredibly exciting, and I dare to say, even unprecedented, as you will read in the next few sections.

On those rare occasions when I eat at a restaurant, no matter what the portion size is, I feel unsatisfied. The reason behind this dissatisfaction is that nutritional value is lacking in the majority of the foods you get when you eat out. Your body responds accordingly by being sluggish, sleepy, tired, dissatisfied, and craves more "bad" stuff. On the other hand, when I finish my meal at home, I feel absolutely satisfied, full of energy, and ready to conquer anything that life throws at me!

TRIALS

Through trial and error I experimented with having a small steak or a piece of fish with a salad on the side. Also, I could no longer use store bought dressings, as the vast majority are loaded with chemicals, preservatives, and flavor enhancers. I had to come up with different ways of making certain that over 60% of my meal consisted of raw food and at the same time had a worthwhile taste. So I tried extra virgin olive oil and vinegar, and that was somewhat OK, but only for a little while. Even lemon juice, balsamic vinegar, and Italian seasonings became boring and unpalatable after a while. But because I saw huge improvements in my health, I had no choice but to continue to experiment until something would actually work, and it certainly did.

THE BASE IS KEY!
LW BASE = LIVING WONDERFULLY RAW VEGETABLE BASE

"Tell me what you eat and I shall tell you what you are"
- Anthelme Brillat-Savarin, 1826 –

Because I recognized the taste and the monotony of the same old stuff to be a problem that could possibly derail my efforts towards improving my health, I devised a very clear way of eating without being tired of boring and redundant foods. The current way of eating is no longer boring or repetitious, but quite exciting. My family and I look forward to our incredible and satisfying nutritious meals.

There are two components to every meal: live food and chemical free cooked food. In other words, we have 60% of our "Living Wonderfully" raw vegetable base or "LW-Base", and 40% of our awesome cooked foods. You will find the list of vegetables in the "LW-Base" along with their nutritional attributes in the "Shopping List" section at the end of this chapter. Here's the way it works:

Once or twice per week we go "greenery" shopping. When we come home, we wash and cut our vegetables in a big, and I mean BIG container as you can see in the picture below.

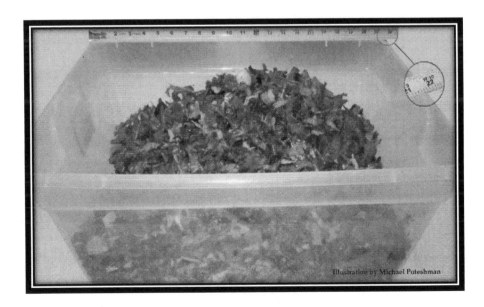

Illustration by Michael Poteshman

Make certain that the container is "food grade", as non-food grade plastics can release BPA's or bisphenol A or Phthalates that are used to make PVC plastics. Studies have shown that there are risks to using products with BPA, which include the disruption of hormone levels, effects on the brain and behavior, cancer, among other problems.[1393]

To speed things up, we use a food processor for hard vegetables such as carrots, celery, and radishes. Leafy vegetables such as kale, collard greens, and herbs such as parsley, cilantro, etc., are cut with a knife. Please don't be alarmed as the entire process from washing to a fully cut "Base" takes less than half an hour.

Once again, this happens <u>only once or twice per week</u>. Even if you're exceedingly busy, it actually takes less time to "Eat-Wonderfully" than to drive to a restaurant and order food. The big difference is that "Eating Wonderfully" food is nourishing you on a cellular level. **With every incredible bite you're absorbing nutrients that are lacking in practically every dish that is served at the majority of restaurants.**

Now that you have your base, let's begin with the meal.

THE MAGIC OF EATING WONDERFULLY

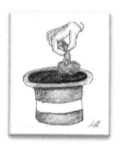

Place the pre-cut 60% portion of your vegetable base into your personal size mixing bowl...and here's where the magic of "Eating-Wonderfully" begins. It is imperative that this portion of vegetables also includes a nice helping of foods that contain probiotics such as sauerkraut, or kimchee, pickles without vinegar, tempeh or miso. We count that as part of 60%, as these garnishes contain live bacteria in order to promote "gut health." Thus, you may end up with a bit more than 60% of raw foods including your rich source of probiotics. Keep experimenting with your favorite probiotic foods and find those that you like the most.

My wife, prefers kimchee and sauerkraut mixed. Don't forget to slice some onion, avocado, and fresh tomato not only for taste, but for the Vitamin, <u>healthy fat</u>, and mineral value.

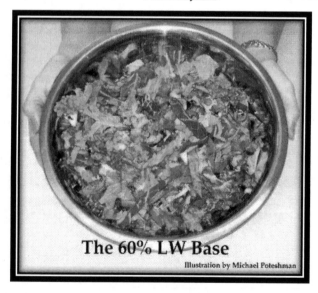

The 60% LW Base

Illustration by Michael Poteshman

Taste is King!

Start piling your favorite unprocessed cooked foods onto your bowl of "greenery", not to exceed 40%. For example, we use hummus, beans (can be baked or boiled, but without sugar,) baked ratatouille, boiled egg, couple of slices of roasted or baked chicken, or beef, turkey, or fish; a tablespoon of cooked quinoa, cooked buckwheat, and/or a small amount of stew. Also **add couple of teaspoons of non-processed organic coconut oil and/or extra virgin olive oil in order to maintain satiety**.

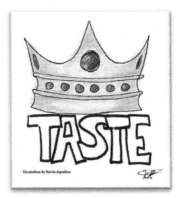

Prepare your favorite beef or chicken stew that does <u>not</u> contain any store bought spice mixes. Instead of the usual ingredients, use vegetables that release beneficial substances when cooked. And yes, there will be a recipe for stew and everything else that I described above in the "Recipes" section at the end of the book. Below is an example of a meal, as food combinations are endless.

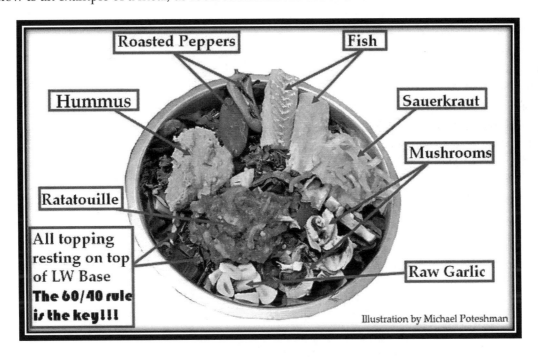

Illustration by Michael Poteshman

The most delightful thing about "Eating-Wonderfully" is that you can adjust the taste to your liking with every meal. Even though the raw "Base" remains the same, with slight variations that you may decide to implement, your cooked portion should constantly change. For example, from time to time we cook chicken with vegetables and Indian spices. Sometimes we prepare awesome Italian or tomato-ginger meatballs with quinoa. That goes on top of the raw "Base" along with the sauce. We use quinoa in meatballs instead of breadcrumbs. Believe it or not, it actually tastes better. As long as all of your cooked toppings do not exceed 40% of the entire meal, you're in business!

Most of the foods described above will keep you full longer without packing on empty calories;[1394] hence, you begin experiencing unexpected weight loss that "comes at you out of the blue!" When my wife and I first began eating this way, we couldn't believe that we could actually lose weight by eating these huge portions, but it's a reality!

Don't think that this way of eating is only confined to "LW-base" with toppings. In Chapter 33 we will be discussing ways to eat cooked foods without abolishing the 60/40 rule or sacrificing your new found "Living Wonderfully" lifestyle.

Chapter 31 TIME TO EAT

Now it's time to eat! We will first talk about lunch and dinner, and then breakfast immediately thereafter.

I eat my lunch at around noon and my dinner at 5:30 PM. That way there is enough time for digestion before going to bed. Please refer to the "SLEEP" chapter.

When preparing lunch or dinner, mix your raw and cooked ingredients to make certain that you coat your greenery with the aforementioned cooked toppings. You can also sprinkle spices such as turmeric, not only for the taste, but for additional anti-inflammatory and cancer fighting properties. Italian spices, Indian spices, or any other spices can be used as long as they're not processed or have any artificial ingredients or propylene glycol. We always use ground flaxseed for added creaminess. By consuming this incredible seed, we absorb Omega-3 fatty acids that are known to reduce risks of cardiovascular disease. The sky is the limit when "Eating Wonderfully!"

Make certain that you chew every bite at least 10 times. For the majority of you, your bodies are not used to such healthful meals, so it will take some time for your entire system to adjust to eating this way. By **chewing slowly**, you're not only feeling fully satisfied at the end of the meal, but you're helping your digestive system to cultivate your soon to be incredible "flora garden" which leads to "happy" gut. When I began eating this way, out of a lifetime habit, I couldn't chew slowly, so I placed a digital timer in front of me for a constant reminder to slow down. Your meal should take no less than 25 to 30 minutes; the longer, the better. In return, the "flora garden" in your gut will thank you by strengthening your immune system, as you gently continue to fertilize its delicate "good bacteria" with proper nutrition.

HALF BREAKFAST?

Since we already discussed lunch and dinner, what remains is breakfast.

You might be wondering "Why half breakfast?" I will respond by saying that if you look at the number of ingredients in this shake, it is equivalent to a nice size meal and a dessert; all in one. Since this sizable meal is in the form of a smoothie, we call it a half breakfast.

Besides packing huge amounts of nutrients and fiber, this shake is extremely timesaving. Trying to consume all of the ingredients that go into the shake in native "salad" form, would be quite an undertaking, especially in the morning when you're trying to get ready for work. Let's also be realistic. If you're eating a combination of these ingredients as a salad, it would not taste as "divine" as in a form of a smoothie.

This particular smoothie does not compare with empty calorie toast, croissant, danish, doughnut, jelly, or any other Insulin spiking or nitrate releasing breakfast food. Instead, this half breakfast packs a punch of nutrients that replenishes and recharges your body with Vitamins and minerals.

Use your already pre-cut "Base" for every meal including breakfast. It is <u>the same raw "greenery"</u> base that I use for my lunch and dinner.

The half breakfast or what I call the "LW Morning Re-charge" smoothie consists of the following:
- 2 cups of the "LW-Base" or the raw medley of vegetables that are loaded with fiber, Vitamins, minerals, and antioxidants.
- ½ banana for Riboflavin, Niacin, Vitamins A, C, B5, B6, potassium, among others. [1395]
- ½ carrot for Vitamin A, B, C, K, Beta-carotene, among others.[1396]
- 1 stalk of celery for foliate, potassium, Vitamins C, K, B1, B2, B6, among other minerals and fiber.[1397]
- 1 <u>whole</u> peeled lemon or lime not only for Vitamin C, but for cancer fighting flavonoids, as well as carotenoids for antioxidant properties. [1398]
- ¼ or <u>less</u> of green apple for fiber, Vitamin C, phytonutrients to help regulate blood sugar, etc.[1399]
- 1 teaspoon of spirulina for antioxidant and anti-inflammatory effects, as well as, protein, iron, copper, calcium, thiamin, riboflavin, pantothenic acid, and a slew of B-complex Vitamins.[1400] [1401] Spirulina is considered to be a superfood.
- If available, 1 strawberry, and/or ¼ cup of raspberries and/or blueberries for a slew of B Vitamins including Foliate, as well as Vitamins C, E, and K, manganese, among a number of others nutrients.[1402] Berries are considered to be a superfood.
- Approximately 1 tablespoon of fresh ginger root for gingerols that help reduce inflammation, inhibit some forms of cancer, and boost immune system.[1403]
- Approximately ½ teaspoon of fresh turmeric root for its anti-inflammatory, antioxidant, DNA damage and cancer preventing properties. [1404]
- Filtered water so the smoothie will be easy to drink and easy to absorb on the cellular level. You can make your smoothie thick or thin; it's a matter of preference. I add more water because I prefer it on the thin side; my wife likes her smoothies thicker.

Depending on your preference, you should end up with approximately 24 - 28 oz. or 680 - 794 g. smoothie. You can vary this shake as long as your "Base" remains constant. For example, you can substitute some of the fruit ingredients above with a chunk of pineapple for Vitamin C, manganese, thiamine, and copper.[1405] You can also use a small piece of cantaloupe for beta carotene, Vitamins A and C, among many other healthful properties including anti-inflammatory and anti-oxidant.[1406] Use ½ of the kiwi fruit with skin for Vitamins C, fiber, copper, calcium, potassium, magnesium, among other Vitamins and minerals.[1407]

Just make certain that your fruit doesn't overpower your base, as the <u>sugar content in fruit is capable of wreaking havoc on your body</u>. **If there is too much sugar from the fruit in your shake, <u>you will begin having cravings for sugar and carbs</u>**. It is something that we're trying to avoid at all costs! I'm saying this because I've experienced this phenomenon, so use caution and common sense when adding fruit to your "LW Morning Re-charge" smoothie. The rule of thumb is that your shake should have <u>very low sugar content</u>. If your shake tastes sweet, then <u>you are not doing yourself any favors as you will be back to where you started in no time</u>. **<u>Limit the fruit to a bare minimum!</u>**

The absorption of nutrients is significant, as your body will not have to work as hard to break down the "LW Morning Re-charge" shake. Unlike juicing, this smoothie retains the necessary dietary fiber.

You're probably thinking that it may take too much time to prepare this shake in the morning when you're rushing out the door to go to work. To remove excuses, you can put all of the ingredients in your favorite blender carafe the night before, leaving the water out. Just add water to the smoothie in the morning to regulate how thick you want it to be.

THE HALF BREAKFAST IS OPTIONAL – INSULIN AGAIN?

The half breakfast that I just described in detail, is <u>completely optional</u>. If you are only hungry twice a day, then by all means, skip this half breakfast. Just make certain to check your hunger levels in order to assess if additional meal is warranted, as a lot of people are not hungry after a full night's sleep. Unfortunately we've been trained to almost blindly accept through our parents, grandparents, processed food manufacturers, breakfast cereal producers in particular, that breakfast is the most important meal of the day, regardless of not being hungry. Even many doctors and nutritionists advocate that despite the lack of appetite in the morning, we should force the meal down our throats. Not true!

In LIVING WONDERFULLY land, we only eat when we're hungry, and we do not snack! Why is that? Please recall our discussion as part of the Insulin chapter, which includes the sentence that I'm about to repeat for the third and final time, I promise. **As a result of very low or no Insulin production, <u>your body uses stored fat for energy instead of glucose</u>**.[1408] That means that after you had your dinner four hours before you retired for the night, and you slept for seven or eight hours, <u>majority</u> of your glycogen (sugar type that's stored in the liver for the times when you don't eat) is depleted. At that point you're almost ready to burn fat, but you decide to ram breakfast down your throat. By doing so, you raise your Insulin level. Once the Insulin hormone is in your system, it is difficult to burn fat that you've been storing for as long as you can remember. But **if you decide to not eat until lunch, <u>not even snacks</u>, and just drink water instead when you feel hunger, you begin to tap into your fat reserves and actually burn fat.**

Please check with a reputable physician if your body is able to tolerate this type of eating pattern. If your physician advises against it, then stick to half breakfast, lunch, and dinner, and **no snacks or coffee.** Once your body is adapted to this type of eating pattern through improvements in your overall state of being, perhaps you may get a green light from your doctor down the road in order to commence skipping breakfast.

My wife and older son, for example, consume two, and rarely 2½ meals per day, while I only eat one, and rarely two meals on any given day. As such, I only drink water until my power meal; **no snacks or coffee!** If you do decide to have the half breakfast or skip breakfast altogether, **do not drink coffee**, at least until lunch. I will be addressing one of the most "painful" subjects of coffee in the next chapter.

Chapter 32 **PORTION SIZE, PORTION CONTROL, DESSERTS, COFFEE, AND SNACKING**

This was an eye opening revelation to the fact that <u>it really wasn't my fault that I was constantly overeating and staying hungry</u> whether on a diet or not!

When my wife and I eat, our portions are enormous as you saw in the photographs earlier. The funny thing is that my wife of 125 pounds practically eats the same amount of food as I do. How is that possible?

The number one question that I get about "Eating-Wonderfully" is portion size, as people are always in awe when they witness how much food we consume, while maintaining a healthy weight. There is a huge difference between what and how much I eat now and what I ate in the past.

<u>What I eat now may not be lower in calories, but is much higher in nutritional content, fiber, and healthy fats</u>. I'm full, and most importantly, satisfied "to the gills!" The reasoning behind this is actually quite simple.

Your stomach has a number of receptors to assess how much you've eaten and how much more food you need to eat.[1409] The caloric density receptors measure the richness of food or how many calories are being consumed, while stretch receptors measure the amount of food eaten. [1410] [1411] [1412]All of these receptors communicate to the brain whether we're full or need to eat more. [1413]

According to Doug Lisle, Ph.D., when we consume 500 calories of plant based natural foods, the stomach fills to <u>capacity,</u> and both stretch and density receptors are activated as in illustration below. [1414]

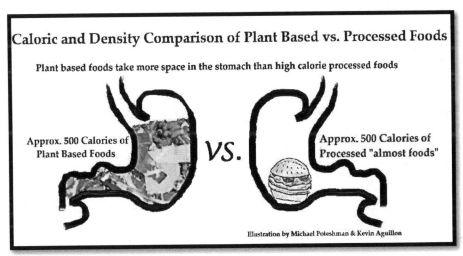

Caloric and Density Comparison of Plant Based vs. Processed Foods

Plant based foods take more space in the stomach than high calorie processed foods

Approx. 500 Calories of Plant Based Foods

VS.

Approx. 500 Calories of Processed "almost foods"

Illustration by Michael Poteshman & Kevin Aguillon

These receptors telegraph to the brain that it's time to stop eating. On the other hand, when we eat processed foods and/or foods that are high in calories that contain simple carbs and bad fats, the stomach receptors barely get stimulated, and respond accordingly. The same 500 calories of processed foods do not fill the stomach up in the same manner as plant based foods. [1415] Therefore, your brain is telegraphed a different a message: "Continue eating." This lack of satiety occurs every time we decide to eat the wrong foods. The receptors in your stomach are fooled in determining that you need to continue to eat. Even though you consumed more than enough "almost food" and its calories, hunger persists and you remain unsatisfied. That was the reason that I was constantly hungry and planning my next meal while I was finishing my current meal.

My present meals occupy more space in my stomach. I stay fuller longer while I let my "gut flora" prosper and my digestion thrive. The end result is I'm full and my excess weight has melted away! Believe it or not, **I actually weigh less now than when I was in high school!** I never thought that it was possible, but it is a clear and undeniable reality. **Just give your body the tools and your body will be happy to comply with your wishes!**

Inadequate portion size is a thing of the past, as every time I eat, I'm a happy boy who can enjoy life without being preoccupied about where and what I'm going to eat during my next meal. In fact, most of the time I can't even finish my bowl of food, so I leave it for the next meal. That is something that I haven't done for the past 30 years. Thus, if you feel full, just cover your leftovers and put them in the refrigerator. With time you will automatically adjust your portion size, as your body will tell you if you had enough. In the past, my body was always a "clean-plate-trash-compactor." I'm finally free of the burden of food! What a relief! Now it's your turn.

PORTION CONTROL? ANOTHER RULE?

Although I hate the notion of portion control, when it comes to "Living Wonderfully", there is a very important caveat. Although portion control is somewhat loose, it is extremely important to **only** consume the 60/40 portion you set for yourself, and

- **Leave the table and/or your kitchen immediately after you've finished eating.**
- **Do not snack after a meal, as you're full and you've gotten all the calories and nutrients your body requires.**

You want to snack after a meal out of habit; I know it too well, as in the past I looked for another piece or an extra morsel of "dead food." We developed this habit due to unsatisfaction and Insulin spikes of our former lifetime of eating like I used to; against your body's needs and nutritional requirements. This is something that you will have to train yourself to overcome. Believe it or not, within couple of weeks, your "eating after eating" will be the thing of the past. Just remember, **do not touch any food or snack after you've finished your bowl of food until your next meal,** which brings me to a very important point…

DESSERT ANYONE?

"Getting into the habit of eating something after a meal is finished may also put you at higher risk of mindless snacking and ignoring fullness signals from your body"
(Schuna, 2014).[1416]

You should **not** have dessert after a meal; **not even a fruit!** If you do, you will spike Insulin and begin to crave more sugar, and then you're back in the same rut as I was in not so long ago. A vicious cycle of looking for something sweet will ensue (please refer to "SUGAR" or "INSULIN" chapters). Believe me, as much as I love sweets, or used to love them, I experimented extensively. **You will only be lying to yourself if you say that sugar, even from a fruit, doesn't affect you. It really does, every single time!** Instead of dessert, here's how I conclude my meal.

I have a cup of warm water with lemon or lime with no sugar. In addition, I may also have one and only one "NOT SO DESSERT-DESSERT TRUFFLE" that you will find in the recipes section at the end of the book.

I don't desire sugar anymore, not only because I'm aware of its health destructing properties, but because I simply no longer crave it. I'm aware that it will be difficult for you to give up this "sweet" taste at first, so try to limit your cup of coffee or tea to a packet of "Stevia" sweetener, but you must exercise extreme caution.

According to a study, Stevia may lower blood pressure level, thus caution should be exercised when taking blood pressure medication and consuming Stevia.[1417] Stevia may also interact with anti-diabetes medications and Lithium. [1418] Furthermore, depending on the company that produces this sweetener, an ingredient called Erythritol, which happens to be sugar alcohol, may be added. A study published in the *Journal of Applied Entomology* showed that Erythritol is deadly to the larvae of fruit flies, and it also impairs reproduction of adult flies.[1419] Even though it's an effective pesticide, Erythritol may cause gastrointestinal disturbances in humans;[1420] therefore, make certain that you read the labels very carefully. So far I haven't found any other literature that would set off additional alarms when it comes to pure Stevia extract. That does not mean that there aren't studies that are being conducted as with Aspartame. So, exercise caution with any processed foods or artificial sweeteners.

In addition to lemon water, I may have a small handful of almonds, macadamia nuts, or pecans; only a small handful, not to exceed 3 oz. or 85 grams per day! If you take more than a handful and continue to eat these nuts, the "mindless snacking" will ensue and you will be back to square one. It's not a good place to be, especially now that you're trying to "Live-Wonderfully" and not be dependent on morsels of food to keep you happy.

SNACKING

All of my life I used to snack uncontrollably. Even with all of the prohibitive dieting that I've been through in the past, there was snacking allowance. "Living Wonderfully" is different, as we snack for a specific purpose only. In "Living Wonderfully" land, snacking means that you are seriously hungry because you were in a circumstance where you missed a meal; otherwise, there is no reason to **spike Insulin** by ramming additional food into your system. If you are hungry in-between meals, every effort should be made to adjust your **good fat intake** in order to maintain satiety. What do I mean by that? Add more good fats to your meals; please refer to chapters 17(Fat) and 24(Insulin). Keep in mind that your half breakfast (optional,) lunch, and dinner pack an incredible amount of nutrients and life-sustaining substances.

If we're **seriously hungry because we missed a meal**, we only snack in order to hold ourselves off until the next awesome nutrient dense meal.

Here's a possible scenario. Four hours after lunch, you're sitting in your office and all of the sudden you feel hungry. But is it really hunger or is your body playing tricks on you? Before snacking on anything, make certain that your body is not dehydrated. First, drink a large glass of water and wait for about 5-7 minutes. **More often than not, the hunger will pass.** Experiment and you'll see that most of the time you are not really hungry.

If drinking water does not solve the problem, then most likely you <u>did not have enough good fats</u> during your meal to keep you full and satisfied. If this is the case, you created a situation that may warrant unnecessary snacking, which inadvertently may slow down your weight loss.

Thus, if you missed a meal, have a handful of in shell nuts such as almonds, pecans, or walnuts. Choose nuts that are raw organic and not roasted in oil. Since <u>hunger keeps your metabolism engaged</u>, have no more than a handful. You don't want to become fuller than you need to be before eating your next meal. Refer to the "Hunger Levels" chapter, as the hunger level in this case is particularly important!

The following are other snack options besides in-shell nuts, although some of them may not be as satisfying or convenient:

- Mix 3 tablespoons of Chia seeds in a glass of water. The seeds absorb more than 10 times their weight, as chia seeds have an incredible ability to hold considerable amount of water. [1421] [1422] Your stomach may feel full, and you will be getting over 10 grams of fiber per ounce besides other extraordinary properties. [1423] Chia seed is considered a superfood.
- Prepare a snack of 4 celery sticks and peanut butter or almond butter spread over the concave side. The peanut butter must be natural without hydrogenated oils.
- Kale chips taste delicious, but require a little prep. Take a few fresh Kale leaves, sprinkle extra virgin olive oil, and a little salt for taste. Bake at 350°F or 176°C for approximately 12 minutes or until crispy. Don't eat the entire bunch of Kale chips as it's no longer live food. Consume only a couple of leaves.
- 1 hardboiled egg with a little Italian spice or non-chemical hot sauce may also do the job of keeping you going until your next meal.

I'm always asked about fruit for snacking? Although neither I nor my family snack, especially on fruits, I still have to answer yes, only because of the amount of nutrients in fruit. But what's more important, is how much fruit, as it contains <u>large amount of sugar</u>. According to Dr. Melina Japolis of CNN, fruit has nearly three and a half times the calories per serving than non-starchy vegetables.[1424] She recommends that in order to break through the weight loss plateau, no more than 1½ cups of fruit per day should be consumed. [1425] That's three ½ cup servings per day. [1426]

If we look at our morning smoothie, we may have already exhausted at least half or more of this quota, as one medium banana is equivalent to approximately ½ cup. While you're trying to reach your weight loss goal, **keep your fruit intake to no more than a maximum of 1 cup per day, or <u>less</u>**. My family and I do not consume fruits unless there is a small amount in a smoothie. We may indulge only on special occasions when we're on vacation, when exotic fruits that we've never tried before are available. Then we're back to our awesome routine.

Although I have achieved my health and weight loss goal, I continue to follow this model. As I mentioned earlier, whenever I eat an extra piece of fruit, I begin to crave sugary and starchy foods, and actually long for more sweet fruit.

I like to "Live-Wonderfully" and there is no fruit in the world that would derail my newly found health that was "misplaced" for almost two decades.

Once again, please remember to **only snack when seriously hungry** in order to hold yourself off until your next fulfilling meal! Better yet, **do not** snack, and make every effort to **adjust the intake of good fats during meals so you won't be hungry in-between**. That way, you will not only keep your Insulin from spiking, but also continue to maximize your weight loss.

COFFEE

Now we come to a dreaded subject of coffee. The majority of people whom I've spoken to or associated with, believe that coffee is a lifeline for their livelihood and they can't live without it. I've been using coffee for many decades in order to get me through the day, especially during those long hours at the office. Note that I said "using" instead of drinking. Indeed, I was hooked, just like a junkie on drugs. What that meant was besides all of the "almost foods and beverages" I was consuming, I was exacerbating my already deteriorating condition with the infusion of coffee and caffeine.

I'm aware that right about now, you want to scream at me through the pages of this book about the benefits of coffee, as you've read studies and articles that show positive aspects of this "heavenly beverage". There are also a myriad of studies that show detrimental effects of drinking this beverage. It can definitely be confusing and frustrating. Because I completely appreciate your sentiment, as I've been there numerous times, all will be explained and backed by scientific research, so you can draw your own conclusion.

Notwithstanding some beneficial qualities of coffee, here are five reasons why one should abstain from drinking it, at least until the desired health objective and weight loss goal are achieved. Only then you can decide whether or not you want to go back to something that may have caused or added to your ailments in the first place.

1. When I begin to talk about the painful coffee subject, most of the time I hear: *"Italians don't just drink coffee, but expresso, all day long. Espresso is much stronger than coffee, and they have no problems. We don't drink espresso, but weak American drip coffee, and only two to four cups per day."* Here's my response that puts the "Italian espresso" issue to rest. Not only do Italians have a problem when drinking espresso, but this problem is much more serious than even I even thought possible.

   A large Italian study entitled, *"Espresso Coffee Consumption and Risk of Coronary Heart Disease in a Large Italian Cohort"*, encompassed 30,449 women and 12,800 men without the history of cardiovascular heart disease or CHD, came up with a conclusion that made my jaw drop.

"Consumption of over 2 cups/day of Italian-style coffee is associated with increased coronary heart disease risk…" (Grioni, Agnoli, Sieri, Pala, Ricceri, Masala, . . . Krogh, 2015).[1427]

   As to the subject of "weak American drip coffee vs. strong espresso", according to Consumer Reports, a typical 8 oz. cup of coffee contains between 95 and 128 mg. of caffeine, while 1 oz. cup of espresso contains 63 mg. of caffeine.[1428] Therefore, if you only drink one cup of coffee, you are actually ingesting almost double the amount of caffeine of the Italian brew. As this book is about reducing the risk or eliminating coronary heart disease altogether, this "coffee model" does not exactly correspond to Living Wonderfully lifestyle.

2. Although coffee may wake you up, its caffeine content will increase your stress hormone level. *"Caffeine elevates cortisol secretion…"* (Lovallo, Farag, Vincent, Thomas, & Wilson, 2006).[1429] Please recall our discussion as part of the Insulin chapter. When cortisol (stress hormone) is secreted, your body is "flooded" with glucose/blood sugar.[1430] [1431]

"Cortisol prepares the body for a fight-or-flight response by flooding it with glucose, supplying an immediate energy source to large muscles"
(Aronson, 2009)[1432]

Cortisol may prevent you from burning fat until it's out of your system. Furthermore, no matter what type of stress you are under, or no stress at all, **caffeine will increase your stress hormone!**

"…caffeine doses increased cortisol levels across the test day without regard to the sex of the subject or type of stressor employed…"
(Lovallo, Farag, Vincent, Thomas, & Wilson, 2006).[1433]

Not only that, but the **Insulin that is released as a result of consistent caffeine ingestion,**[1434] may cause inflammation. I believe that you are already aware of what happens then.

3. Unfortunately when you drink coffee, it affects the absorption of some medications, vitamins, and minerals. A prime example would be the absorption of thyroid medication that has to do with T4 thyroid hormone. As we discussed earlier, thyroid function affects almost every aspect of your system. Well, here's a conclusion of yet another study:

"Coffee should be added to the list of interferers of T4 intestinal absorption, and T4 to the list of compounds whose absorption is affected by coffee."
(Benvenga, Bartolone, Pappalardo, Russo, Lapa, Giorgianni, . . . Trimarchi, 2008)[1435]

Besides this scary thyroid example above, coffee interferes with the absorption of iron. Only one cup of coffee decreased iron absorption from a hamburger meal by 39%.[1436] The tea fared even worse, as the absorption of iron was decreased by a whopping 64%, as you read earler.[1437] This should raise a red flag for every man, and especially, every woman who is reading this book.

I can go on and on, as there are other examples of this beverage interfering with the absorption of vitamins and minerals, but I believe that you recognize the pattern.

One other thing to remember is the **excretion of vitamins**[1438] **and minerals** through urine when drinking coffee, as caffeine elevates production of urine. [1439] [1440] [1441]

4. *"Coffee promotes gastro-esophageal reflux…"* (Boekema, Samsom, & Van Be, 1999). [1442] Please recall our discussion in the SLEEP chapter. To refresh your memory, when you swallow your food or beverage, it travels down to your stomach through the esophagus or a tube that connects your throat to your stomach. Once the food is passed to the stomach, the valve or a tight ring of muscles that are called lower esophageal sphincter, close and do not allow food and acidic stomach juices from seeping back into the esophagus. But if you consistently drink coffee, alcohol, as well as other "almost foods and beverages" discussed in earlier chapters, you are running a risk of having your esophageal sphincter either not close all the way, or remain in a partially open position. This

condition may not only cause heart burn, but a more serious problems such as damage to the esophagus, as well as getting your gut flora out of balance, and the worst case scenario of esophageal cancer. You know what happens then, after reading the GUT HEALTH chapter earlier.

Some may believe that caffeine may promote the gastro-esophageal reflux, but studies show that components of coffee itself are responsible for this condition.

"Coffee, in contrast to tea, increases gastro-esophageal reflux... Caffeine does not seem to be responsible for gastro-esophageal reflux which must be attributed to other components of coffee."
(Wendl, Pfeiffer, Pehl, Schmidt, & Kaess, 2007).[1443]

As for me, as well as my family and friends who have gotten off coffee, booze, and "almost foods" described in this book, no longer suffer from gastro-esophageal reflux! How liberating!

5. ***"Caffeine is the most commonly used drug in the world. "***
(Meredith, Juliano, Hughes, & Griffiths, 2013)[1444]

If you're hooked on coffee as I was, or think you might be, just try to abstain from it for three or four days, and see if you have withdrawal symptoms. Studies show that out of the 49 categories of symptoms identified, the top ten as listed below validate the caffeine withdrawal criteria.[1445] Drum roll please.

1. Irritability,
2. Decreased contentedness,
3. Headache,
4. Decreased energy/activeness,
5. Depressed mood,
6. Fatigue,
7. Drowsiness,
8. Difficulty concentrating,
9. Decreased alertness, and
10. Foggy/not clearheaded. [1446]

Without even knowing, I suffered from a self-induced caffeine-withdrawal syndrome, which is now an official diagnosis!

"Caffeine Withdrawal is now an officially recognized diagnosis..."
(Addicott, M. A., Ph.D, 2014)[1447]

The symptoms begin to manifest within 12 to 24 hours after you stopped drinking coffee (cold turkey) or any beverage that contain caffeine.[1448] According to a study, you begin to feel the intensity of caffeine withdrawal between 20 and 51 hours. [1449] Only then you will be able to observe if you are suffering from withdrawal symptoms. If you don't suffer from any of these symptoms, congratulations! That means that you can stop coffee cold turkey in order to effectively reach the desired health objective and/or weight loss.

If you're addicted to coffee, as I was, <u>you are no longer relying on your own energy, but are using caffeine (drug) as a crutch, to get you through the day</u>. Being hooked on any type of a substance to induce energy or to feel better is not what the Living Wonderfully lifestyle is all about, but goes completely against it. As you continue to implement the lifestyle changes as outlined in this book, it will be easier to kick this addiction. Here is a small pointer that may help quit.

- Quitting cold turkey may put somewhat of a strain on your system, and you may feel miserable. To avoid this, begin slowly in order to quit this addiction within two weeks. Cut your coffee intake by a quarter, and parse your reduced coffee dosages throughout the times when you usually indulge.

Everything else is outlined in the book, i.e. drinking plenty of water, eliminating chemicals in food and anything that comes in touch with your skin, detox, and exercise will make quitting coffee that much easier. You should feel the withdrawal symptoms get better after the first week, and by the second week they may completely taper off.

Chapter 33 EATING WONDERFULLY ON THE GO

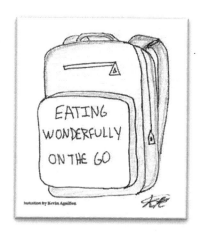

As my son is working full time in addition to being a full time college student, he complained of difficulty "Eating-Wonderfully" even though he saw tremendous changes with his health, improved cognitive functions, including concentration level and clear thinking. He "commissioned" me to come up with a way to eat these awesome nutritious meals on the go. Because he is at work and then in school for the entire day, his criteria were to have two meals and snacks on-the-go.

You already know what to do for breakfast. To jog your memory, put all of the ingredients in your favorite blender carafe the night before and place it in the refrigerator, leaving out the water. Just add water to the smoothie in the morning.

The rest of your meals require a purchase of couple of items available at your local superstore or supermarket:

- Portable cooler
- Ice packs; the largest size that would fit into your cooler or two smaller packs
- 2 lunch containers with lockable-lids, or a three-compartment flat container to separate foods
- 1 or 2 small glass container(s) with lid that seals for one of the toppings that you may want to heat up
- Small container or zip lock bag for nuts

1. Put your ice packs into the freezer the night before.
2. Fill up your flat containers with the LW-Base and put toppings either on top of the "greenery", or if you purchased a three compartment container, in the compartments.
3. If you decide that you have another topping that you want to heat up, fill one of your small containers with that topping. From time to time, I enjoy eating my meals warm.
4. Fill up your other small container with any nuts, in case you miss a meal or decide to have a handful after your meal is complete. Remember, we only eat snacks to hold ourselves off until the next meal; otherwise, no snacking.

5. Before you leave for work, insert all of the filled containers into your cooler, and place the ice pack(s) on top for optimal cooling. If you wish, you can keep your container with nuts out of the cooler. I leave mine in for convenience.

With a little planning ahead, you now have two absolutely awesome and nutritious meals; the same food that you'd eat at home.

EATING OUT

Once I was able to resolve my son's dilemma with his work/school day, he asked me what he should eat when he's invited to a restaurant, or goes out to his friends' homes.

Let's be realistic, from time to time you will be invited to a picnic, work function, or family celebration. Unless your family or friends understand the concept of eating chemical-free food, more often than not you will be consuming chemicals, flavor enhancers, and preservatives. Let's look at how we can take control over what we're eating when Living Wonderfully food is not available:

SOUP

As a rule, I don't order any soup at a restaurant, as the majority of the soup bases have added MSG, "natural flavors", modified yeast, hydrolyzed protein, and/or "spices" that we talked about earlier. If you are thinking about ordering soup, I recommend that you inquire with the restaurant chef about the ingredients. Order soup only after you're 100% certain that it has no "added garbage", and the soup base/stock is actually made out of vegetables and/or meats, and not processed broth. If the chef sounds iffy, don't risk it. Your health is more important than a bowl of liquid with chemicals. Doesn't sound appetizing.

If you're being served soup at your friends' or relatives' homes, ask if store-bought stock was used. Also inquire about added mixes, as a majority of soup mixes possess the same "chemical soup" outlined above. If you believe that it's not tactful to ask such questions, then don't eat the soup or have one spoon just to show that you've at least tried.

SALAD

Don't expect organic vegetables on your salad when ordering at a restaurant unless the menu specifically states that they are using all organic ingredients. Nonetheless, even if the salad is not organic, I'd still order and pick at it, as long as there is no added dressing. Please recollect the GMO and glyphosate section earlier.

Most store-bought salad dressings are loaded with all sorts of chemicals as discussed in the MSG chapter. If you order a salad, ask the waiter for olive oil and white or balsamic vinegar, or lemon. Salt and pepper should already be on the table. Make certain that the balsamic vinegar doesn't have any added "flavors" or sugar. If you can't verify, go with regular white table vinegar. The same rule applies when going to your friends' homes or to picnics. When ordering, a better choice would be a vegetarian Cobb salad without added dressing. The avocados provide a delicious and satiating fat for your food, and the tomatoes and other ingredients add flavor. With such a salad, all that is needed is a little oil and vinegar. For most other salads, when eating out, rely on mostly vegetables to deliver flavor. Most restaurants have tomato wedges or slices, and onions. Adding these ingredients to any salad instantly makes them richer and more flavorful.

ENTRÉES

Just as with our discussion about vegetables above, don't expect steak and/or poultry to be organic. The only thing that you may be able to control is the amount of "stuff" they flavor your entrees with. Keeping this in mind, make certain to inquire if the meat was marinated. If so, a lot of marinades contain chemicals to tenderize the meat and enhance its flavor. Even some "meat/chicken rub" brands contain similar chemicals. Therefore, try to order steak or poultry that has only been flavored with salt and pepper. All you have to do is ask. In a lot of upscale restaurants you get flavor out of aged meat rather than chemically spiked marinades with flavor enhancers. Some Middle Eastern restaurants that marinate meat with onions and native spices that are actually "spices" and not the laundry list in appendices A-F at the end of the book. I wouldn't have a problem ordering this type of meat or poultry; the quality and source is another story. You are already aware what to look for from sections where we talked about hormones, arsenic, and antibiotics.

SIDE DISHES

The safest choice for a side dish at a restaurant would be steamed or grilled vegetables. If possible, ask the staff to briefly steam vegetables so they don't get fully processed and become dead carbs that are devoid of nutrients and fiber. Also ask your server not to add the usual spice/butter mix as you will flavor your vegetables with salt, pepper, and olive oil instead. Sometimes the spice mixes that are added to the steamed vegetables contain harmful chemicals and flavor enhancers.

DESSERT

It's better not to have any dessert, but if you're with your boss, or you really can't wiggle out of a particular situation, the following would be marginally acceptable.

You already know what's in cookies, cakes, and ice cream as you've read all about this stuff in "WHAT NOT TO EAT" section. So, which dessert is safer when going to a restaurant or out on your friends' patio? How about a couple of small pieces of fresh fruit, or an assortment of berries without the addition of chemical syrups or whipped cream? How about few raisins and nuts? Just make certain that the nuts are not prepared with added oils. With the exception of a few brands, oil hydrogenation or partial hydrogenation is almost certain. You can also have one or two pieces of dehydrated fruit, while keeping in mind that before this fruit was dehydrated, it was whole, and contains just as much sugar. As many brands add "stuff" to their dehydrated products, validate that it doesn't have added sugars, chemicals, or preservatives.

There are also some gluten free cakes that are made out of almond or coconut flour. Make certain that they are not sweetened with anything other than dried/dehydrated or fresh fruit.

If you decide to have a fruit based chemical-free dessert, make certain that you have a very small amount. As discussed earlier, even an extra piece of fruit can stimulate the **uncontrollable urge to snack or crave sweets.** Remember, sugar is sugar is sugar, no matter what form it is in. **An extra piece of dessert**

is one step back to the old and unhappy way of life. Dessert should be optional, at best, and **only** in situations that you cannot "wiggle out of."

BEVERAGES

You already know about sodas, whether made with sugar or with artificial sweetener, are bad, especially the ones with Aspartame.

Instead of soda, order plain water with a wedge of lemon or lime. I know, the sweet stuff tastes better, but at what cost? Eventually you'll get used to drinking a better alternative.

In terms of alcohol, you are already familiar with calories, Ethanol, and chemical content in different alcoholic beverages from the "BOOZE AND CALORIES" section earlier. If you decide to have a mixed drink, have one without the added sugary mixers that are mostly loaded with chemicals. If you have no other alternative but to have alcoholic beverage, choose one ounce or 28 grams of alcohol with club soda and a wedge of lemon or lime.

Be careful with beer and wine, as in most cases they contain added sulfites and nitrates as we discussed in the "ALCOHOL" chapter earlier.

WHEN BRINGING YOUR OWN FOOD TO WORK ISN'T AN OPTION

I presented the "On the Go" solutions to my son. Although grateful, he said to me, "Dad, I'm constantly in lunch meetings or meeting with potential clients. In addition, I may have other situations that make carrying food difficult. What should I do in these scenarios?"

My fatherly advice was that if you absolutely cannot bring food to work that your body will thrive upon, do the best you can while following some simple rules:

THE BASICS FOR EATING WONDERFULLY ON THE GO

1. Toxins – If you have gotten this far in the book, you already know what kind of foods are toxic. Try not to eat or drink anything that contains toxins. Remember that water is always available to drink.
2. Simple Sugars and Carbs - DO NOT EAT SIMPLE SUGARS, no white breads, pastas, pastries, white rice, etc.
3. Avoid Dairy

UNAVOIDABLE FOOD SITUATIONS

Unfortunately since much of the world is unenlightened about the poisons we feed ourselves, we are often stuck in its confines. Consider this example of a bagged lunch my son was given in a departmental meeting:

- Ham sandwich, bottled water, apple, cookie and a bag of chips.

After reading this book you might think that organization he works for is deliberately trying to poison him. But he, as many of us, is stuck in a situation as part of a group where you do not want to ostracize yourself by certain food choices, or by not eating lunch at all. What did he do?

- He set aside the apple as okay to eat. Despite containing sugar, it has nutrients and fiber to promote satiety and is probably the least harmful of the options above.

- He took the ham and lettuce out of the sandwich and ate that separately, leaving the bread behind.
- Everything else was given to co-workers who had no problem taking his "junk food" and were even grateful.

Ultimately in that meal he consumed sugar and a large amount of toxins, but it was the best he could do in this particular circumstance. The point is to maintain balance and consume as small an amount of unbalanced foods as possible. With this meal he consumed sugar (from the apple) without completely overdosing. Instead of eating bread which would have given him an Insulin spike and left him with sugar cravings for the rest of the day, he had the ham. While toxic with nitrates and other "stuff", he was able to process this ham through a sauna session and some of the other toxin removal remedies suggested in the book.

Keep in mind that this solution is only for this specific scenario. Continued ingestion of this stuff will eventually lead you back to where you started - "Living Dead."

Chapter 34 IMPORTANT "WHAT IF" SCENARIOS

When I speak at different venues, I'm grateful that people ask me important questions that I can pass along to my readers:

- ❖ "If I just want a bowl of soup, how do I eat the 60% of the LW-Base raw foods?"
- ❖ "How about if I just want beef and bean chili and I don't want to add this chili to the raw salad?"

The answer is quite simple. Your meal, once again, should always consist of 60% raw and 40% cooked food; that's non-negotiable. By all means, have yourself a bowl with the understanding that it's not going to be a huge serving of chili or soup because **the cooked portion cannot exceed 40%.**

As for the other 60% of your meal, you can consume it as a salad, which will not be as exciting without the cooked toppings that you just devoured.

To counteract this situation, put LW-Base greenery into your blender, add a few slices of fruits, nuts, water, and drink it as a smoothie. Although your 60% greenery is in liquid form, you will still be full. The difference is that you're going to speed up the absorption of nutrients.

On those rare occasions when I just want a bowl of soup, I follow this method. **It is crucial to remember that <u>60% raw food or LW-Base is mandatory</u>!**

- ❖ "What if my boss orders carry-out, and in solidarity of team spirit I have no other alternative but to join my workgroup for lunch?"

If you are at work, your boss decides to get carry-out, and you have no other alternative but be part of the team, you can follow the same principle as above. The only difference is it would require you to bring blender from home or just purchase another inexpensive blender for your office. Before going to work, fill your blender with LW-Base and other ingredients as we discussed earlier. That way, on those rare occasions, you will still get your 40% or less of the "dead" carry-out food, and at the same time continue to get your 60% of cancer fighting/inflammation reducing greenery!

Notice that I regarded carry-out food as dead. Indeed I have, because I've worked in an office environment, and seen that most carry-out meals consist of "processed almost-foods." This scenario only applies if you have no other alternative but to eat this "stuff" so your boss doesn't think that you're not a team player. I completely understand your predicament.

Play it by ear while remembering that health is your number one asset. Your boss will not replace your health. **Your well-being is worth much more than a morsel of "dead food."**

I hope that with this chapter, every excuse for not Eating Wonderfully has been eliminated. So, my dear reader, as the new saying goes, "Eat, drink, prosper, and Live Wonderfully!" You now know what to do!

We're not done yet. Next, we are headed to your favorite store, fresh produce market, or farm.

Chapter 35 THE SHOPPING LIST

VEGETABLE SHOPPING LIST

Before going shopping, please keep one thing in mind. Even if fruits and vegetables are labeled as organic, the manure that may have been used to fertilize the crop could have been compromised.

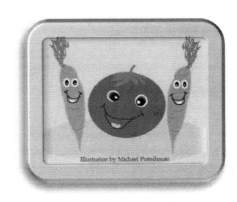

"Unfortunately, arsenic-laced chicken manure can still be used to grow organic produce"
(Greger, 2012).[1450]

In order to avoid using produce that's laced with arsenic, make certain to question your purveyors. Reputable establishments should have staff who respond truthfully. Since my family consumes a lot of greenery, we verify that no arsenic-laced manure or other chemicals are used to grow the crop that makes its way into our food. We either ask the produce manager for a phone number of the grower, or if produce is grown locally, we visit the farm. We also check multiple sources on the Internet before purchasing produce. This procedure is not as tedious as it sounds. You only have to verify this information once in order to ensure that you're not ingesting toxic chemicals or feeding them to your kids.

Now that we know what to look for and what to avoid, we can move on to the shopping list for the most important component of **every meal**, the "LW-Base." I added a properties section that comprises of Vitamins and minerals for each vegetable, which includes the main and few trace nutrients that are contained within these power packed foods. Also, for your reference, B Vitamin names[1451] [1452] are used interchangeably:

- Vitamin B1=Thiamine
- Vitamin B2=Riboflavin
- Vitamin B3=Niacin
- Vitamin B4=Choline
- Vitamin B5=Pantothenic acid
- Vitamin B6=Pyridoxine
- Vitamin B7=Biotin
- Vitamin B8=Inositol

- Vitamin B9=Folate/folic acid
- Vitamin B10=Paba
- Vitamin B11=Salicylic acid
- Vitamin B12=Cobalamin

Asparagus	Copper, selenium, fiber, manganese, potassium, Vitamins A, B1, B2, B3, C, E, K,[1453]
Avocado	Pantothenic acid, fiber, Vitamin K, copper, folate, Vitamin B6, potassium, magnesium, Vitamin E, Vitamin C[1454]
Beets	Has the potential to improve cerebral and cardiovascular blood flow and restoration of endothelial function.[1455] Contains high amounts of folic acid to protect against cancer and heart attacks[1456]
Broccoli	Fiber, zinc, selenium, iron, polyphenols such as quercetin glucosides, kaempferol, and isorhamnetin, Vitamins A, C, K, B9 [1457]
Cabbage	Manganese, fiber, potassium, Vitamins B6, C, K [1458]
Carrots	Iron, zinc, potassium, manganese, fiber, β-carotene, Vitamins A, C, B6, K, biotin (B7) [1459]
Cauliflower	Phosphorous, calcium, iron, Vitamins A, C, thiamine, niacin, riboflavin [1460]
Cilantro	Magnesium, phosphorus, potassium, zinc, Vitamins A, K, C, riboflavin, niacin
Collard Greens	Fiber, calcium, potassium, iron, zinc, Vitamins A, B1, B2, B3, B6, B9, C, E, K
Dill	Vitamins A, C, Niacin, B6, Folate, magnesium, phosphorus, potassium, zinc
Garlic	Vitamins B1, B2, B3, B6, D, K, calcium, iron, magnesium, phosphorus, potassium, zinc
Ginger Root	Potassium, magnesium, phosphorus, Vitamins B1, B2 B3, B6, C, E
Jalapeno Peppers	Phosphorus, calcium, potassium, magnesium, Vitamins A, C, E, K, B6, niacin, folate
Jicama	Calcium, iron, potassium, phosphorus, magnesium, Vitamins A, C, B1, B2, B3, B6, B9
Kale	Calcium, iron, magnesium, phosphorus, potassium, zinc, Vitamins A, C, K, B1, B2, B3, B6, B9

Leeks	Calcium, iron, magnesium, phosphorus, potassium, zinc , Vitamins A, C, K, niacin, B6, folate
Mustard greens	Magnesium, iron, calcium, potassium, zinc, Vitamins C, E, folate, riboflavin, niacin, thiamin
Onion	Calcium, potassium, magnesium, phosphorus, Vitamins C, B1, B2, B3, B6, B9
Parsley	Calcium, iron, potassium, magnesium, zinc, phosphorus, Vitamins A, C, K, niacin, folate[1461]
Parsnips	Potassium, zinc, calcium, phosphorus, Vitamins C, K, E, folate
Radishes	Potassium, zinc, calcium, phosphorus, iron, Vitamins C ,A, K, B3
Rutabaga	Potassium, phosphorus, calcium, magnesium, iron, Vitamins B1, B3, B9, C, E
Spinach	Potassium, iron, calcium, magnesium, phosphorus, zinc, Vitamins A, B1, B2, B6, B9, C, E, K
Tomatoes	Potassium, magnesium, phosphorus, iron, zinc, Vitamins A, C, K, E, niacin, folate, pyridoxine
Turnip	Calcium, potassium, phosphorous, magnesium, Vitamins C, folate, niacin, pyridoxine
Turnip greens	Iron, calcium, potassium, magnesium, phosphorus Vitamins A, C, B3, B6, B9, E, K
Unless specified by the end note numbers contained within this table, the properties of each vegetable are based on information obtained from the United States Department of Agriculture - Agricultural Research Service, USDA Food Composition Databases/National Nutrient Database for Standard Reference[1462]	

You can add more vegetables or vary your LW-Base. For example, the addition of cucumbers infuses Vitamin K, molybdenum, and pantothenic acid, among others[1463] into your system. You are only limited by your imagination!

ANIMAL BASED PRODUCTS SHOPPING LIST

PORK, CHICKEN, TURKEY, AND FOWL

As discussed in the "WHAT NOT TO EAT" section, most standard store bought poultry contains arsenic and antibiotics. In order to reduce the consumption of arsenic, look for USDA Organic labels.[1464] [1465]
According to Michael Greger, M.D., only one-third of organic or "premium" chicken or chicken parts have a detectable arsenic level. This is considerably less than non-organic chicken.[1466]

If a label on pork, bison, chicken, turkey, fowl, or any bird parts states, "No steroid hormones added", or "we don't use growth hormones in our chicken" or "hormone free product", or something along those lines, understand that regardless of those statements, <u>food producers are not allowed to use any of these drugs anyway</u>. In reality they are trying to boost their reputation by stating the obvious. To a consumer who doesn't know better, this bunch of nonsense may seem that a particular food company is selling drug-free meats. But are they really drug-free?

Steroid hormones are not permitted by USDA for the usage in pork, chicken, or other birds.[1467]

Don't even waste your time reading this obvious and useless information. Instead, look for a label that clearly states "antibiotic-free", "no antibiotics used", or "USDA Organic" label.

<u>Even if the label just states "antibiotic-free", arsenic may be used</u>. To avoid arsenic drugs in your bird, "USDA Organic" would be a wiser choice. Here are some examples of what you need to look for when shopping for pork or any type of bird:

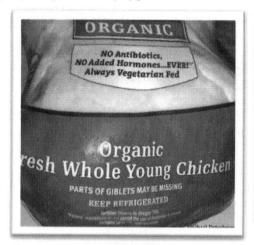
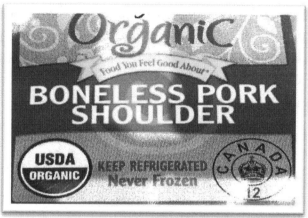

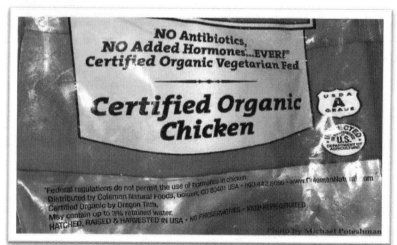

BEEF AND LAMB

Cow and sheep farmers are allowed to use steroid hormones as well as antibiotics, so look for the labels that clearly state "No steroid hormones used", "Antibiotic-free", "USDA Organic", and "USDA Process Verified." USDA defines organic as following:

"Organic meat, poultry, eggs, and dairy products come from animals that are given no antibiotics or growth hormones."
(USDA, 2004).[1468]

Some manufacturers use labels that masquerade as healthful but can be quite deceiving. If the information on the package is sketchy, ask a simple question of a purveyor in order to verify whether or not antibiotics or hormones were used. If you can't get a satisfactory answer, most of the time there's a web address or phone number on the package. Since you only have one question, it shouldn't take more than a few minutes to get a satisfactory answer. If you're still in doubt, here's a sure bet label when buying beef or lamb:

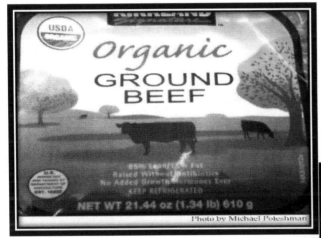

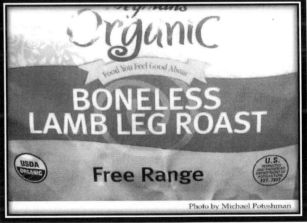

Although we're at the end of the book, this is only the beginning of the rest of your life! You now have knowledge for a lifetime of great health! Go back to the beginning and review chapters as many times as necessary until the "Living Wonderfully" routine becomes an effortless and pleasurable habit.

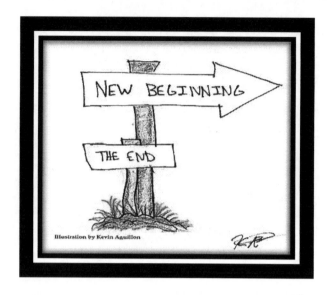

Illustration by Kevin Aguillon

Chapter 36 LIVING WONDERFULLY RECIPES

Before we begin making Living Wonderfully recipes, make certain that <u>all</u> of the ingredients are organic. Good luck…

ROASTED VEGETABLES

1 small acorn or butternut squash, cubed and peeled
1 large yam, cubed and unpeeled
1 green bell pepper, coarsely sliced
1 red bell pepper, coarsely sliced
1 onion, quartered and separated
4 tablespoons extra virgin olive oil
3 tablespoons balsamic vinegar
½ teaspoon black pepper or to taste
1 tablespoon dried rosemary
Salt to taste
1 tablespoon fresh minced garlic or use garlic press

1. *Leaving garlic out, combine all of the ingredients in a large bowl and mix well making certain that all of the vegetables are coated evenly*
2. *Spread evenly on a large roasting pan; preferably in a single layer without overlap*
3. *Bake for 30 to 40 minutes depending on the texture that you prefer in 425°F or 218°C preheated oven*
4. *After 20 minutes of baking stir in minced/crushed garlic and mix well on the roasting pan. Return to oven for the remaining time*

QUINOA SALAD

1 cup uncooked quinoa

2 cups water

2 avocados peeled and coarsely diced

1 cup thinly sliced green onions

1 cup of seeded and diced cherry or plum tomatoes

1 cup sweet corn

Extra virgin olive oil

White or balsamic vinegar

2 cloves of minced or crushed garlic

1 cup cilantro chopped

½ teaspoon black pepper

Salt to taste

1. *Cook 1 cup of quinoa in 2 cups of water using rice cooker or cook on stove top at low heat until water is absorbed. Let cool in the refrigerator 30 minutes*
2. *Combine cooked quinoa and all of remaining ingredients in a bowl*
3. *Drizzle olive oil and vinegar to taste and toss lightly so the avocado breakage is at a minimum*
4. *Serve immediately. Don't let salad sit for long as vinegar will be absorbed and the taste will change drastically*

I recommend dividing the undressed salad into parts and only using the amount that will be consumed

BEEF JERKY

1½ Lbs. flank steak or any low fat organic beef. Any meat cut will work because there will be no need for tenderizing. Inexpensive cuts will do the job.

1 tablespoons salt

1 teaspoon crushed red pepper flakes

2 cloves crushed garlic

1 tablespoon white vinegar

1 tablespoon paprika

1. *Trim fat off of the meat*
2. *Freeze the defatted meat for 4 hours for easier slicing. Make certain that the meat doesn't fully freeze.*
3. *Cut meat against the grain into 1/8" (0.32 cm.) slices to a maximum of 3/16" (0.45 cm.) thickness. The thicker the cut the chewier the beef jerky will be. Also, if you decide to cut with the grain, the meat will seem chewier as well.*
4. *Note: Majority of commercial jerky brands cut their meat with the grain. Try both and see which one you prefer.*
5. *In a bowl combine all of the ingredients. Mix or toss thoroughly, making certain that every sliver of meat is covered.*
6. *Refrigerate for 24 hours*
7. *Mix again thoroughly*
8. *Arrange meat slices on a dehydrator trays while making certain that there is space in-between for thorough drying.*
9. *Depending on your dehydrator model, it may take between 5 to 9 hours to achieve the final product.*
10. *Refrigerate*

POTATO FREE SPAGHETTI SQUASH HASH

1 small spaghetti squash

2 eggs

1 large coarsely chopped onion

1 clove crushed garlic

1 teaspoon chopped parsley

3 tablespoons of extra virgin coconut oil

½ teaspoon black pepper

Salt to taste

1. *Bake spaghetti squash until soft and remove skin*
2. *Using cheese cloth or thin cloth squeeze excess water out of the squash. Put aside.*
3. *In a large pan, sauté onion in coconut oil until golden brown*
4. *Combine all of the ingredients in the large pan where you just sautéed onion and mix thoroughly*
5. *Keep sautéing while stirring frequently until golden brown, i.e. 8-12 minutes*

BEEF STEW

2 Lbs. Cubed stew beef. Chicken or turkey can be used as well

3 tablespoons of extra virgin coconut oil

2 large onions sliced to medium thinness using food processor

1 medium acorn, butternut, or spaghetti squash cubed and peeled

3 large carrots

5 stalks of celery

½ cup raw tomato paste

2 cups of organic beef or chicken stock, or water

½ teaspoon cumin powder

½ teaspoon coriander powder

½ teaspoon ground black pepper

1 teaspoon crushed garlic

Himalayan salt to taste

1. *Sauté onions in coconut oil until golden brown*
2. *Add beef and sauté until slightly brown*
3. *Add stock, cumin, coriander, black pepper, and salt. Bring to simmer*
4. *Cook for 1 hour on low heat under closed lid. If using chicken or turkey, cook for 10 minutes*
5. *Add celery, carrots, and squash. Simmer for additional 40 minutes. If using chicken or turkey, simmer for only for 20 minutes.*
6. *Add tomato paste and stir until dissolved. If stew is too thick, add additional stock or water. Bring to simmer. Cook for 10 minutes on low heat.*
7. *Turn off heat and stir in fresh crushed garlic. Mix well.*

ROASTED BRUSSELS SPROUTS

1½ lbs. or 0.68 kg. fresh Brussels sprouts

3 tablespoons extra virgin coconut oil

3 cloves crushed garlic

1 teaspoon Hymalayan salt

1. *Preheat oven to 400°F or 205°C*
2. *In a mixing bowl combine Brussels sprouts with salt and coconut oil. Coat evenly. If coconut oil is solid, dissolve on stove top to make it easier to combine*
3. *Roast in a preheated oven for 30 min*
4. *Stir every 5 minutes for even roasting*
5. *Add garlic to roasted Brussels sprouts. Coat evenly*
6. *Return to the oven and roast for 5 additional minutes. Stir before serving*

If you desire softer consistency, roast for additional 5 minutes or until the desired consistency is achieved. Keep in mind, the longer you cook, the further you break down the fiber

GRAIN-FREE-GLUTEN-FREE-WHEAT-FREE-CHEESE-FREE PIZZA

The crust is unfortunately not light or fluffy, but tastes almost like pizza, except this pizza is not toxic.

1 head of cauliflower

2 eggs

2 cloves crushed garlic

½ teaspoon dried oregano

½ teaspoon dried basil

½ cup coconut flour or ½ cup bean flour

Salt to taste

1. *Cut your entire cauliflower head including stem into medium size florets*
2. *Using food processor rice or pulse the pre-cut florets and stem pieces into fine crumbles. Do not cream. If you don't have food processor, use the large hole size on your cheese grater.*
3. *Place cauliflower crumbs in a microwavable dish and cook in a microwave for 6-7 minutes.*
4. *Using a cheese cloth or thin towel squeeze moisture out the of the cooked cauliflower crumbles*
5. *Transfer back into the bowl and add all of the crust ingredients. Mix well. Divide into four portions*
6. *Flatten the ingredients to the desired thickness on baking sheet or cookie sheet lined with parchment paper that is lightly oiled until evenly flat. You should end up with four 7" round crusts. Brush olive oil on top of crust.*
7. *Bake at 400°F or 205°C for 20-25 min or until golden brown*
8. *Let cool for 15 minutes*
9. *Apply sauce or toppings of your choice such as roasted vegetables and/or pizza sauce as in the recipe below*

QUICK AND EASY NO COOK PIZZA SAUCE

1 16 oz. (473 ml.) can crushed tomatoes

1 6 oz. (178 ml.) can tomato paste

1 tablespoon fresh minced garlic or use garlic press

1 teaspoon dried oregano leaves

1 teaspoon dried basil leaves

½ teaspoon pepper flakes or to taste

Salt to taste

Water

1. *Combine all ingredients and mix well*

2. *Add water for desired consistency*

MARINATED MUSHROOMS – THE OLD WORLD RECIPE

24 oz.-680 grams common button mushrooms or 24 oz. large common mushrooms quartered
2 cups water
4 cloves garlic crushed in garlic press
4 whole bay leaves
4 tablespoons distilled white vinegar
1 teaspoon whole peppercorn
1 tablespoon Himalayan salt

1. *Add water, peppercorns, bay leaves, and salt to a medium size pot. Bring to boil*
2. *Add vinegar and return to boil*
3. *Add mushrooms. Do not be concerned if water is not covering mushrooms. Return to boil*
4. *Boil on high setting for 1 minute*
5. *Add garlic, stir well, and remove from heat*
6. *Let cool before transferring into glass jar*
7. *Make certain that when mushrooms are transferred into the jar, they are fully covered by the liquid that they were cooked in*
8. *Marinade in the refrigerator overnight*
9. *Serve cold*

SPICY QUINOA MEATBALLS IN GINGER TOMATO SAUCE

1 lb. ground beef or ground chicken, or any organic meat you prefer
2 tablespoons quinoa whole
3 tablespoons quinoa ground (you can grind it in a basic coffee grinder)
1 egg
1/2 cup chopped parsley or cilantro
1 minced onion
1 tablespoon minced ginger
1 tablespoon minced garlic
1/2 teaspoon cumin powder
1/2 teaspoon coriander powder
1 tablespoon olive oil
Salt to taste
Cayenne pepper to taste

SAUCE:

1/2 tablespoon coconut oil
1 large finely chopped onion
1½ tablespoons ginger
1 tablespoon minced garlic
20 oz. of crushed tomatoes or 12 oz. tomato paste diluted in water to thick consistency
1 teaspoon cumin powder

1 tablespoon coriander powder

Additional water to adjust the thickness of the sauce

Salt to taste

Cayenne pepper to taste

1. *Mix all of the meat ingredient together in a large bowl including oil and quinoa.*
2. *Roll into balls and place them on oiled baking tray or parchment paper*
3. *Bake for 30-35 min. in 350°F or 177°C preheated oven. Let rest for 15 minutes*

Sauce and final dish preparation process:

1. *Sauté onions in coconut oil until golden brown*
2. *Add ginger and garlic and cook for 1 minute*
3. *Add spices and crushed tomatoes or tomato paste mixture; bring to very slow boil, and simmer for 10 minutes. If the sauce is too thick, add water to thin it out*
4. *Add meatballs to tomato sauce and simmer for another 15 minutes. Turn off the burner, and let meatballs sit in the sauce for at least 15 min before serving. That way, they will absorb more sauce*

EGGPLANT DIP

3 medium common eggplants or 3 large Chinese eggplants

1 cup walnuts

1 or 2 slices of raw red beet for color; add more if you prefer more intense color

4 cloves garlic

1 tablespoon and 1 teaspoon of white vinegar

¼ cup extra virgin olive oil

1 teaspoon Himalayan salt

¼ teaspoon ground black pepper

¼ bunch parsley chopped

1. *Bake eggplants 30 to 40 min. or until soft in 350°F or 177°C preheated oven. Let cool for 20 minutes*
2. *Cut cooled eggplants into chunks*
3. *Place all of the ingredients into food processor leaving parsley out*
4. *Process until the mixture is smooth or semi-smooth in accordance with your taste*
5. *If the mixture is too thick for your taste, add a tablespoon or two of chilled boiled water or until the dip reaches desired consistency*
6. *Process until the mixture is even*
7. *Transfer into serving dish and garnish with chopped parsley*

INDIAN OR ITALIAN STYLE QUINOA MEATBALLS IN TOMATO SAUCE

Indian: *Use the same recipe as above and just add 1 teaspoon of garam masala Indian spice to the meat and 2 teaspoons to the sauce.*

Italian: *Substitute ginger, cumin, and coriander with ½ teaspoon dried basil leaves and ½ teaspoon dried oregano in meat, and 1 teaspoon dried basil leaves and 1 teaspoon dried oregano in sauce*

SAUERKRAUT WITH OR WITHOUT FERMENTED VEGETABLES

If you don't feel like making it yourself, several small companies are producing "boutique" raw sauerkraut in small batches. Just make certain that the package states "Raw and unpasteurized." That way you will be assured that you're getting live probiotic bacteria…. Or you can make a small batch yourself with only two to three ingredients:

1 medium head of cabbage – 3 to 4 lbs.
3 carrots
1 ½-2 tablespoons Himalayan Salt
10 peppercorns (optional)
Large mixing bowl
Large mason jar or cooking pot
Plate that fits snuggly inside the jar
Weight such as 2-3 lbs. dumbbell plate or a heavy stone

1. *Slice cabbage into ribbons and place in a large mixing bowl*
2. *Grate carrots with the large grater; add to the mixing bowl*
3. *Add salt; with time you will be able to adjust the salt amount to your liking*
4. *Work salt into cabbage by squeezing and massaging it with your hands until it releases juice. This step is the most important for fermentation; should take approximately 8-10 minutes to complete this process.*
5. *Mix in the peppercorns; you can also crack peppercorns for more flavor*
6. *(This step is optional) You can also add sliced radishes, carrots, beets, rutabaga, or other hard vegetables to your cabbage and salt mixture. Just make certain to compensate with additional salt as your volume will increase.*
7. *Place your mixture into the mason jar or cooking pot*
8. *Cover with plate face down, and put weight on top of the plate. I recommend using additional plate or even a small bowl to put the weight in. That way, the weight will not come in contact with cabbage juice as it begins to rise.*
9. *Ferment cabbage for 4 days at room temperature at approximately 70°F or 21°C. If after 4 days you believe that sauerkraut is not ready, let ferment for another 1 to 2 days. During the fermentation period you will observe bubbles and bubble foam that are rising to the top; it's absolutely normal. What that means is that fermentation process is working.*
10. *Transfer sauerkraut and juice into jars with lids and place in the refrigerator. It will continue to ferment and will actually taste better with time. Because it's fermented, it can stay in the fridge as long as two months.*

By the way, the fermented cabbage juice is one of the most potent probiotic carriers, so don't pour it out; use it as salad dressing. Just make certain that you don't use too much as it is high in sodium.

EASY KIMCHEE

Although traditional Korean kimchee requires multitude of steps and ingredients that include sugar, the following is a simplified recipe. Thus, follow the same procedure as above for the exception of the following:
Use 1 medium size Napa or Bok Choi cabbage *cabbage head instead of regular cabbage*
Substitute peppercorns with 1 tablespoon of dried pepper flakes and/or 1 teaspoon of cayenne pepper.
2 cloves garlic pushed through garlic press
1 teaspoon finely minced ginger

Mix kimchee on the second day of the fermentation process
Place the plate back on top of the kimchi and apply weight for additional two days

PICKLES

Medium size glass container or a jar

Small or medium pickling cucumbers; purchase enough to fill a glass or porcelain jar where you will be fermenting cucumbers

Fresh filtered water

4 cloves garlic pushed through garlic press

½ bunch dill weed coarsely chopped (optional)

3 bay leaves

1 teaspoon peppercorns

½-1 tablespoon Himalayan salt per one cup of water (adjust to taste as you see fit)

½ teaspoon coriander seeds

Salt to taste

1. *Prepare brine by combining water with all of the ingredients as listed above except for dill.*
2. *Put cucumbers in the pickling jar making certain to place pieces of dill weed in-between cucumber layers. Note: You may also put few sliced carrots, cauliflower florets, string beans, mushroom, ginger, and even cherry tomatoes. Just make certain that you keep all vegetables within the volume of the pickling jar. If you wish to have larger yield of pickled vegetables and cucumbers, double the brine recipe.*
3. *Pour your prepared brine over cucumbers to fully cover them. If not completely covered by brine, place a small ramekin on top and poor brine into ramekin as additional weight.*
4. *Cover with lid, but make certain that no air tight seal was created.*
5. *Ferment for a minimum of seven days in the refrigerator. If you like a more pronounced taste, ferment for additional seven or more days.*

ZUCCHINI AND YELLOW SQUASH FRIES

2 zucchini

2 yellow squash

1 cup bean flour (you can purchase bean flour or use food processor or spice grinder to achieve similar results)

2 eggs

2 cloves finely chopped garlic

1 teaspoon salt or to taste

Salt in a shaker for garnish

1 teaspoon black pepper

1 teaspoon paprika

½ teaspoon cayenne pepper

1. *Combine bean flour, salt, paprika, black pepper, and cayenne pepper in the wide bowl. Mix thoroughly*
2. *Cut zucchini and yellow squash into thick French fries; approximately twice the size of standard French fries.*
3. *Whisk eggs and chopped garlic in a separate bowl*
4. *Dip 5 fries at a time into bean flour mixture*

5. *Dip into egg mixture*
6. *Dip again into bean flour mixture*
7. *Transfer into greased baking sheet;*
8. *Repeat steps 4-7 until completed*
9. *Preheat oven*
10. *Bake for 30-35 min. or until golden brown in 400°F or 204°C*

ADJIKA SPICY DIP – AN OLD GEORGIAN RECIPE

This is a family sized recipe. If you want to make lesser amount, divide all of the ingredients in half.

4 cups walnuts minced
4 cups tomato paste
1 cup boiled water chilled to room temperature
8 cloves garlic crushed in garlic press
½ bunch cilantro minced
1½ cups distilled white vinegar
2 cups extra virgin olive oil
*1 tablespoon cayenne pepper
*1 teaspoon crushed red pepper
*2 jalapeno peppers fresh finely minced
1 teaspoon cumin
1 teaspoon coriander
1½ tablespoon Himalayan salt

8. *Combine all of the ingredients in the mixing bowl*
9. *Mix well until mixture is even*
10. *If the mixture is too thick, add more chilled boiled water until the dip reaches the desired consistency*
11. *If you prefer to have spicier Adjika, add more cayenne and crushed red pepper*
*If you are not a fan of spicy foods, leave out peppers or divide the amount outlined in half

MEDITERRANEAN CHICKPEAS SALAD

1 lb. dry chickpeas
3 large cloves of garlic
1 tablespoon coconut oil for cooking
2 tablespoons extra virgin olive oil for dressing
¼ cup cilantro minced
White vinegar to taste
½ teaspoon ground cumin
½ teaspoon ground coriander
Ground cayenne pepper to taste
Salt to taste

1. *Soak chickpeas in filtered water overnight, i.e. 8+ hours. Make certain that the level of water is 1.5 times higher than dry chickpeas. The next day drain old water and refill the pot with fresh water.*

2. *Add salt to water, bring to a boil and set on low heat. Simmer until chickpeas are soft. May take 40+ minutes depending on the texture that you prefer. Drain when ready, and put aside.*
3. *In an iron skillet sauté cumin and coriander in 1 table spoon of olive oil or coconut oil for 2 minutes.*
4. *Add garlic and sauté for 20 seconds*
5. *Combine chickpeas and the spice mixture you just created*
6. *Add 2 tablespoons of extra virgin olive oil as dressing*
7. *Add ground cayenne pepper to taste*
8. *Add vinegar to taste*
9. *Use potato masher to partially mash the entire dish. Leave at least 25% chickpeas whole for texture.*
10. *Add 1 clove of minced uncooked garlic if you prefer*
11. *Garnish with fresh cilantro*

TROPICAL JICAMA SLAW

2 medium-large jicamas julienned
1 ripe banana mashed
3 tablespoons lemon or lime juice
2 green onions finely chopped
1 tablespoon extra-virgin olive oil
1 tablespoon extra-virgin coconut oil
¼ cup cilantro chopped
Ground cayenne pepper to taste
Salt to taste

1. *Combine banana, lemon/lime juice, coconut and olive oil, cayenne pepper, and salt in a bowl and whisk until smooth*
2. *Add jicama, green onion, and cilantro and mix thoroughly*
3. *Let stand for twenty minutes before serving in order for the lemon juice to get obsorbed*

NOT SO DESSERT - DESSERT TRUFFLES

1 lb. crunchy unsalted almond butter or peanut butter
1 cup dried unsweetened coconut flakes (thinly shredded)
1 cup raw sunflower seeds
1½ ripe bananas mashed
½ teaspoon Himalayan salt
½ cup raw cacao powder

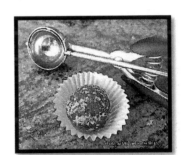

1. *Combine all of the ingredients in a bowl for the exception of raw cacao powder*
2. *Mix well until even consistency is achieved*
3. *Scoop out ingredients using candy size small cookie scoop (approximately 45 portions)*
4. *Form a ball*
5. *Pour raw cacao powder in a separate bowl*
6. *Roll each ball in cacao powder until evenly coated*
7. *Place truffles into small baking cups*

8. *Refrigerate or freeze*

EASY TOOTHPASTE

½ cup baking soda

5 tablespoons xylitol

2 teaspoons peppermint extract

4 tablespoons or ¼ cup coconut oil

*You may also double the ingredients for larger amount of toothpaste

1. *Combine all ingredients in the stainless steel bowl*
2. *Mix thoroughly until all ingredients are blended and toothpaste is formed*
   The mixing process may take as long as three minutes

APPENDIX 1

OTHER CAUSES OF HYPOGLYCEMIA

According to Mayo Clinic, non-diabetic hypoglycemia can also be caused by excessive alcohol consumption, kidney disorder, pancreatic tumor, anorexia, fasting, etc. In addition, people who had gastric bypass surgery may suffer from post-meal hypoglycemia.[1469]

APPENDIX I

Vitamins – Function, Sources, and Solubility. Obtained from MedlinePlus, a service for the U.S. National Library of Medicine, National Institutes of Health (NIH) http://www.nlm.nih.gov/medlineplus/ency/article/002399.htm.[1470] The text in the publication as described above was arranged into a chart form below:

Name	Function	Food Sources	Fat/Water Soluble
Vitamin A	Helps form and maintain healthy teeth, bones, soft tissue, mucus membranes, and skin	•Dark-colored fruit •Dark leafy vegetables •Egg yolk •Fortified milk and dairy products (cheese, yogurt, butter, and cream) •Liver, beef, and fish	Fat Soluble
Vitamin B6	Also called pyridoxine. Vitamin B6 helps form red blood cells and maintain brain function. This vitamin also plays an important role in the proteins that are part of many chemical reactions in the	•Avocado •Banana •Legumes (dried beans) •Meat •Nuts •Poultry	Water Soluble

	body. Eating larger amounts of protein may reduce Vitamin B6 levels in the body.	•Whole grains (milling and processing removes a lot of this Vitamin)	
Vitamin B12	Like the other B Vitamins, is important for metabolism. It also helps form red blood cells and maintain the central nervous system.	•Meat •Eggs •Fortified foods such as soymilk •Milk and milk products •Organ meats (liver and kidney) •Poultry •Shellfish	Water Soluble
Vitamin C	Also called ascorbic acid, is an antioxidant that promotes healthy teeth and gums. It helps the body absorb iron and maintain healthy tissue. It also promotes wound healing.	•Bell Peppers •Broccoli •Brussels sprouts •Cabbage •Cauliflower •Citrus fruits •Potatoes •Spinach •Strawberries •Tomato juice •Tomatoes	Water Soluble
Vitamin D	Also known as the "sunshine Vitamin", since it is made by the body after being in the sun. Ten to 15 minutes of sunshine three times a week is enough to produce the body's requirement of Vitamin D. People who do not live in sunny places may not make enough Vitamin D. It is very difficult to get enough Vitamin D from food sources alone. Vitamin D helps the body absorb calcium, which you need for normal development and maintenance of healthy teeth and bones. It also helps maintain proper blood levels of calcium and phosphorus.	•Fish (fatty fish such as salmon, mackerel, herring, and orange roughy) •Fish liver oils (cod's liver oil) •Fortified cereals •Fortified milk and dairy products (cheese, yogurt, butter, and cream)	Fat Soluble
Vitamin E	An antioxidant also known as tocopherol. It plays a role in the formation of red blood cells and helps the body use Vitamin K.	•Avocado •Dark green vegetables (spinach, broccoli, asparagus, turnip greens) •Oils (safflower, corn, and sunflower) •Papaya and mango •Seeds and nuts	Fat Soluble

		•Wheat germ and wheat germ oil	
Vitamin K	Not listed among the essential Vitamins, but without it blood would not stick together (coagulate). Some studies suggest that it is important for promoting bone health.	•Cabbage •Cauliflower •Cereals •Dark green vegetables (broccoli, Brussels sprouts, asparagus) •Dark leafy vegetables (spinach, kale, collards, turnip greens) •Fish, liver, beef, eggs	Fat Soluble
Biotin (Vitamin B7)	Essential for the metabolism of proteins and carbohydrates, and in the production of hormones and cholesterol. Also for hair and nails health.	•Chocolate •Cereal •Egg yolk •Legumes •Milk •Nuts •Organ meats (liver, kidney) •Pork •Yeast	Water Soluble
Niacin (Vitamin B3)	B Vitamin that helps maintain healthy skin and nerves. It also has cholesterol-lowering effects.	•Avocado •Eggs •Enriched breads and fortified cereals •Fish (tuna and salt-water fish) •Lean meats •Legumes •Nuts •Potato •Poultry	Water Soluble
Folate (Vitamin B9)	Works with Vitamin B12 to help form red blood cells. It is needed for the production of DNA, which controls tissue growth and cell function. Any woman who is pregnant should be sure to get enough folate. Low levels of folate are linked to birth defects such as spinabifida. Many foods are now fortified with folic acid.	•Asparagus and broccoli •Beets •Brewer's yeast •Dried beans (cooked pinto, navy, kidney, and lima) •Fortified cereals •Green, leafy vegetables (spinach and romaine lettuce) •Lentils •Oranges and orange juice •Peanut butter •Wheat germ	Water Soluble

Pantothenic acid (Vitamin B5)	Essential for the metabolism of food. It is also plays a role in the production of hormones and cholesterol.	•Avocado •Broccoli, kale, and other vegetables in the cabbage family •Eggs •Legumes and lentils •Milk •Mushroom •Organ meats •Poultry •White and sweet potatoes •Whole-grain cereals	Water Soluble
Riboflavin (Vitamin B2)	(Vitamin B2) works with the other B Vitamins. It is important for body growth and the production of red blood cells.	•Dairy products •Eggs •Green leafy vegetables •Lean meats •Legumes •Milk •Nuts	Water Soluble
Thiamine (Vitamin B1)	Helps the body cells change carbohydrates into energy. Getting plenty of carbohydrates is very important during pregnancy and breast-feeding. It is also essential for heart function and healthy nerve cells.	•Avocado •Banana •Legumes (dried beans) •Meat •Nuts •Poultry •Whole grains (milling and processing removes a lot of this Vitamin)	Water Soluble

APPENDIX II

ACE inhibitors by name
Obtained from the U.S. Food and Drug Administration[1471]

Lisinopril (Prinivil, Zestril)
Ramipril (Altace)
Enalapril (Vasotec, Epaned)
Benazepril (Lotensin)
Captopril (Capoten)
Trandolapril (Mavik)
Moexipril (Univasc)
Quinapril (Accupril)
Enalapril (Vasotec, Epaned)
Fosinopril (Monopril)
Perindopril (Aceon)

APPENDIX III

Beta blockers by name
Obtained from U.S. Food and Drug Administration[1472]

Atenolol (Tenormin)
Metoprolol (Lopressor, Toprol XL)
Propranolol (Hemangeol, Inderal LA, Inderal XL, InnoPran XL)
Nadolol (Corgard)
Esmolol (Brevibloc)
Betaxolol (Kerlone)
Carvedilol (Coreg)
Nebivolol (Bystolic)
Penbutolol (Levatol)
Sotalol (Betapace, Sorine)
Acebutolol (Sectral)
Betaxolol
Bisoprolol fumarate (ZIAC)

APPENDIX IV

Defining the term natural flavor or natural flavoring

The quote below was obtained from
http://www.accessdata.fda.gov/scripts/cdrh/cfdocs/cfcfr/cfrsearch.cfm?fr=101.22
[Code of Federal Regulations]
[Title 21, Volume 2]
[Revised as of April 1, 2014]
[CITE: 21CFR101.22]
TITLE 21--FOOD AND DRUGS
CHAPTER I--FOOD AND DRUG ADMINISTRATION
DEPARTMENT OF HEALTH AND HUMAN SERVICES
SUBCHAPTER B--FOOD FOR HUMAN CONSUMPTION

"(3) The term natural flavor or natural flavoring means the essential oil, oleoresin, essence or extractive, protein hydrolysate, distillate, or any product of roasting, heating or enzymolysis, which contains the flavoring constituents derived from a spice, fruit or fruit juice, vegetable or vegetable juice, edible yeast, herb, bark, bud, root, leaf or similar plant material, meat, seafood, poultry, eggs, dairy products, or fermentation products thereof, whose significant function in food is flavoring rather than nutritional. Natural flavors include the natural essence or extractives obtained from plants listed in 182.10, 182.20, 182.40, and 182.50 and part 184 of this chapter, and the substances listed in 172.510 of this chapter" (FDA, 2014).[1473]

APPENDIX A

Code of Federal Regulations - 172.510 Natural flavoring substances and natural substances used in conjunction with flavors - 21CFR172.510. [1474] Obtained from
http://www.accessdata.fda.gov/scripts/cdrh/cfdocs/cfcfr/CFRSearch.cfm?fr=172.510

[Code of Federal Regulations]
[Title 21, Volume 3]
[Revised as of April 1, 2013]
[CITE: 21CFR172.510]

TITLE 21--FOOD AND DRUGS
CHAPTER I--FOOD AND DRUG ADMINISTRATION
DEPARTMENT OF HEALTH AND HUMAN SERVICES
SUBCHAPTER B--FOOD FOR HUMAN CONSUMPTION (CONTINUED)

PART 172 -- FOOD ADDITIVES PERMITTED FOR DIRECT ADDITION TO FOOD FOR HUMAN CONSUMPTION

Subpart F--Flavoring Agents and Related Substances

Sec. 172.510 Natural flavoring substances and natural substances used in conjunction with flavors.

Natural flavoring substances and natural adjuvants may be safely used in food in accordance with the following conditions.

(a) They are used in the minimum quantity required to produce their intended physical or technical effect and in accordance with all the principles of good manufacturing practice.

(b) In the appropriate forms (plant parts, fluid and solid extracts, concentrates, absolutes, oils, gums, balsams, resins, oleoresins, waxes, and distillates) they consist of one or more of the following, used alone or in combination with flavoring substances and adjuvants generally recognized as safe in food, previously sanctioned for such use, or regulated in any section of this part.

Common name	Scientific name
Aloe	*Aloe perryi*Baker,*A. barbadensis*Mill.,*A. ferox*Mill., and hybrids of this sp. with*A. africana*Mill. and*A. spicata*Baker
Althea root and flowers	*Althea officinalis*L
Amyris (West Indian sandalwood)	*Amyris balsamifera*L
Angola weed	*Roccella fuciformis*Ach
Arnica flowers	*Arnica montana*L.,*A. fulgens*Pursh,*A. sororia*Greene, or*A. cordifolia*Hooker
Artemisia (wormwood)	*Artemisia*spp
Artichoke leaves	*Cynara scolymus*L
Benzoin resin	*Styrax benzoin*Dryander,*S. paralleloneurus*Perkins,*S. tonkinensis*(Pierre) Craib ex Hartwich, or other spp. of the Section *Anthostyrax*of the genus *Styrax*
Blackberry bark	*Rubus,*Section *Eubatus*
Boldus (boldo) leaves	*Peumus boldus* Mol

Boronia flowers	*Boronia megastigma* Nees
Bryonia root	*Bryonia alba* L., or *B. Diocia* Jacq
Buchu leaves	*Barosma betulina* Bartl. et Wendl., *B. crenulata* (L.) Hook. or *B. serratifolia* Willd
Buckbean leaves	*Menyanthes trifoliata* L
Cajeput	*Melaleuca leucadendron* L. and other *Melaleuca* spp
Calumba root	*Jateorhiza palmata* (Lam.) Miers
Camphor tree	*Cinnamomum camphora* (L.) Nees et Eberm
Cascara sagrada	*Rhamnus purshiana* DC
Cassie flowers	*Acacia farnesiana* (L.) Willd
Castor oil	*Ricinus communis* L
Catechu, black	*Acacia catechu* Willd
Cedar, white (aborvitae), leaves and twigs	*Thuja occidentalis* L
Centuary	*Centaurium umbellatum* Gilib
Cherry pits	*Prunus avium* L. or *P. cerasus* L
Cherry-laurel leaves	*Prunus laurocerasus* L
Chestnut leaves	*Castanea dentata* (Marsh.) Borkh
Chirata	*Swertia chirata* Buch.-Ham
Cinchona, red, bark	*Cinchona succirubra* Pav. or its hybrids
Cinchona, yellow, bark	*Cinchona ledgeriana* Moens, *C. calisaya* Wedd., or hybrids of these with other spp. of *Cinchona.*
Copaiba	South American spp. of *Copaifera* L
Cork, oak	*Quercus suber* L., or *Q. occidentalis* F. Gay
Costmary	*Chrysanthemum balsamita* L
Costus root	*Saussurea lappa* Clarke
Cubeb	*Piper cubeba* L. f
Currant, black, buds and leaves	*Ribes nigrum* L
Damiana leaves	*Turnera diffusa* Willd
Davana	*Artemisia pallens* Wall
Dill, Indian	*Anethum sowa* Roxb. (*Peucedanum graveolens* Benth et Hook., *Anethum graveolens* L.)
Dittany (fraxinella) roots	*Dictamnus albus* L
Dittany of Crete	*Origanum dictamnus* L
Dragon's blood (dracorubin)	*Daemonorops* spp
Elder tree leaves	*Sambucus nigra* L
Elecampane rhizome and roots	*Inula helenium* L
Elemi	*Canarium commune* L. or *C. luzonicum* Miq

Erigeron	*Erigeron canadensis*L
Eucalyptus globulus leaves	*Eucalyptus globulus*Labill
Fir ("pine") needles and twigs	*Abies sibirica*Ledeb.,*A. alba*Mill.,*A. sachalinesis*Masters or*A. mayriana*Miyabe et Kudo
Fir, balsam, needles and twigs	*Abies balsamea*(L.) Mill
Galanga, greater	*Alpinia galanga*Willd
Galbanum	*Ferula galbaniflua*Boiss. et Buhse and other*Ferula*spp
Gambir (catechu, pale)	*Uncaria gambir*Roxb
Genet flowers	*Spartium junceum*L
Gentian rhizome and roots	*Gentiana lutea*L
Gentian, stemless	*Gentiana acaulis*L
Germander, chamaedrys	*Teucrium chamaedrys*L
Germander, golden	*Teucrium polium*L
Guaiac	*Guaiacum officinale*L.,*G. santum*L.,*Bulnesia sarmienti*Lor
Guarana	*Paullinia cupana*HBK
Haw, black, bark	*Viburnum prunifolium*L
Hemlock needles and twigs	*Tsuga canadensis*(L.) Carr. or*T. heterophylla*(Raf.) Sarg
Hyacinth flowers	*Hyacinthus orientalis*L
Iceland moss	*Cetraria islandica*Ach
Imperatoria	*Peucedanum ostruthium*(L.). Koch (*Imperatoria ostruthium*L.)
Iva	*Achillea moschata*Jacq
Labdanum	*Cistus*spp
Lemon-verbena	*Lippia citriodora*HBK
Linaloe wood	*Bursera delpechiana*Poiss. and other*Bursera*spp
Linden leaves	*Tillia*spp
Lovage	*Levisticum officinale*Koch
Lungmoss (lungwort)	*Sticta pulmonacea*Ach
Maidenhair fern	*Adiantum capillus-veneris*L
Maple, mountain	*Acer spicatum*Lam
Mimosa (black wattle) flowers	*Acacia decurrens*Willd. var.*dealbata*
Mullein flowers	*Verbascum phlomoides*L. or*V. thapsiforme*Schrad
Myrrh	*Commiphora molmol*Engl.,*C. abyssinica*(Berg) Engl., or other*Commiphora*spp
Myrtle leaves	*Myrtus communis*L
Oak, English, wood	*Quercus robur*L
Oak, white, chips	*Quercus alba*L

Oak moss	*Evernia prunastri*(L.) Ach.,*E. furfuracea*(L.) Mann, and other lichens
Olibanum	*Boswellia carteri*Birdw. and other*Boswellia*spp
Opopanax (bisabolmyrrh)	*Opopanax chironium*Koch (true opopanax) of*Commiphora erythraea*Engl. var.*Llabrescens*
Orris root	*Iris germanica*L. (including its variety*florentina*Dykes) and*I. pallida*Lam
Pansy	*Viola tricolor*L
Passion flower	*Passiflora incarnata*L
Patchouly	*Pogostemon cablin*Benth. and*P. heyneanus*Benth
Peach leaves	*Prunus persica*(L.) Batsch
Pennyroyal, American	*Hedeoma pulegioides*(L.) Pers
Pennyroyal, European	*Mentha pulegium*L
Pine, dwarf, needles and twigs	*Pinus mugo*Turra var.*pumilio*(Haenke) Zenari
Pine, Scotch, needles and twigs	*Pinus sylvestris*L
Pine, white, bark	*Pinus strobus*L
Pine, white oil	*Pinus palustris*Mill., and other*Pinus*spp
Poplar buds	*Populus balsamifera*L. (*P. tacamahacca*Mill.),*P. candicans*Ait., or*P. nigra*L
Quassia	*Picrasma excelsa*(Sw.) Planch, or*Quassia amara*L
Quebracho bark	*Aspidosperma quebracho-blanco*Schlecht, or (*Quebrachia lorentzii*(Griseb))
Quillaia (soapbark)	*Quillaja saponaria*Mol
Red saunders (red sandalwood)	*Pterocarpus san alinus*L
Rhatany root	*Krameria triandra*Ruiz et Pav. or*K. argentea*Mart
Rhubarb, garden root	*Rheum rhaponticum*L
Rhubarb root	*Rheum officinale*Baill.,*R. palmatum*L., or other spp. (excepting*R. rhaponticum*L.) or hybrids of*Rheum*grown in China
Roselle	*Hibiscus sabdariffa*L
Rosin (colophony)	*Pinus palustris*Mill., and other*Pinus*spp
St. Johnswort leaves, flowers, and caulis	*Hypericum perforatum*L
Sandalwood, white (yellow, or East Indian)	*Santalum album*L
Sandarac	*Tetraclinis articulata*(Vahl.), Mast
Sarsaparilla	*Smilax aristolochiaefolia*Mill., (Mexican sarsaparilla),*S. regelii*Killip et Morton (Honduras sarsaparilla),*S. febrifuga*Kunth (Ecuadorean sarsaparilla), or undetermined*Smilax*spp. (Ecuadorean or Central American sarsaparilla)
Sassafras leaves	*Sassafras albidum*(Nutt.) Nees
Senna, Alexandria	*Cassia acutifolia*Delile

Serpentaria (Virginia snakeroot)	*Aristolochia serpentaria*L
Simaruba bark	*Simaruba amara*Aubl
Snakeroot, Canadian (wild ginger)	*Asarum canadense*L
Spruce needles and twigs	*Picea glauca*(Moench) Voss or*P. mariana*(Mill.) BSP
Storax (styrax)	*Liquidambar orientalis*Mill. or*L. styraciflua*L
Tagetes (marigold)	*Tagetes patula*L.,*T. erecta*L., or*T. minuta*L. (*T. glandulifera*Schrank)
Tansy	*Tanacetum vulgare*L
Thistle, blessed (holy thistle)	*Onicus benedictus*L
Thymus capitatus(Spanish "origanum")	*Thymus capitatus*Hoffmg. et Link
Tolu	*Myroxylon balsamum*(L.) Harms
Turpentine	*Pinus palustris*Mill. and other*Pinus*spp. which yield terpene oils exclusively
Valerian rhizome and roots	*Valeriana officinalis*L
Veronica	*Veronica officinalis*L
Vervain, European	*Verbena officinalis*L
Vetiver	*Vetiveria zizanioides*Stapf
Violet, Swiss	*Viola calcarata*L
Walnut husks (hulls), leaves, and green nuts	*Juglans nigra*L. or*J. regia*L
Woodruff, sweet	*Asperula odorata*L
Yarrow	*Achillea millefolium*L
Yerba santa	*Eriodictyon californicum*(Hook, et Arn.) Torr
Yucca, Joshua-tree	*Yucca brevifolia*Engelm
Yucca, Mohave	*Yucca schidigera*Roezl ex Ortgies (*Y. mohavensis*Sarg.)

[1]As determined by using the method (or, in other than alcoholic beverages, a suitable adaptation thereof) in section 9.129 of the "Official Methods of Analysis of the Association of Official Analytical Chemists", 13th Ed. (1980), which is incorporated by reference. Copies may be obtained from the AOAC INTERNATIONAL, 481 North Frederick Ave., suite 500, Gaithersburg, MD 20877, or may be examined at the National Archives and Records Administration (NARA). For information on the availability of this material at NARA, call 202-741-6030, or go to:*http://www.archives.gov/federal_register/code_of_federal_regulations/ibr_locations.html*.

[42 FR 14491, Mar. 15, 1977, as amended at 43 FR 14644, Apr. 7, 1978; 49 FR 10104, Mar. 19, 1984; 54 FR 24897, June 12, 1989; 69 FR 24511, May 4, 2004; 72 FR 10357, Mar. 8, 2007]

APPENDIX B

Code of Federal Regulations - Sec. 182.10 Spices and other natural seasonings and flavorings - 21CFR182.10.[1475] Obtained from

http://www.accessdata.fda.gov/scripts/cdrh/cfdocs/cfcfr/CFRSearch.cfm?fr=182.10

```
[Code of Federal Regulations]
[Title 21, Volume 3]
[Revised as of April 1, 2013]
[CITE: 21CFR182.10]
```

TITLE 21--FOOD AND DRUGS
CHAPTER I--FOOD AND DRUG ADMINISTRATION
DEPARTMENT OF HEALTH AND HUMAN SERVICES
SUBCHAPTER B--FOOD FOR HUMAN CONSUMPTION (CONTINUED)

PART 182 -- SUBSTANCES GENERALLY RECOGNIZED AS SAFE

Subpart A--General Provisions

Sec. 182.10 Spices and other natural seasonings and flavorings.

Spices and other natural seasonings and flavorings that are generally recognized as safe for their intended use, within the meaning of section 409 of the Act, are as follows:

Common name	Botanical name of plant source
Alfalfa herb and seed	Medicago sativa L.
Allspice	Pimenta officinalis Lindl.
Ambrette seed	Hibiscus abelmoschus L.
Angelica	Angelica archangelica L. or other spp. of Angelica.
Angelica root	Do.
Angelica seed	Do.
Angostura (cusparia bark)	Galipea officinalis Hancock.
Anise	Pimpinella anisum L.
Anise, star	Illicium verum Hook. f.
Balm (lemon balm)	Melissa officinalis L.
Basil, bush	Ocimum minimum L.
Basil, sweet	Ocimum basilicum L.
Bay	Laurus nobilis L.
Calendula	Calendula officinalis L.
Camomile (chamomile), English or Roman	Anthemis nobilis L.
Camomile (chamomile), German or Hungarian	Matricaria chamomilla L.
Capers	Capparis spinosa L.

Capsicum	Capsicum frutescens L. or Capsicum annuum L.
Caraway	Carum carvi L.
Caraway, black (black cumin)	Nigella sativa L.
Cardamom (cardamon)	Elettaria cardamomum Maton.
Cassia, Chinese	Cinnamomum cassia Blume.
Cassia, Padang or Batavia	Cinnamomum burmanni Blume.
Cassia, Saigon	Cinnamomum loureirii Nees.
Cayenne pepper	Capsicum frutescens L. or Capsicum annuum L.
Celery seed	Apium graveolens L.
Chervil	Anthriscus cerefolium (L.) Hoffm.
Chives	Allium schoenoprasum L.
Cinnamon, Ceylon	Cinnamomum zeylanicum Nees.
Cinnamon, Chinese	Cinnamomum cassia Blume.
Cinnamon, Saigon	Cinnamomum loureirii Nees.
Clary (clary sage)	Salvia sclarea L.
Clover	Trifolium spp.
Coriander	Coriandrum sativum L.
Cumin (cummin)	Cuminum cyminum L.
Cumin, black (black caraway)	Nigella sativa L.
Elder flowers	Sambucus canadensis L.
Fennel, common	Foeniculum vulgare Mill.
Fennel, sweet (finocchio, Florence fennel)	Foeniculum vulgare Mill. var. duice (DC.) Alex.
Fenugreek	Trigonella foenum-graecum L.
Galanga (galangal)	Alpinia officinarum Hance.
Geranium	Pelargonium spp.
Ginger	Zingiber officinale Rosc.
Grains of paradise	Amomum melegueta Rosc.
Horehound (hoarhound)	Marrubium vulgare L.
Horseradish	Armoracia lapathifolia Gilib.
Hyssop	Hyssopus officinalis L.
Lavender	Lavandula officinalis Chaix.
Linden flowers	Tilia spp.
Mace	Myristica fragrans Houtt.
Marigold, pot	Calendula officinalis L.
Marjoram, pot	Majorana onites (L.) Benth.
Marjoram, sweet	Majorana hortensis Moench.
Mustard, black or brown	Brassica nigra (L.) Koch.
Mustard, brown	Brassica juncea (L.) Coss.
Mustard, white or yellow	Brassica hirta Moench.
Nutmeg	Myristica fragrans Houtt.

Oregano (oreganum, Mexican oregano, Mexican sage, origan)	Lippia spp.
Paprika	Capsicum annuum L.
Parsley	Petroselinum crispum (Mill.) Mansf.
Pepper, black	Piper nigrum L.
Pepper, cayenne	Capsicum frutescens L. or Capsicum annuum L.
Pepper, red	
Pepper, white	Piper nigrum L.
Peppermint	Mentha piperita L.
Poppy seed	Papayer somniferum L.
Pot marigold	Calendula officinalis L.
Pot marjoram	Majorana onites (L.) Benth.
Rosemary	Rosmarinus officinalis L.
Saffron	Crocus sativus L.
Sage	Salvia officinalis L.
Sage, Greek	Salvia triloba L.
Savory, summer	Satureia hortensis L. (Satureja).
Savory, winter	Satureia montana L. (Satureja).
Sesame	Sesamum indicum L.
Spearmint	Mentha spicata L.
Star anise	Illicium verum Hook. f.
Tarragon	Artemisia dracunculus L.
Thyme	Thymus vulgaris L.
Thyme, wild or creeping	Thymus serpyllum L.
Turmeric	Curcuma longa L.
Vanilla	Vanilla planifolia Andr. or Vanilla tahitensis J. W. Moore.
Zedoary	Curcuma zedoaria Rosc.

[42 FR 14640, Mar. 15, 1977, as amended at 43 FR 3705, Jan. 27, 1978; 44 FR 3963, Jan. 19, 1979; 50 FR 21044, May 22, 1985; 61 FR 14246, Apr. 1, 1996]

APPENDIX C

Code of Federal Regulations - Sec. 182.20 Essential oils, oleoresins (solvent-free), and natural extractives (including distillates) - 21CFR182.20.[1476] Obtained from
http://www.accessdata.fda.gov/scripts/cdrh/cfdocs/cfcfr/CFRSearch.cfm?fr=182.20

```
[Code of Federal Regulations]
[Title 21, Volume 3]
[Revised as of April 1, 2013]
[CITE: 21CFR182.20]
```

PART 182 -- SUBSTANCES GENERALLY RECOGNIZED AS SAFE

Subpart A--General Provisions

Sec. 182.20 Essential oils, oleoresins (solvent-free), and natural extractives (including distillates).

Essential oils, oleoresins (solvent-free), and natural extractives (including distillates) that are generally recognized as safe for their intended use, within the meaning of section 409 of the Act, are as follows:

Common name	Botanical name of plant source
Alfalfa	Medicago sativa L.
Allspice	Pimenta officinalis Lindl.
Almond, bitter (free from prussic acid)	Prunus amygdalus Batsch, Prunus armeniaca L., or Prunus persica (L.) Batsch.
Ambrette (seed)	Hibiscus moschatus Moench.
Angelica root	Angelica archangelica L.
Angelica seed	Do.
Angelica stem	Do.
Angostura (cusparia bark)	Galipea officinalis Hancock.
Anise	Pimpinella anisum L.
Asafetida	Ferula assa-foetida L. and related spp. of Ferula.
Balm (lemon balm)	Melissa officinalis L.
Balsam of Peru	Myroxylon pereirae Klotzsch.
Basil	Ocimum basilicum L.
Bay leaves	Laurus nobilis L.
Bay (myrcia oil)	Pimenta racemosa (Mill.) J. W. Moore.
Bergamot (bergamot orange)	Citrus aurantium L. subsp. bergamia Wright et Arn.
Bitter almond (free from prussic acid)	Prunus amygdalus Batsch, Prunus armeniaca L., or Prunus persica (L.) Batsch.
Bois de rose	Aniba rosaeodora Ducke.
Cacao	Theobroma cacao L.
Camomile (chamomile) flowers, Hungarian	Matricaria chamomilla L.
Camomile (chamomile) flowers, Roman or English	Anthemis nobilis L.
Cananga	Cananga odorata Hook. f. and Thoms.
Capsicum	Capsicum frutescens L. and Capsicum annuum L.
Caraway	Carum carvi L.

Cardamom seed (cardamon)	Elettaria cardamomum Maton.
Carob bean	Ceratonia siliqua L.
Carrot	Daucus carota L.
Cascarilla bark	Croton eluteria Benn.
Cassia bark, Chinese	Cinnamomum cassia Blume.
Cassia bark, Padang or Batavia	Cinnamomum burmanni Blume.
Cassia bark, Saigon	Cinnamomum loureirii Nees.
Celery seed	Apium graveolens L.
Cherry, wild, bark	Prunus serotina Ehrh.
Chervil	Anthriscus cerefolium (L.) Hoffm.
Chicory	Cichorium intybus L.
Cinnamon bark, Ceylon	Cinnamomum zeylanicum Nees.
Cinnamon bark, Chinese	Cinnamomum cassia Blume.
Cinnamon bark, Saigon	Cinnamomum loureirii Nees.
Cinnamon leaf, Ceylon	Cinnamomum zeylanicum Nees.
Cinnamon leaf, Chinese	Cinnamomum cassia Blume.
Cinnamon leaf, Saigon	Cinnamomum loureirii Nees.
Citronella	Cymbopogon nardus Rendle.
Citrus peels	Citrus spp.
Clary (clary sage)	Salvia sclarea L.
Clover	Trifolium spp.
Coca (decocainized)	Erythroxylum coca Lam. and other spp. of Erythroxylum.
Coffee	Coffea spp.
Cola nut	Cola acuminata Schott and Endl., and other spp. of Cola.
Coriander	Coriandrum sativum L.
Cumin (cummin)	Cuminum cyminum L.
Curacao orange peel (orange, bitter peel)	Citrus aurantium L.
Cusparia bark	Galipea officinalis Hancock.
Dandelion	Taraxacum officinale Weber and T. laevigatum DC.
Dandelion root	Do.
Dog grass (quackgrass, triticum)	Agropyron repens (L.) Beauv.
Elder flowers	Sambucus canadensis L. and S. nigra I.
Estragole (esdragol, esdragon, tarragon)	Artemisia dracunculus L.
Estragon (tarragon)	Do.
Fennel, sweet	Foeniculum vulgare Mill.
Fenugreek	Trigonella foenum-graecum L.
Galanga (galangal)	Alpinia officinarum Hance.
Geranium	Pelargonium spp.
Geranium, East Indian	Cymbopogon martini Stapf.
Geranium, rose	Pelargonium graveolens L'Her.

Ginger	Zingiber officinale Rosc.
Grapefruit	Citrus paradisi Macf.
Guava	Psidium spp.
Hickory bark	Carya spp.
Horehound (hoarhound)	Marrubium vulgare L.
Hops	Humulus lupulus L.
Horsemint	Monarda punctata L.
Hyssop	Hyssopus officinalis L.
Immortelle	Helichrysum augustifolium DC.
Jasmine	Jasminum officinale L. and other spp. of Jasminum.
Juniper (berries)	Juniperus communis L.
Kola nut	Cola acuminata Schott and Endl., and other spp. of Cola.
Laurel berries	Laurus nobilis L.
Laurel leaves	Laurus spp.
Lavender	Lavandula officinalis Chaix.
Lavender, spike	Lavandula latifolia Vill.
Lavandin	Hybrids between Lavandula officinalis Chaix and Lavandula latifolin Vill.
Lemon	Citrus limon (L.) Burm. f.
Lemon balm (see balm)	
Lemon grass	Cymbopogon citratus DC. and Cymbopogon lexuosus Stapf.
Lemon peel	Citrus limon (L.) Burm. f.
Lime	Citrus aurantifolia Swingle.
Linden flowers	Tilia spp.
Locust bean	Ceratonia siliqua L,
Lupulin	Humulus lupulus L.
Mace	Myristica fragrans Houtt.
Mandarin	Citrus reticulata Blanco.
Marjoram, sweet	Majorana hortensis Moench.
Mate	Ilex paraguariensis St. Hil.
Melissa (see balm)	
Menthol	Mentha spp.
Menthyl acetate	Do.
Molasses (extract)	Saccarum officinarum L.
Mustard	Brassica spp.
Naringin	Citrus paradisi Macf.
Neroli, bigarade	Citrus aurantium L.
Nutmeg	Myristica fragrans Houtt.
Onion	Allium cepa L.
Orange, bitter, flowers	Citrus aurantium L.
Orange, bitter, peel	Do.

Orange leaf	Citrus sinensis (L.) Osbeck.
Orange, sweet	Do.
Orange, sweet, flowers	Do.
Orange, sweet, peel	Do.
Origanum	Origanum spp.
Palmarosa	Cymbopogon martini Stapf.
Paprika	Capsicum annuum L.
Parsley	Petroselinum crispum (Mill.) Mansf.
Pepper, black	Piper nigrum L.
Pepper, white	Do.
Peppermint	Mentha piperita L.
Peruvian balsam	Myroxylon pereirae Klotzsch.
Petitgrain	Citrus aurantium L.
Petitgrain lemon	Citrus limon (L.) Burm. f.
Petitgrain mandarin or tangerine	Citrus reticulata Blanco.
Pimenta	Pimenta officinalis Lindl.
Pimenta leaf	Pimenta officinalis Lindl.
Pipsissewa leaves	Chimaphila umbellata Nutt.
Pomegranate	Punica granatum L.
Prickly ash bark	Xanthoxylum (or Zanthoxylum) Americanum Mill. or Xanthoxylum clava-herculis L.
Rose absolute	Rosa alba L., Rosa centifolia L., Rosa damascena Mill., Rosa gallica L., and vars. of these spp.
Rose (otto of roses, attar of roses)	Do.
Rose buds	Do.
Rose flowers	Do.
Rose fruit (hips)	Do.
Rose geranium	Pelargonium graveolens L'Her.
Rose leaves	Rosa spp.
Rosemary	Rosmarinus officinalis L.
Saffron	Crocus sativus L.
Sage	Salvia officinalis L.
Sage, Greek	Salvia triloba L.
Sage, Spanish	Salvia lavandulaefolia Vahl.
St. John's bread	Ceratonia siliqua L.
Savory, summer	Satureia hortensis L.
Savory, winter	Satureia montana L.
Schinus molle	Schinus molle L.
Sloe berries (blackthorn berries)	Prunus spinosa L.
Spearmint	Mentha spicata L.
Spike lavender	Lavandula latifolia Vill.

Tamarind	Tamarindus indica L.
Tangerine	Citrus reticulata Blanco.
Tarragon	Artemisia dracunculus L.
Tea	Thea sinensis L.
Thyme	Thymus vulgaris L. and Thymus zygis var. gracilis Boiss.
Thyme, white	Do.
Thyme, wild or creeping	Thymus serpyllum L.
Triticum (see dog grass)	
Tuberose	Polianthes tuberosa L.
Turmeric	Curcuma longa L.
Vanilla	Vanilla planifolia Andr. or Vanilla tahitensis J. W. Moore.
Violet flowers	Viola odorata L.
Violet leaves	Do.
Violet leaves absolute	Do.
Wild cherry bark	Prunus serotina Ehrh.
Ylang-ylang	Cananga odorata Hook. f. and Thoms.
Zedoary bark	Curcuma zedoaria Rosc.

[42 FR 14640, Mar. 15, 1977, as amended at 44 FR 3963, Jan. 19, 1979; 47 FR 29953, July 9, 1982; 48 FR 51613, Nov. 10, 1983; 50 FR 21043 and 21044, May 22, 1985]

APPENDIX D

Code of Federal Regulations - Sec. 182.40 Natural extractives (solvent-free) used in conjunction with spices, seasonings, and flavorings - 21CFR182.40.[1477] Obtained from
http://www.accessdata.fda.gov/scripts/cdrh/cfdocs/cfcfr/CFRSearch.cfm?fr=182.40

```
[Code of Federal Regulations]
[Title 21, Volume 3]
[Revised as of April 1, 2013]
[CITE: 21CFR182.40]


                    TITLE 21--FOOD AND DRUGS
            CHAPTER I--FOOD AND DRUG ADMINISTRATION
          DEPARTMENT OF HEALTH AND HUMAN SERVICES
        SUBCHAPTER B--FOOD FOR HUMAN CONSUMPTION (CONTINUED)


PART 182 -- SUBSTANCES GENERALLY RECOGNIZED AS SAFE


Subpart A--General Provisions
```

Sec. 182.40 Natural extractives (solvent-free) used in conjunction with spices, seasonings, and flavorings.

Natural extractives (solvent-free) used in conjunction with spices, seasonings, and flavorings that are generally recognized as safe for their intended use, within the meaning of section 409 of the Act, are as follows:

Common name	Botanical name of plant source
Apricot kernel (persic oil)	Prunus armeniaca L.
Peach kernel (persic oil)	Prunus persica Sieb. et Zucc.
Peanut stearine	Arachis hypogaea L.
Persic oil (see apricot kernel and peach kernel)	
Quince seed	Cydonia oblonga Miller.

[42 FR 14640, Mar. 15, 1977, as amended at 47 FR 47375, Oct. 26, 1982]

APPENDIX E

Code of Federal Regulations - Sec. 182.50 Certain other spices, seasonings, essential oils, oleoresins, and natural extracts - 21CFR182.50.[1478] Obtained from
http://www.accessdata.fda.gov/scripts/cdrh/cfdocs/cfcfr/CFRSearch.cfm?fr=182.50

[Code of Federal Regulations]
[Title 21, Volume 3]
[Revised as of April 1, 2013]
[CITE: 21CFR182.50]

TITLE 21--FOOD AND DRUGS
CHAPTER I--FOOD AND DRUG ADMINISTRATION
DEPARTMENT OF HEALTH AND HUMAN SERVICES
SUBCHAPTER B--FOOD FOR HUMAN CONSUMPTION (CONTINUED)

PART 182 -- SUBSTANCES GENERALLY RECOGNIZED AS SAFE

Subpart A--General Provisions

Sec. 182.50 Certain other spices, seasonings, essential oils, oleoresins, and natural extracts.

Certain other spices, seasonings, essential oils, oleoresins, and natural extracts that are generally recognized as safe for their intended use, within the meaning of section 409 of the Act, are as follows:

Common name	Derivation
Ambergris	Physeter macrocephalus L.
Castoreum	Castor fiber L. and C. canadensis Kuhl.
Civet (zibeth, zibet, zibetum)	Civet cats, Viverra civetta Schreber and Viverra zibetha Schreber.
Cognac oil, white and green	Ethyl oenanthate, so-called.
Musk (Tonquin musk)	Musk deer, Moschus moschiferus L.

APPENDIX F

Code of Federal Regulations - Part 184 Direct Food Substances Affirmed as Generally Recognized as Safe.[1479]

Obtained from http://www.accessdata.fda.gov/scripts/cdrh/cfdocs/cfcfr/CFRSearch.cfm?CFRPart=184

TITLE 21--FOOD AND DRUGS
CHAPTER I--FOOD AND DRUG ADMINISTRATION
DEPARTMENT OF HEALTH AND HUMAN SERVICES
SUBCHAPTER B--FOOD FOR HUMAN CONSUMPTION (CONTINUED)

PART 184   DIRECT FOOD SUBSTANCES AFFIRMED AS GENERALLY RECOGNIZED
AS SAFE

Subpart A--General Provisions
§ 184.1 - Substances added directly to human food affirmed as generally recognized as safe (GRAS).

Subpart B--Listing of Specific Substances Affirmed as GRAS
§ 184.1005 - Acetic acid.
§ 184.1007 - Aconitic acid.
§ 184.1009 - Adipic acid.
§ 184.1011 - Alginic acid.
§ 184.1012 - [alpha]-Amylase enzyme preparation from Bacillus stearothermophilus.
§ 184.1021 - Benzoic acid.
§ 184.1024 - Bromelain.
§ 184.1025 - Caprylic acid.
§ 184.1027 - Mixed carbohydrase and protease enzyme product.
§ 184.1033 - Citric acid.
§ 184.1034 - Catalase (bovine liver).
§ 184.1061 - Lactic acid.
§ 184.1063 - Enzyme-modified lecithin.
§ 184.1065 - Linoleic acid.
§ 184.1069 - Malic acid.
§ 184.1077 - Potassium acid tartrate.
§ 184.1081 - Propionic acid.
§ 184.1090 - Stearic acid.
§ 184.1091 - Succinic acid.
§ 184.1095 - Sulfuric acid.
§ 184.1097 - Tannic acid.
§ 184.1099 - Tartaric acid.
§ 184.1101 - Diacetyl tartaric acid esters of mono- and diglycerides.
§ 184.1115 - Agar-agar.
§ 184.1120 - Brown algae.
§ 184.1121 - Red algae.
§ 184.1133 - Ammonium alginate.
§ 184.1135 - Ammonium bicarbonate.

§ 184.1137 - Ammonium carbonate.
§ 184.1138 - Ammonium chloride.
§ 184.1139 - Ammonium hydroxide.
§ 184.1140 - Ammonium citrate, dibasic.
§ 184.1141a - Ammonium phosphate, monobasic.
§ 184.1141b - Ammonium phosphate, dibasic.
§ 184.1143 - Ammonium sulfate.
§ 184.1148 - Bacterially-derived carbohydrase enzyme preparation.
§ 184.1150 - Bacterially-derived protease enzyme preparation.
§ 184.1155 - Bentonite.
§ 184.1157 - Benzoyl peroxide.
§ 184.1165 - n-Butane and iso-butane.
§ 184.1185 - Calcium acetate.
§ 184.1187 - Calcium alginate.
§ 184.1191 - Calcium carbonate.
§ 184.1193 - Calcium chloride.
§ 184.1195 - Calcium citrate.
§ 184.1199 - Calcium gluconate.
§ 184.1201 - Calcium glycerophosphate.
§ 184.1205 - Calcium hydroxide.
§ 184.1206 - Calcium iodate.
§ 184.1207 - Calcium lactate.
§ 184.1210 - Calcium oxide.
§ 184.1212 - Calcium pantothenate.
§ 184.1221 - Calcium propionate.
§ 184.1229 - Calcium stearate.
§ 184.1230 - Calcium sulfate.
§ 184.1240 - Carbon dioxide.
§ 184.1245 - Beta-carotene.
§ 184.1250 - Cellulase enzyme preparation derived from Trichoderma longibrachiatum.
§ 184.1257 - Clove and its derivatives.
§ 184.1259 - Cocoa butter substitute.
§ 184.1260 - Copper gluconate.
§ 184.1261 - Copper sulfate.
§ 184.1262 - Corn silk and corn silk extract.
§ 184.1265 - Cuprous iodide.
§ 184.1271 - L-Cysteine.
§ 184.1272 - L-Cysteine monohydrochloride.
§ 184.1277 - Dextrin.
§ 184.1278 - Diacetyl.
§ 184.1282 - Dill and its derivatives.
§ 184.1287 - Enzyme-modified fats.
§ 184.1293 - Ethyl alcohol.
§ 184.1295 - Ethyl formate.
§ 184.1296 - Ferric ammonium citrate.
§ 184.1297 - Ferric chloride.
§ 184.1298 - Ferric citrate.
§ 184.1301 - Ferric phosphate.
§ 184.1304 - Ferric pyrophosphate.
§ 184.1307 - Ferric sulfate.
§ 184.1307a - Ferrous ascorbate.
§ 184.1307b - Ferrous carbonate.
§ 184.1307c - Ferrous citrate.
§ 184.1307d - Ferrous fumarate.
§ 184.1308 - Ferrous gluconate.
§ 184.1311 - Ferrous lactate.
§ 184.1315 - Ferrous sulfate.
§ 184.1316 - Ficin.
§ 184.1317 - Garlic and its derivatives.

§ 184.1318 - Glucono delta-lactone.
§ 184.1321 - Corn gluten.
§ 184.1322 - Wheat gluten.
§ 184.1323 - Glyceryl monooleate.
§ 184.1324 - Glyceryl monostearate.
§ 184.1328 - Glyceryl behenate.
§ 184.1329 - Glyceryl palmitostearate.
§ 184.1330 - Acacia (gum arabic).
§ 184.1333 - Gum ghatti.
§ 184.1339 - Guar gum.
§ 184.1343 - Locust (carob) bean gum.
§ 184.1349 - Karaya gum (sterculia gum).
§ 184.1351 - Gum tragacanth.
§ 184.1355 - Helium.
§ 184.1366 - Hydrogen peroxide.
§ 184.1370 - Inositol.
§ 184.1372 - Insoluble glucose isomerase enzyme preparations.
§ 184.1375 - Iron, elemental.
§ 184.1386 - Isopropyl citrate.
§ 184.1387 - Lactase enzyme preparation from Candida pseudotropicalis.
§ 184.1388 - Lactase enzyme preparation from Kluyveromyces lactis.
§ 184.1400 - Lecithin.
§ 184.1408 - Licorice and licorice derivatives.
§ 184.1409 - Ground limestone.
§ 184.1415 - Animal lipase.
§ 184.1420 - Lipase enzyme preparation derived from Rhizopus niveus.
§ 184.1425 - Magnesium carbonate.
§ 184.1426 - Magnesium chloride.
§ 184.1428 - Magnesium hydroxide.
§ 184.1431 - Magnesium oxide.
§ 184.1434 - Magnesium phosphate.
§ 184.1440 - Magnesium stearate.
§ 184.1443 - Magnesium sulfate.
§ 184.1443a - Malt.
§ 184.1444 - Maltodextrin.
§ 184.1445 - Malt syrup (malt extract).
§ 184.1446 - Manganese chloride.
§ 184.1449 - Manganese citrate.
§ 184.1452 - Manganese gluconate.
§ 184.1461 - Manganese sulfate.
§ 184.1472 - Menhaden oil.
§ 184.1490 - Methylparaben.
§ 184.1498 - Microparticulated protein product.
§ 184.1505 - Mono- and diglycerides.
§ 184.1521 - Monosodium phosphate derivatives of mono- and diglycerides.
§ 184.1530 - Niacin.
§ 184.1535 - Niacinamide.
§ 184.1537 - Nickel.
§ 184.1538 - Nisin preparation.
§ 184.1540 - Nitrogen.
§ 184.1545 - Nitrous oxide.
§ 184.1553 - Peptones.
§ 184.1555 - Rapeseed oil.
§ 184.1560 - Ox bile extract.
§ 184.1563 - Ozone.
§ 184.1583 - Pancreatin.
§ 184.1585 - Papain.
§ 184.1588 - Pectins.
§ 184.1595 - Pepsin.

§ 184.1610 - Potassium alginate.
§ 184.1613 - Potassium bicarbonate.
§ 184.1619 - Potassium carbonate.
§ 184.1622 - Potassium chloride.
§ 184.1625 - Potassium citrate.
§ 184.1631 - Potassium hydroxide.
§ 184.1634 - Potassium iodide.
§ 184.1635 - Potassium iodate.
§ 184.1639 - Potassium lactate.
§ 184.1643 - Potassium sulfate.
§ 184.1655 - Propane.
§ 184.1660 - Propyl gallate.
§ 184.1666 - Propylene Glycol.
§ 184.1670 - Propylparaben.
§ 184.1676 - Pyridoxine hydrochloride.
§ 184.1685 - Rennet (animal-derived) and chymosin preparation (fermentation-derived).
§ 184.1695 - Riboflavin.
§ 184.1697 - Riboflavin-5'-phosphate (sodium).
§ 184.1698 - Rue.
§ 184.1699 - Oil of rue.
§ 184.1702 - Sheanut oil.
§ 184.1721 - Sodium acetate.
§ 184.1724 - Sodium alginate.
§ 184.1733 - Sodium benzoate.
§ 184.1736 - Sodium bicarbonate.
§ 184.1742 - Sodium carbonate.
§ 184.1751 - Sodium citrate.
§ 184.1754 - Sodium diacetate.
§ 184.1763 - Sodium hydroxide.
§ 184.1764 - Sodium hypophosphite.
§ 184.1768 - Sodium lactate.
§ 184.1769a - Sodium metasilicate.
§ 184.1784 - Sodium propionate.
§ 184.1792 - Sodium sesquicarbonate.
§ 184.1801 - Sodium tartrate.
§ 184.1804 - Sodium potassium tartrate.
§ 184.1807 - Sodium thiosulfate.
§ 184.1835 - Sorbitol.
§ 184.1845 - Stannous chloride (anhydrous and dihydrated).
§ 184.1848 - Starter distillate.
§ 184.1851 - Stearyl citrate.
§ 184.1854 - Sucrose.
§ 184.1857 - Corn sugar.
§ 184.1859 - Invert sugar.
§ 184.1865 - Corn syrup.
§ 184.1866 - High fructose corn syrup.
§ 184.1875 - Thiamine hydrochloride.
§ 184.1878 - Thiamine mononitrate.
§ 184.1890 - [alpha]-Tocopherols.
§ 184.1901 - Triacetin.
§ 184.1903 - Tributyrin.
§ 184.1911 - Triethyl citrate.
§ 184.1914 - Trypsin.
§ 184.1923 - Urea.
§ 184.1924 - Urease enzyme preparation from Lactobacillus fermentum.
§ 184.1930 - Vitamin A.
§ 184.1945 - Vitamin B12..
§ 184.1950 - Vitamin D.
§ 184.1973 - Beeswax (yellow and white).

§ 184.1976 - Candelilla wax.
§ 184.1978 - Carnauba wax.
§ 184.1979 - Whey.
§ 184.1979a - Reduced lactose whey.
§ 184.1979b - Reduced minerals whey.
§ 184.1979c - Whey protein concentrate.
§ 184.1983 - Bakers yeast extract.
§ 184.1984 - Zein.
§ 184.1985 - Aminopeptidase enzyme preparation derived from lactococcus lactis.

Authority: 21 U.S.C. 321, 342, 348, 371.
Source: 42 FR 14653, Mar 15, 1977, unless otherwise noted.

REFERENCES

[1] Anglesey, D.L. (2011). Symptoms of MSG Toxicity Chart. *Home - MSGMYTH*. Retrieved October 9, 2015 from http://msgmyth.com/msg_symptoms.html

[2] Yelp. (n.d.). Pho Nam Restaurant, Reviews and Ratings. *Yelp*. Retrieved January 5, 2014 from www.yelp.com/biz/pho-nam-restaurant-gaithersburg?start=40

[3] Yelp. (n.d.). Pho Nam Restaurant, Reviews and Ratings. *Yelp*. Retrieved October 12, 2016 from https://www.yelp.com/biz/pho-nam-restaurant-gaithersburg?start=20

[4] Yelp. (n.d.). Pho Nam Restaurant, Reviews and Ratings. *Yelp*. Retrieved October 12, 2016 from https://www.yelp.com/biz/pho-nam-restaurant-gaithersburg?start=40

[5] Yelp. (n.d.). Pho Nam Restaurant, Reviews and Ratings. *Yelp*. Retrieved Retrieved September 16, 2016 from https://www.yelp.com/biz/pho-nam-restaurant-gaithersburg?start=160

[6] Yelp. (n.d.). Pho Nam Restaurant, Reviews and Ratings. *Yelp*. Retrieved September 16, 2016 from https://www.yelp.com/biz/pho-nam-restaurant-gaithersburg?start=140

[7] Yelp. (n.d.). Pho Nam Restaurant, Reviews and Ratings. *Yelp*. Retrieved September 16, 2016 from https://www.yelp.com/biz/pho-nam-restaurant-gaithersburg?start=60

[8] Yelp. (n.d.). Pho Nam Restaurant, Reviews and Ratings. *Yelp*. Retrieved September 16, 2016 from http://www.yelp.com/biz/pho-nam-restaurant-gaithersburg?start=100

[9] Yelp. (n.d.). Pho Nam Restaurant, Reviews and Ratings. *Yelp*. Retrieved September 16, 2016 from https://www.yelp.com/biz/pho-nam-restaurant-gaithersburg?start=100

[10] Juan, S. (2006, September 29). Why are people so often in denial?. *The Register: Sci/Tech News for the World*. Retrieved October 9, 2015 from http://www.theregister.co.uk/2006/09/29/the_odd_body_denial/

[11] Ibid

[12] Blaylock, R. L. (1998). *Excitotoxins: The Taste That Kills*. Santa Fe, N.M.: Health Press.

[13] Steffens, A. B., Leuvenink, H., & Scheurink, A. J. (1994). Effects of monosodium glutamate (Umami taste) with and without guanosine 5′-monophosphate on rat autonomic responses to meals. *Physiology & Behavior*, 56(1), 59-63. doi:10.1016/0031-9384(94)90261-5

[14] Blaylock, R. (2012, October 31). MSG Excitotoxins: The Taste That Kills - Nutrition . *Life Enthusiast*. Retrieved October 9, 2015 from http://www.life-enthusiast.com/msg-excitotoxins-the-taste-that-kills-a-935.html

[15] Ibid

[16] Khalaf, H. A., & Arafat, E. A. (2015). Effect of different doses of monosodium glutamate on the thyroid follicular cells of adult male albino rats: a histological study. *International Journal of Clinical and Experimental Pathology*, 8(12), 15498–15510.

[17] Svidnicki, P. V., Leite, N. D., Venturelli, A. C., Camargo, R. L., Vicari, M. R., Almeida, M. C., . . . Grassiolli, S. (2013). Swim training restores glucagon-like peptide-1 insulinotropic action in pancreatic islets from monosodium glutamate-obese rats. *Acta Physiologica*, 209(1), 34-44. doi:10.1111/apha.12128

[18] Savcheniuk, O. A., Virchenko, O. V., Falalyeyeva, T. M., Beregova, T. V., Babenko, L. P., Lazarenko, L. M., . . . Spivak, M. Y. (2014). The efficacy of probiotics for monosodium glutamate-induced obesity: dietology concerns and opportunities for prevention. *EPMA Journal*, 5(1). doi:10.1186/1878-5085-5-2

[19] UT Southwestern Medical Center. (2011, March 1). Signaling path in brain may prevent that 'I'm full' message. *ScienceDaily*. Retrieved October 9, 2015 from www.sciencedaily.com/releases/2011/03/110301122146.htm

[20] Ibid

[21] Ibid

[22] Marcus, A. (2011, May 27). MSG linked to weight gain| Reuters. *Business & Financial News, Breaking US & International News | Reuters.com*. Retrieved October 9, 2015 from http://www.reuters.com/article/2011/05/27/us-msg-linked-weight-gain-idUSTRE74Q5SJ20110527

[23] Ibid

[24] Richards, B. (2009, January 12). What is Leptin? | Weight Loss News. *Wellness Resources*. Retrieved October 9, 2015 from http://www.wellnessresources.com/weight/articles/what_is_Leptin/

[25] Ibid

[26] Blaylock, R. Interview by Adams, M. (2006, September 27). Interview with Dr. Russell Blaylock on devastating health effects of MSG, Aspartame and excitotoxins. *Natural health news*. Retrieved October 9, 2015 from http://www.naturalnews.com/020550.html

[27] Ibid

[28] Ibid

[29] Marcus, A. (2011, May 27). MSG linked to weight gain| Reuters. *Business & Financial News, Breaking US & International News | Reuters.com*. Retrieved October 9, 2015 from http://www.reuters.com/article/2011/05/27/us-msg-linked-weight-gain-idUSTRE74Q5SJ20110527

[30] Ibid

[31] Richards, B. (2009, January 12). What is Leptin? | Weight Loss News. *Wellness Resources*. Retrieved October 9, 2015 from http://www.wellnessresources.com/weight/articles/what_is_Leptin/

[32] He, K., Zhao, L., Daviglus, M. L., Dyer, A. R., Horn, L. V., Garside, D., . . . Stamler, J. (2008). Association of Monosodium Glutamate Intake With Overweight in Chinese Adults: The INTERMAP Study. *Obesity*,16(8), 1875-1880. doi:10.1038/oby.2008.274

[33] Ibid

[34] Ibid

[35] Ibid

[36] Dhindsa, K. S., Omran, R. G., & Bhup, R. (1981). Histological changes in the thyroid gland induced by monosodium glutamate in mice. *Acta Anatomica*. 109(2):97-102. PMID: 7246043

[37] Khalaf, H. A., & Arafat, E. A. (2015). Effect of different doses of monosodium glutamate on the thyroid follicular cells of adult male albino rats: a histological study. *International Journal of Clinical and Experimental Pathology*, 8(12), 15498–15510.

[38] National Library of Medicine PubMed Health Glossary. (2016, September 29). Hypothyroidism. *National Library of Medicine NIH - National Cancer Institute*. Retrieved September 06, 2017, from https://www.ncbi.nlm.nih.gov/pubmedhealth/PMHT0022776/

[39] El-Shafie, K. T. (2003). CLINICAL PRESENTATION OF HYPOTHYROIDISM. *Journal of Family & Community Medicine*, 10(1), 55–58.

[40] Ibid

[41] Shi, Z., Yuan, B., Taylor, A. W., Dai, Y., Pan, X., Gill, T. K., & Wittert, G. A. (2011). Monosodium glutamate is related to a higher increase in blood pressure over 5 years: findings from the Jiangsu Nutrition Study of Chinese adults. *Journal of Hypertension*, 29(5), 846-853. doi:10.1097/hjh.0b013e328344da8e

[42] Ibid

[43] Ibid

[44] Allen, R. P., Barker, P. B., Horska, A., & Earley, C. J. (2013). Thalamic glutamate/glutamine in restless legs syndrome: Increased and related to disturbed sleep. *Neurology*, 80(22), 2028-2034. doi:10.1212/wnl.0b013e318294b3f6

[45] Johns Hopkins News and Publications. (2013, May 7). Restless Legs Syndrome, Insomnia And Brain Chemistry: A Tangled Mystery Solved?. *Johns Hopkins Medicine*. Retrieved October 9, 2015, from http://www.hopkinsmedicine.org/news/media/releases/restless_legs_syndrome_insomnia_and_brain_chemistry_a_tangled_mystery_solved

[46] Ibid

[47] Ibid

[48] Finkelstein, Y., Meshorer, A., Talmi, Y. P., Zohar, Y., Brenner, J., & Gal, R. (1992). The Riddle of the Uvula. *Otolaryngology-Head and Neck Surgery*, 107(3), 444-450. doi:10.1177/019459989210700318

[49] Bawaskar, H., Bawaskar, P., & Bawaskar, P. (2017). Chinese restaurant syndrome. *Indian Journal of Critical Care Medicine*, 21(1), 49. doi:10.4103/0972-5229.198327

[50] Ibid

[51] Schwartz, G. R. (1999). *In bad taste the MSG symptom complex : how Monosodium Glutamate is a major cause of treatable and preventable illnesses, such as headaches, asthma, epilepsy, heart irregularities, depression, rage reactions, and attention deficit hyperactivity disorder*. Santa Fe, NM: Health Press.

[52] U-T San Diego. (1984, July 19). San Ysidro massacre: July 18, 1984. *San Diego Union-Tribune*. Retrieved October 13, 2015, from http://www.utsandiego.com/news/1984/jul/19/san-ysidro-massacre/

[53] Schwartz, G. R. (1999). *In bad taste the MSG symptom complex : how Monosodium Glutamate is a major cause of treatable and preventable illnesses, such as headaches, asthma, epilepsy, heart irregularities, depression, rage reactions, and attention deficit hyperactivity disorder*. Santa Fe, NM: Health Press.

[54] Ibid

[55] Quizlet. (2010, December 2). Psychology- the brain chapter 3. *Quizlet*. Retrieved from http://quizlet.com/2991133/psychology-the-brain-chapter-3-flash-cards/

[56] Bowen, R. (1998, September 20). Adrenocorticotropic Hormone (ACTH). *Colorado State University*. Retrieved October 13, 2015, from http://www.vivo.colostate.edu/hbooks/pathphys/endocrine/hypopit/acth.html

[57] Topiwala, S., MD. (2012, November 20). Pituitary gland – Anatomy - MedlinePlus Medical Encyclopedia. *U.S National Library of Medicine*. Retrieved October 13, 2015, from http://www.nlm.nih.gov/medlineplus/ency/anatomyvideos/000099.htm

[58] American Association for Clinical Chemistry. (2014, August 7). ACTH: Related tests: Cortisol, Cortrosyn (ACTH) Stimulation Test, Dexamethasone Suppression Test, Androstenedione. AACC | Lab Tests Online. Retrieved October 13, 2015, from http://labtestsonline.org/understanding/analytes/acth/tab/test

[59] Gong, S., Xia, F., Wei, J., Li, X., Sun, T., Lu, Z., et al. (1995, December 1). Harmful effects of MSG on function of hypothalamus-pituitary-target gland system. *Biomedical and Environmental Science*. PMID: 8719172 8(4):310-7

[60] Schwartz, G. R. (1999). *In bad taste the MSG symptom complex : how Monosodium Glutamate is a major cause of treatable and preventable illnesses, such as headaches, asthma, epilepsy, heart irregularities, depression, rage reactions, and attention deficit hyperactivity disorder*. Santa Fe, NM: Health Press.

[61] Shin, J., Seo, Y., Cho, N., & Noh, G. (2004). Modulation of intracellular gene expression toward Th2 predominant profile by monosodium glutamate in Jurkat cell line. *Journal of Allergy and Clinical Immunology*, 113(2). doi:10.1016/j.jaci.2004.01.220

[62] Asero, R. (2002). Food additives intolerance: A possible cause of perennial rhinitis. *Journal of Allergy and Clinical Immunology*, 110(6), 937-938. doi:10.1067/mai.2002.130054,

[63] Farombi, E. O., & Onyema, O. O. (2006). Monosodium glutamate-induced oxidative damage and genotoxicity in the rat: modulatory role of Vitamin C, Vitamin E and quercetin. *Human & Experimental Toxicology*, 25(5), 251-259. doi:10.1191/0960327106ht621oa

[64] Arees, E. A., & Mayer, J. (1970). Monosodium Glutamate-Induced Brain Lesions: Electron Microscopic Examination. *Science*, 170(3957), 549-550.

[65] Nakanishi, Y., Tsuneyama, K., Fujimoto, M., Salunga, T. L., Nomoto, K., An, J., . . . Gershwin, M. E. (2008). Monosodium glutamate (MSG): A villain and promoter of liver inflammation and dysplasia. *Journal of Autoimmunity*, 30(1-2), 42-50. doi:10.1016/j.jaut.2007.11.016

[66] Shimada, A., Cairns, B. E., Vad, N., Ulriksen, K., Pedersen, A. M., Svensson, P., & Baad-Hansen, L. (2013). Headache and mechanical sensitization of human pericranial muscles after repeated intake of monosodium glutamate (MSG). The Journal of Headache and Pain, 14(1), 2. doi:10.1186/1129-2377-14-2

[67] Livingstone, V. (1981). Current Clinical Findings on Monosodium Glutamate. *US National Library of Medicine National Institutes of Health*. Retrieved March 1, 2017, from https://www.ncbi.nlm.nih.gov/pmc/articles/PMC2306064/pdf/canfamphys00256-0096.pdf

[68] Goyal, A., Dureja, A., Sharma, D., & Dhiman, K. (2012, February). A Comprehensive Insight into the Development of Animal Models for Obesity Research, Double Blind Peer Reviewed International Research. *Global Journal ofMedical research*, 12(1), 1. ISSN : 0975-5888

[69] Nigg, J. T., & Holton, K. (2014). Restriction and Elimination Diets in ADHD Treatment. Child and Adolescent Psychiatric Clinics of North America, 23(4), 937-953. doi:10.1016/j.chc.2014.05.010

[70] Schwartz, G. R. (1999). *In bad taste the MSG symptom complex : how Monosodium Glutamate is a major cause of treatable and preventable illnesses, such as headaches, asthma, epilepsy, heart irregularities, depression, rage reactions, and attention deficit hyperactivity disorder*. Santa Fe, NM: Health Press.

[71] Goyal, A., Dureja, A., Sharma, D., & Dhiman, K. (2012, February). A Comprehensive Insight into the Development of Animal Models for Obesity Research, Double Blind Peer Reviewed International Research. *Global Journal ofMedical research*, 12(1), 1. ISSN : 0975-5888

[72] Simmons, A. L., Schlezinger, J. J., & Corkey, B. E. (2014). What Are We Putting in Our Food That Is Making Us Fat? Food Additives, Contaminants, and Other Putative Contributors to Obesity. *Current Obesity Reports*, Table 1., 3(2), 273-285. doi:10.1007/s13679-014-0094-y

[73] Farombi, E. O., & Onyema, O. O. (2006). Monosodium glutamate-induced oxidative damage and genotoxicity in the rat: modulatory role of Vitamin C, Vitamin E and quercetin. *Human & Experimental Toxicology*, 25(5), 251-259. doi:10.1191/0960327106ht621oa

[74] Schwartz, G. R. (1999). *In bad taste the MSG symptom complex : how Monosodium Glutamate is a major cause of treatable and preventable illnesses, such as headaches, asthma, epilepsy, heart irregularities, depression, rage reactions, and attention deficit hyperactivity disorder*. Santa Fe, NM: Health Press.

[75] Ibid

[76] Shi, Z., Yuan, B., Taylor, A. W., Dai, Y., Pan, X., Gill, T. K., & Wittert, G. A. (2011). Monosodium glutamate is related to a higher increase in blood pressure over 5 years: findings from the Jiangsu Nutrition Study of Chinese adults. Journal of Hypertension, 29(5), 846-853. doi:10.1097/hjh.0b013e328344da8e

[77] Goyal, A., Dureja, A., Sharma, D., & Dhiman, K. (2012, February). A Comprehensive Insight into the Development of Animal Models for Obesity Research, Double Blind Peer Reviewed International Research. *Global Journal ofMedical research*, 12(1), 1. ISSN : 0975-5888

[78] Simmons, A. L., Schlezinger, J. J., & Corkey, B. E. (2014). What Are We Putting in Our Food That Is Making Us Fat? Food Additives, Contaminants, and Other Putative Contributors to Obesity. *Current Obesity Reports*, 3(2), 273-285. doi:10.1007/s13679-014-0094-y

[79] The New York Times. (1993, April 11). Government to Weigh Restrictions on M.S.G.. *The New York Times*. Retrieved February 11, 2015, from http://www.nytimes.com/1993/04/11/us/government-to-weigh-restrictions-on-msg.html

[80] FDA. (2014, March 1). CFR - Code of Federal Regulations Sec. 101.22 Foods; labeling of spices, flavorings, colorings and chemical preservatives. *U.S. Food and Drug Administration*. Retrieved September 9, 2015, from http://www.accessdata.fda.gov/scripts/cdrh/cfdocs/cfcfr/cfrsearch.cfm?fr=101.22

[81] CBS News Film. (2011, November 27). The Flavorists: Tweaking tastes and creating cravings; Morley Safer, correspondent, Ruth Streeter, producer. *Film - CBS News*. Retrieved October 13, 2015, from http://www.cbsnews.com/news/the-flavorists-tweaking-tastes-and-creating-cravings-27-11-2011/

[82] Nicole, W. (2013). Secret Ingredients: Who Knows Whats in Your Food? *Environmental Health Perspectives, 121*(4). doi:10.1289/ehp.121-a126

[83] Burdock, G. A. (2007). Safety Assessment of Castoreum Extract as a Food Ingredient. *International Journal of Toxicology, 26*(1), 51-55. doi:10.1080/10915810601120145

[84] Ibid

[85] Ibid

[86] Marcus, A. (2011, May 27). MSG linked to weight gain| Reuters. *Business & Financial News, Breaking US & International News | Reuters.com*. Retrieved October 13, 2015, from http://www.reuters.com/article/2011/05/27/us-msg-linked-weight-gain-idUSTRE74Q5SJ20110527

[87] Schwartz, G. R. (1999). *In bad taste the MSG symptom complex : how Monosodium Glutamate is a major cause of treatable and preventable illnesses, such as headaches, asthma, epilepsy, heart irregularities, depression, rage reactions, and attention deficit hyperactivity disorder*. Santa Fe, NM: Health Press.

[88] FDA. (2015, April 1). CFR - Code of Federal Regulations Title 21 - Sec. 102.22 Protein hydrolysates, *U.S. Food and Drug Administration*. Retrieved September 9, 2015, from http://www.accessdata.fda.gov/scripts/cdrh/cfdocs/cfcfr/CFRSearch.cfm?fr=102.22

[89] Ibid

[90] Schwartz, G. R. (1999). *In bad taste the MSG symptom complex : how Monosodium Glutamate is a major cause of treatable and preventable illnesses, such as headaches, asthma, epilepsy, heart irregularities, depression, rage reactions, and attention deficit hyperactivity disorder*. Santa Fe, NM: Health Press.

[91] Ibid

[92] FDA. (2014, July 22). Questions and Answers on Monosodium Glutamate (MSG). *U.S. Food and Drug Administration*. Retrieved October 13, 2015, from http://www.fda.gov/Food/IngredientsPackagingLabeling/FoodAdditivesIngredients/ucm328728.htm

[93] FDA. (2015, April 1). CFR - Code of Federal Regulations Title 21 - Sec. 102.22 Protein hydrolysates, *U.S. Food and Drug Administration*. Retrieved September 9, 2015, from http://www.accessdata.fda.gov/scripts/cdrh/cfdocs/cfcfr/CFRSearch.cfm?fr=102.22

[94] FDA. (2015, April 1). CFR - Code of Federal Regulations Title 21 - Sec. 102.22 Protein hydrolysates, *U.S. Food and Drug Administration*. Retrieved September 9, 2015, from http://www.accessdata.fda.gov/scripts/cdrh/cfdocs/cfcfr/CFRSearch.cfm?fr=102.22

[95] Schwartz, G. R. (1999). *In bad taste the MSG symptom complex : how Monosodium Glutamate is a major cause of treatable and preventable illnesses, such as headaches, asthma, epilepsy, heart irregularities, depression, rage reactions, and attention deficit hyperactivity disorder*. Santa Fe, NM: Health Press.

[96] Blaylock, R. L. (1998). *Excitotoxins: The Taste That Kills*. Santa Fe, N.M.: Health Press.

[97] Schwartz, G. R. (1999). *In bad taste the MSG symptom complex : how Monosodium Glutamate is a major cause of treatable and preventable illnesses, such as headaches, asthma, epilepsy, heart irregularities, depression, rage reactions, and attention deficit hyperactivity disorder*. Santa Fe, NM: Health Press.

[98] Samuels, A., Ph.D. (2013). *It Wasn't Alzheimer's. It Was MSG*. Solana Beach, CA. doi:B00EODF4YQ. ISBN: 978-0-9885584-1-0

[99] Ibid

[100] PubChem Compound Database . (n.d.). MONOSODIUM GLUTAMATE Names and Identifiers. National Center for Biotechnology Information, *U.S. National Library of Medicine*. CID: 23672308. Retrieved December 28, 2017, from https://pubchem.ncbi.nlm.nih.gov/compound/monosodium_glutamate#section=Names-and-Identifiers

[101] Ibid

[102] Samuels, A., Ph.D. (2013). *It Wasn't Alzheimer's. It Was MSG*. Solana Beach, CA. doi:B00EODF4YQ. ISBN: 978-0-9885584-1-0

[103] Blaylock, R. L. (1998). *Excitotoxins: The Taste That Kills*. Santa Fe, N.M.: Health Press.

[104] Schwartz, G. R. (1999). *In bad taste the MSG symptom complex : how Monosodium Glutamate is a major cause of treatable and preventable illnesses, such as headaches, asthma, epilepsy, heart irregularities, depression, rage reactions, and attention deficit hyperactivity disorder*. Santa Fe, NM: Health Press.

[105] Ibid

[106] Kurihara, K. (2015). Umami the Fifth Basic Taste: History of Studies on Receptor Mechanisms and Role as a Food Flavor. *BioMed Research International, 2015*, 1-10. doi:10.1155/2015/189402

[107] Du Bois, C., Tan, C., & Mintz, S. (2008). *The world of soy*. Urbana, Ill: University of Illinois Press.

[108] Kurihara, K. (2015). Umami the Fifth Basic Taste: History of Studies on Receptor Mechanisms and Role as a Food Flavor. *BioMed Research International, 2015*, 1-10. doi:10.1155/2015/189402

[109] Ibid

[110] Ibid

[111] Sano, C. (2009). History of glutamate production. *American Journal of Clinical Nutrition, 90*(3). doi:10.3945/ajcn.2009.27462f

[112] Schwartz, G. R. (1999). *In bad taste the MSG symptom complex : how Monosodium Glutamate is a major cause of treatable and preventable illnesses, such as headaches, asthma, epilepsy, heart irregularities, depression, rage reactions, and attention deficit hyperactivity disorder*. Santa Fe, NM: Health Press.

[113] Schwartz, G. R. (1999). *In bad taste the MSG symptom complex : how Monosodium Glutamate is a major cause of treatable and preventable illnesses, such as headaches, asthma, epilepsy, heart irregularities, depression, rage reactions, and attention deficit hyperactivity disorder*. Santa Fe, NM: Health Press.

[114] Blaylock, R. L. (1998). *Excitotoxins: The Taste That Kills*. Santa Fe, N.M.: Health Press.

[115] Ibid

[116] Ibid

[117] Lucas, D. R., & Newhouse, J. P. (1957). The Toxic Effect of Sodium L-Glutamate on the Inner Layers of the Retina. *Archives of Ophthalmology*, 58(2), 193-201. doi:10.1001/archopht.1957.00940010205006

[118] Ibid

[119] Blaylock, R. L. (1998). *Excitotoxins: The Taste That Kills*. Santa Fe, N.M.: Health Press.

[120] Ibid

[121] Olney, J. W. (1969). Brain Lesions, Obesity, and Other Disturbances in Mice Treated with Monosodium Glutamate. *Science, 164*(3880), 719-721. doi:10.1126/science.164.3880.719

[122] Blaylock, R. L. (1998). *Excitotoxins: The Taste That Kills*. Santa Fe, N.M.: Health Press.

[123] The Harvard Crimson. (1969, October 27). Baby Food Manufacturers Will Suspend Use of MSG. *News | The Harvard Crimson*. Retrieved March 01, 2017, from http://www.thecrimson.com/article/1969/10/27/baby-food-manufacturers-will-suspend-use/

[124] Blaylock, R. L. (1998). *Excitotoxins: The Taste That Kills*. Santa Fe, N.M.: Health Press.

[125] Palmnäs, M. S., Cowan, T. E., Bomhof, M. R., Su, J., Reimer, R. A., Vogel, H. J., . . . Shearer, J. (2014). Low-Dose Aspartame Consumption Differentially Affects Gut Microbiota-Host Metabolic Interactions in the Diet-Induced Obese Rat. *PLoS ONE, 9*(10). doi:10.1371/journal.pone.0109841

[126] Gold, M. (2003, January 12). Aspartame as a Neurotoxic Drug: File #4: Reported Aspartame Toxicity Reactions . FDA Dockets: Submittal Docket # 02P-0317. *Aspartame Toxicity Information Center*, Concord, NH.

[127] Samuels, A., Ph.D. (2013). *It Wasn't Alzheimer's. It Was MSG*. Solana Beach, CA. doi:B00EODF4YQ. ISBN: 978-0-9885584-1-0

[128] Carper, J. (1993). *Food - your miracle medicine*. New York, NY: HarperCollins.

[129] Jacob, S., & Stechschulte, S. (2008, May). Formaldehyde, Aspartame, and Migraines: A Possible Connection. *Dermatitis*. 19(3):E10-1. PMID: 18627677

[130] The Editors of Encyclopædia Britannica. (2017, October 23). Formaldehyde. Encyclopædia Britannica. Retrieved January 07, 2018, from https://www.britannica.com/science/formaldehyde

[131] Mercola, J. (2010, July 6). America's Deadliest Sweetener Betrays Millions, Then Hoodwinks You With Name Change. *The Huffington Post*. Retrieved October 13, 2015, from http://www.huffingtonpost.com/dr-mercola/americas-deadliest-sweete_b_630549.html

[132] Palmnäs, M. S., Cowan, T. E., Bomhof, M. R., Su, J., Reimer, R. A., Vogel, H. J., . . . Shearer, J. (2014). Low-Dose Aspartame Consumption Differentially Affects Gut Microbiota-Host Metabolic Interactions in the Diet-Induced Obese Rat. *PLoS ONE, 9*(10). doi:10.1371/journal.pone.0109841

[133] Yang, Q. (2010). Gain weight by "going diet?" Artificial sweeteners and the neurobiology of sugar cravings: Neuroscience 2010. *The Yale Journal of Biology and Medicine*, 83(2), 101–108.

[134] Ibid

[135] Patterson Neubert, A. (2013, July 11). Susan E. Swithers - Prof: Diet drinks are not the sweet solution to fight obesity, health problems. *Purdue News*. Retrieved October 13, 2015, from http://www.purdue.edu/newsroom/releases/2013/Q3/prof-diet-drinks-are-not-the-sweet-solution-to-fight-obesity,-health-problems.html

[136] Ibid

[137] Ibid

[138] Nettleton, J. A., Lutsey, P. L., Wang, Y., Lima, J. A., Michos, E. D., & Jacobs, D. R. (2009). Diet Soda Intake and Risk of Incident Metabolic Syndrome and Type 2 Diabetes in the Multi-Ethnic Study of Atherosclerosis (MESA). *Diabetes Care*, 32(4), 688–694. http://doi.org/10.2337/dc08-1799

[139] Ibid

[140] Yang, Q. (2010). Gain weight by "going diet?" Artificial sweeteners and the neurobiology of sugar cravings: Neuroscience 2010. *The Yale Journal of Biology and Medicine*, 83(2), 101–108.

[141] Palmnäs, M. S., Cowan, T. E., Bomhof, M. R., Su, J., Reimer, R. A., Vogel, H. J., . . . Shearer, J. (2014). Low-Dose Aspartame Consumption Differentially Affects Gut Microbiota-Host Metabolic Interactions in the Diet-Induced Obese Rat. *PLoS ONE, 9*(10). doi:10.1371/journal.pone.0109841

[142] Nettleton, J. A., Lutsey, P. L., Wang, Y., Lima, J. A., Michos, E. D., & Jacobs, D. R. (2009). Diet Soda Intake and Risk of Incident Metabolic Syndrome and Type 2 Diabetes in the Multi-Ethnic Study of Atherosclerosis (MESA). *Diabetes Care*, 32(4), 688–694. http://doi.org/10.2337/dc08-1799

[143] Soffritti, M., Belpoggi, F., Esposti, D. D., Lambertini, L., Tibaldi, E., & Rigano, A. (2005). First Experimental Demonstration of the Multipotential Carcinogenic Effects of Aspartame Administered in the Feed to Sprague-Dawley Rats. *Environmental Health Perspectives*, 114(3), 379-385. doi:10.1289/ehp.8711

[144] Warner, M. (2006, February 11). The Lowdown on Sweet?. *The New York Times*. Retrieved October 13, 2015, from http://www.nytimes.com/2006/02/12/business/yourmoney/12sweet.html?pagewanted=all&_r=2&

[145] Soffritti, M., Belpoggi, F., Esposti, D. D., Lambertini, L., Tibaldi, E., & Rigano, A. (2005). First Experimental Demonstration of the Multipotential Carcinogenic Effects of Aspartame Administered in the Feed to Sprague-Dawley Rats. *Environmental Health Perspectives*, 114(3), 379-385. doi:10.1289/ehp.8711

[146] Ibid

[147] Ibid

[148] Ibid

[149] Warner, M. (2006, February 11). The Lowdown on Sweet?. *The New York Times*. Retrieved October 13, 2015, from http://www.nytimes.com/2006/02/12/business/yourmoney/12sweet.html?pagewanted=all&_r=2&

[150] Ibid

[151] PubChem Compound Database . (n.d.). Aspartame Names and Identifiers. *National Center for Biotechnology Information, U.S. National Library of Medicine*. CID: 134601. Retrieved January 07, 2018, from https://pubchem.ncbi.nlm.nih.gov/compound/aspartame#section=Synonyms

[152] Ibid

[153] OFW. (2016, September 1). Aspartame Potentially Subject to Prop 65 Listing. Law Firm of Olsson, Frank, Weeda, Terman, Matz. Retrieved February 26, 2017, from http://www.ofwlaw.com/2016/09/01/aspartame-potentially-subject-prop-65-listing/

[154] Sleight, E. (2013, July 26). Why Are We So Addicted To Sugar?. UK News and Opinion - *The Huffington Post United Kingdom*. Retrieved October 13, 2015, from http://www.huffingtonpost.co.uk/2013/07/26/why-is-sugar-so-addictive_n_3643965.html

[155] CBS News. (2012, August 5). Is sugar toxic? . *60 Minutes - CBS News Documentary Film*. Retrieved October 15, 2015, from http://www.cbsnews.com/video/watch/?id=7417238n

[156] Avena, N. M., Rada, P., & Hoebel, B. G. (2008). Evidence for sugar addiction: Behavioral and neurochemical effects of intermittent, excessive sugar intake. *Neuroscience & Biobehavioral Reviews*, 32(1), 20-39. doi:10.1016/j.neubiorev.2007.04.019

[157] Ahmed, S. H., Guillem, K., & Vandaele, Y. (2013). Sugar addiction: pushing the drug-sugar analogy to the limit. *Current Opinion in Clinical Nutrition and Metabolic Care*, 16(4), 434-439. doi:10.1097/mco.0b013e328361c8b8

[158] Gupta., S. (2012, April 28). Is Sugar Toxic?. *CNN Transcripts | CNN*. Retrieved November 19, 2016, from http://transcripts.cnn.com/TRANSCRIPTS/1204/28/hcsg.01.html

[159] 10News. (2012, April 2). Sugar, is it toxic? | wtsp.com. Tampa Bay News | *Connect to 10 News in Tampa, Sarasota, Clearwater, St. Petersburg, Florida | WTSP.com* . Retrieved October 15, 2015, from http://www.wtsp.com/news/article/248439/250/Sugar-is-it-toxic

[160] Avena, N. M., Rada, P., & Hoebel, B. G. (2008). Evidence for sugar addiction: Behavioral and neurochemical effects of intermittent, excessive sugar intake. *Neuroscience & Biobehavioral Reviews*,32(1), 20-39. doi:10.1016/j.neubiorev.2007.04.019

[161] Ibid

[162] CBS News. (2012, August 5). Is sugar toxic? . *60 Minutes - CBS News Documentary Film*. Retrieved October 15, 2015, from http://www.cbsnews.com/video/watch/?id=7417238n

[163] Ibid

[164] Ibid

[165] Stanhope, K. L., Bremer, A. A., Medici, V., Nakajima, K., Ito, Y., Nakano, T., . . . Havel, P. J. (2011). Consumption of Fructose and High Fructose Corn Syrup Increase Postprandial Triglycerides, LDL-Cholesterol, and Apolipoprotein-B in Young Men and Women. *The Journal of Clinical Endocrinology & Metabolism*, 96(10). doi:10.1210/jc.2011-1251

[166] CBS News. (2012, August 5). Is sugar toxic? . *60 Minutes - CBS News Documentary Film*. Retrieved October 15, 2015, from http://www.cbsnews.com/video/watch/?id=7417238n

[167] Ibid

[168] Stanhope, K. L., Bremer, A. A., Medici, V., Nakajima, K., Ito, Y., Nakano, T., . . . Havel, P. J. (2011). Consumption of Fructose and High Fructose Corn Syrup Increase Postprandial Triglycerides, LDL-Cholesterol, and Apolipoprotein-B in Young Men and Women. *The Journal of Clinical Endocrinology & Metabolism*, 96(10). doi:10.1210/jc.2011-1251

[169] Lamarche, B., Lemieux, I., & Després, J. (1999, September 25). The small, dense LDL phenotype and the risk of coronary heart disease: epidemiology, patho-physiology and therapeutic aspects. *Diabetes and Metabolism*. 25(3):199-211 PMID: 10499189

[170] Warburg, O. H. (1966). The Prime Cause and Prevention of Cancer - Part 1. *Total Health Associates*. Retrieved October 15, 2015, from http://healingtools.tripod.com/primecause1.html/

[171] Brand, R. A. (2010). Biographical Sketch: Otto Heinrich Warburg, PhD, MD. *Clinical Orthopaedics and Related Research®*, 468(11), 2831-2832. doi:10.1007/s11999-010-1533-z

[172] CBS News. (2012, August 5). Is sugar toxic? . *60 Minutes - CBS News Documentary Film*. Retrieved October 15, 2015, from http://www.cbsnews.com/video/watch/?id=7417238n

[173] Vigneri, R., Goldfine, I. D., & Frittitta, L. (2016). Insulin, insulin receptors, and cancer. *Journal of Endocrinological Investigation*, 39(12), 1365-1376. doi:10.1007/s40618-016-0508-7

[174] Klement, R. J., & Kämmerer, U. (2011). Is there a role for carbohydrate restriction in the treatment and prevention of cancer? *Nutrition & Metabolism*, 8(1), 75. doi:10.1186/1743-7075-8-75

[175] Donaldson, M. S. (2004). Nutrition and cancer: A review of the evidence for an anti-cancer diet. *Nutrition Journal*, 3(1). doi:10.1186/1475-2891-3-19

[176] BBC Science. (2013, March 22). BBC Science - Why is sugar so addictive?. *BBC* . Retrieved October 15, 2015, October from http://www.bbc.co.uk/science/0/21835302

[177] Roberts, C. K., Hevener, A. L., & Barnard, R. J. (2013). Metabolic Syndrome and Insulin Resistance: Underlying Causes and Modification by Exercise Training. *Comprehensive Physiology*. doi:10.1002/cphy.c110062

[178] Ibid

[179] Diabetes Association. (n.d.). Insulin. *American Diabetes Association - Planet D*. Retrieved October 15, 2015, from http://www.diabetes.org/living-with-diabetes/parents-and-kids/planet-d/new-to-diabetes/Insulin/

[180] Ibid

[181] Guyton, A. C., & Hall, J. E. (2000). *Textbook of medical physiology*. Philadelphia: Saunders.

[182] Gkogkolou, P., & Böhm, M. (2012). Advanced glycation end products: Key players in skin aging?. *Dermato-Endocrinology, 4*(3), 259-270. doi:10.4161/derm.22028

[183] Uribarri, J., Woodruff, S., Goodman, S., Cai, W., Chen, X., Pyzik, R., . . . Vlassara, H. (2010). Advanced Glycation End Products in Foods and a Practical Guide to Their Reduction in the Diet. *Journal of the American Dietetic Association, 110*(6). doi:10.1016/j.jada.2010.03.018

[184] Shape Magazine. (2013, September 13). Glycation, GlyTerra, and Aging: Does Sugar Cause Wrinkles?. *Shape Magazine*. Retrieved October 15, 2015, from http://www.shape.com/lifestyle/beauty-style/sugar-giving-you-wrinkles

[185] Ibid

[186] Long, A. (2012, February 1). Sugar and Aging - The Truth About Glycation. *ELLE*. Retrieved October 15, 2013, from http://www.elle.com/beauty/makeup-skin-care/sugar-aging-how-to-fight-glycation-614621

[187] Draelos, Z. D. (2010, May 1). Oxidation, glycation main culprits of skin damage . Dermatology Times. Retrieved October 15, 2015, from http://dermatologytimes.modernmedicine.com/dermatology-times/news/modernmedicine/modern-medicine-now/oxidation-glycation-main-culprits-skin-dam

[188] Gkogkolou, P., & Böhm, M. (2012). Advanced glycation end products: Key players in skin aging?. *Dermato-Endocrinology, 4*(3), 259-270. doi:10.4161/derm.22028

[189] The Editors of Encyclopedia Britannica. (2015, September 16). Sucrose organic compound. *Encyclopedia Britannica*. Retrieved June 12, 2017, from https://www.britannica.com/science/sucrose

[190] Wolever, T. M. (2006). *The glycemic index a physiological classification of dietary carbohydrate*. Wallingford, UK: CABI.

[191] Woollen, A., Sharples, J., Gill, M. (1998, May 2). Agriculture and Food Supplies: Year In Review 1997 : Sugar . *Encyclopedia Britannica*. Retrieved October October 15, 2015, from http://www.britannica.com/EBchecked/topic/9652/Agriculture-and-Food-Supplies-Year-In-Review-1997/91998/Sugar

[192] The Editors of Encyclopedia Britannica. (2001, February 1). Fructose (chemical compound). *Encyclopedia Britannica*. Retrieved October 15, 2015, from http://www.britannica.com/EBchecked/topic/220981/fructose

[193] Forshee, R. (2007, July 24). UM. Study - Not Enough Evidence to Indict High Fructose Corn Syrup in Obesity: University Communications Newsdesk. *University of Maryland*. Retrieved June 12, 2017, from http://archive.li/T9BWT

[194] The Editors of Encyclopedia Britannica. (2001, February 1). Glucose (biochemistry) . *Encyclopedia Britannica*. Retrieved October 16, 2015, from http://www.britannica.com/EBchecked/topic/235853/glucose

[195] The Editors of Encyclopedia Britannica. (2003, March 1). Sucrose (organic compound) . *Encyclopedia Britannica*. Retrieved October 16, 2015, from http://www.britannica.com/EBchecked/topic/1386564/sucrose

[196] The Editors of Encyclopedia Britannica. (2001, February 1). Fructose (chemical compound). *Encyclopedia Britannica*. Retrieved October 16, 2015, from http://www.britannica.com/EBchecked/topic/220981/fructose

[197] Campbell, M. K., & Farrell, S. O. (2006). *Biochemistry* (5th international student ed.). Pacific Grove, Calif.: Brooks/Cole.

[198] Mercola, J. (2010, April 15). Dr. Joseph Mercola: This Sweetener Is Far Worse Than High Fructose Corn Syrup. *The Huffington Post*. Retrieved October 16, 2015, from http://www.huffingtonpost.com/dr-mercola/agave-this-sweetener-is-f_b_537936.html

[199] O'connor, A. (2007, June 11). The Claim: Brown Sugar Is Healthier Than White Sugar. *The New York Times*. Retrieved October 16, 2015, from http://www.nytimes.com/2007/06/12/health/nutrition/12real.html?_r=0

[200] Olaitan, P. B., Adeleke, O. E., & Ola, I. O. (2007). Honey: a reservoir for microorganisms and an inhibitory agent for microbes. *African Health Sciences*, 7(3), 159–165.

[201] Nutritionistic. (2013, June 24). Calories In Honey & Nutrition Facts. *Nutritionistic- Natural health for better life*. Retrieved October 16, 2015, from http://nutritionistic.blogspot.com/2013/06/calories-in-honey-nutrition-facts.html

[202] Raatz, S. K., Johnson, L. K., & Picklo, M. J. (2015). Consumption of Honey, Sucrose, and High-Fructose Corn Syrup Produces Similar Metabolic Effects in Glucose-Tolerant and -Intolerant Individuals. *Journal of Nutrition, 145*(10), 2265-2272. doi:10.3945/jn.115.218016

[203] Lamarche, B., Lemieux, I., & Després, J. (1999, September 25). The small, dense LDL phenotype and the risk of coronary heart disease: epidemiology, patho-physiology and therapeutic aspects. *Diabetes and Metabolism*. 25(3):199-211 PMID: 10499189

[204] Calorie Count. (n.d.). Calories in Syrups, Corn, High-fructose | Nutrition and Health Facts. *Calorie Counter | Food Nutrition Data*. Retrieved October 16, 2015, from http://caloriecount.about.com/calories-syrups-corn-high-fructose-i19351

[205] Source:University of Maryland, College Park. (2007, July 30). Not Enough Evidence To Indict High Fructose Corn Syrup In Obesity. *ScienceDaily*. Retrieved October 16, 2015, from http://www.sciencedaily.com/releases/2007/07/070727172644.htm

[206] Bowden, J. B., PhD. (2010, February 15). Debunking The Blue Agave Myth. *Huffpost Healthy Living*. Retrieved October 16, 2015, from www.huffingtonpost.com/dr-jonny-bowden/debunking-the-blue-agave_b_450144.html

[207] Horton, J. (2014, July 22). The Truth About Agave | Agave: Calories, Nutrition Facts, and More. *WebMD*. Retrieved October 16, 2015, from http://www.webmd.com/diet/features/the-truth-about-agave

[208] Bowden, J. B., PhD. (2010, February 15). Debunking The Blue Agave Myth. *Huffpost Healthy Living*. Retrieved October 16, 2015, from www.huffingtonpost.com/dr-jonny-bowden/debunking-the-blue-agave_b_450144.html

[209] Ibid

[210] WebMD. (2014, November 18). Food Dye and ADHD: Food Coloring, Sugar, and Diet | Does sugar cause symptoms of ADHD?. *WebMD*. Retrieved October 16, 2015, from http://www.webmd.com/add-adhd/childhood-adhd/food-dye-adhd?page=2

[211] FDA. (2014, December 31). Raw Fruits Poster (Text Version / Accessible Version) | Nutrition Information on Raw Fruits for Restaurants & Retail Establishments. *U.S. Food and Drug Administration*. Retrieved November 19, 2016, from http://www.fda.gov/Food/IngredientsPackagingLabeling/LabelingNutrition/ucm063482.htm

[212] Nelson, J. (2014, January 30). Juicing: What are the health benefits? | Is juicing healthier than eating whole fruits or vegetables?. *Mayo Clinic*. Retrieved October 16, 2015, from http://www.mayoclinic.com/health/juicing/AN02107

[213] Sanchez, A., Reeser, J. L., Lau, H. S., Yahiku, P. Y., Willard, R. E., McMillan, P. J., et al. (1973). Role of sugars in human neutrophilic phagocytosis. *The American Journal of Clinical Nutrition*. vol. 26, 11 1180-1184

[214] Ibid

[215] Plesman, J. (2011, October 30). Hypoglycemic Health Association of Australia - What is Hypoglycemia. *Hypoglycemic Health Association of Australia*. Retrieved October 16, 2015, from http://www.hypoglycemia.asn.au/2011/what-is-hypoglycemia/

[216] Ibid

[217] Plesman, J. (2011, October 30). Hypoglycemic Health Association of Australia - What is Hypoglycemia. *Hypoglycemic Health Association of Australia*. Retrieved October 16, 2015, from http://www.hypoglycemia.asn.au/2011/what-is-hypoglycemia/

[218] NIH-National Institute of Diabetes and Digestive and Kidney Diseases. (2016, September 29). Hypoglycemia: Symptoms. *National Library of Medicine - PubMed Health*. Retrieved July 05, 2017, from https://www.ncbi.nlm.nih.gov/pubmedhealth/PMHT0024700/

[219] Ibid

[220] Plesman, J. (2011, October 30). Hypoglycemic Health Association of Australia - What is Hypoglycemia. *Hypoglycemic Health Association of Australia*. Retrieved October 16, 2015, from http://www.hypoglycemia.asn.au/2011/what-is-hypoglycemia/

[221] Harvard Medical School. (Updated 2015, August 27). Glycemic index and glycemic load for 100+ foods. *Harvard Health Publications | Harvard Medical School*. Retrieved October 16, 2015, from http://www.health.harvard.edu/newsweek/Glycemic_index_and_glycemic_load_for_100_foods.htm

[222] FDA. (2016, June 15). Nutrition Glossary. *US Food and Drug Administration*. Retrieved March 12, 2017, from https://www.accessdata.fda.gov/scripts/InteractiveNutritionFactsLabel/glossary.html
Also see https://www.accessdata.fda.gov/scripts/InteractiveNutritionFactsLabel/factsheets/Glossary.pdf

[223] FDA. (2016, July 11). Dietary Fiber. *US Food and Drug Administration*. Retrieved March 16, 2017, from https://www.accessdata.fda.gov/scripts/InteractiveNutritionFactsLabel/dietary-fiber.html

[224] Ibid

[225] Ibid

[226] EUFIC. (2000, March). The Origins of our Daily Bread. *(EUFIC) European Food Information Council*. Retrieved October 22, 2015, from http://www.eufic.org/article/en/nutrition/understanding-food/artid/origins-of-bread/

[227] Ibid

[228] The college of Agricultural, Food and Environmental Sciences. (Modified 2004, December 6). The Beginning of the Green Revolution. *University of Minnesota*. Retrieved November 22, 2016, from https://web.archive.org/web/20041227090100/http://www.coafes.umn.edu/The_Beginning_of_the_Green_Revolution.html

[229] Eng, M. (2011, October 26). Against the grain | 'Wheat Belly' author claims staple is destructive to the body. *Chicago Tribune - Tribune Newspapers*. Retrieved October 22, 2015, from http://articles.chicagotribune.com/2011-10-26/features/sc-food-1021-wheat-belly-book-20111026_1_wheat-products-gluten-sensitivity-blood-sugar

[230] Ibid

[231] Perlmutter, D., MD. (2015). *Grain brain: The surprising truth about wheat, carbs, and sugar--your brain's silent killers*. New York, Boston, London: Little Brown.
The quote can also be found at Hampton, D. (2016, June 11). Fat Is Your Brain's Friend. *The Best Brain Possible*. Retrieved March 19, 2017, from https://www.thebestbrainpossible.com/fat-is-your-friend/

[232] Glycemic Research Institute. (2006, February 27). Glycemic Index Defined | Glycemic Index Testing | Glycemic | Glycemic Load. *Glycemic Research Institute* . Retrieved October 22, 2015, from http://www.glycemic.com/GlycemicIndex-LoadDefined.htm

[233] Glycemic Research Institute. (2006, February 27). Glycemic Index Defined | Glycemic Index Testing | Glycemic | Glycemic Load. *Glycemic Research Institute* . Retrieved October 22, 2015, from http://www.glycemic.com/GlycemicIndex-LoadDefined.htm

[234] The Nutrition Source. (2013, August 5). Carbohydrates and Blood Sugar. *Harvard School of Public Health*. Retrieved November 22, 2016, from https://www.hsph.harvard.edu/nutritionsource/carbohydrates/carbohydrates-and-blood-sugar/

[235] Ibid

[236] Weil, A. (2006, June 23). What is the Glycemic Index?. *Dr. Weil - Q & A Library | Dr. Andrew Weil*. Retrieved October 22, 2015, from http://www.drweil.com/drw/u/QAA367357/The-Glycemic-Index-Dr-Weil.html

[237] Ibid

[238] Ibid

[239] Ibid

[240] Higdon, Ph.D., J., Drake, Ph.D., V., & Delage, Ph.D., B. (2017, January 03). Glycemic Index and Glycemic Load. *Oregon State University Micronutrient Information Center*. Retrieved March 17, 2017, from http://lpi.oregonstate.edu/mic/food-beverages/glycemic-index-glycemic-load#table-1

[241] University of Sidney. (2004, January 12). Glycemic Index. Glycemic index and international *GI database | Human Nutrition Unit, School of Molecular Bioscience, University of Sydney*. Retrieved March 17, 2017, from http://www.glycemicindex.com/foodSearch.php

[242] Davis, W. (2012, November 30). Are You Addicted to Wheat? Pt 1 Dr. Oz interviews Dr. William Davis . *The Dr. Oz Show*. Retrieved October 22, 2015, from http://www.doctoroz.com/videos/are-you-addicted-wheat-pt-1

[243] Ibid

[244] Snyder, K. (2013, August 6). Are You Addicted to Wheat?. *Kimberly Snyder*. Retrieved October 22, 2015, from http://kimberlysnyder.net/blog/2013/08/06/are-you-addicted-to-wheat/

[245] Davis, W. (2013, September 27). Surviving wheat withdrawal. *Wheat Belly | The New York Times Best Seller*. Retrieved October 22, 2015, from http://www.wheatbellyblog.com/2013/09/surviving-wheat-withdrawal/

[246] Ibid

[247] Medical-Dictionary. (2005, August 27). Gliadin definition. *Medical-Dictionary | TheFreeDictionary.com*. Retrieved October 22, 2015, from http://medical-dictionary.thefreedictionary.com/gliadin

[248] NIH - National Institute of Diabetes and Digestive and Kidney Diseases. (2011, March 16). Celiac Disease (Gluten Intolerance). *National Library of Medicine - PubMed Health*. Retrieved March 18, 2017, from https://www.ncbi.nlm.nih.gov/pubmedhealth/PMHT0024528/

[249] FDA. (2015, January 30). What is Gluten-Free? FDA Has an Answer. *FDA U.S. Food and Drug Administration | U.S. Department of Health and Human Services*. Retrieved October 22, 2015, from http://www.fda.gov/ForConsumers/ConsumerUpdates/ucm363069.htm

[250] Ibid

[251] WebMD. (2005, April 12). Celiac Disease Diagnosis: Tests & Results. WebMD. Retrieved October 22, 2015, from http://www.webmd.com/digestive-disorders/celiac-disease/celiac-disease-diagnosis-tests

[252] Carrasco, A. (2012, November 28). Why You Might Have a Gluten Sensitivity and Not Even Know It. *MindBodyGreen*. Retrieved October 22, 2015, from http://www.mindbodygreen.com/0-6950/Why-You-Might-Have-a-Gluten-Sensitivity-and-Not-Even-Know-It.html

[253] Kam, K. (2013, July 19). Gluten Intolerance, Sensitivity, & Gluten-Free Diets | What to know about celiac disease, gluten sensitivity, and gluten-free diets. *WebMD*. Retrieved October 22, 2015, from http://www.webmd.com/digestive-disorders/celiac-disease/features/gluten-intolerance-against-grain

[254] Carrasco, A. (2012, November 28). Why You Might Have a Gluten Sensitivity and Not Even Know It. *MindBodyGreen*. Retrieved October 22, 2015, from http://www.mindbodygreen.com/0-6950/Why-You-Might-Have-a-Gluten-Sensitivity-and-Not-Even-Know-It.html

[255] Ibid

[256] Punder, K. D., & Pruimboom, L. (2013). The Dietary Intake of Wheat and other Cereal Grains and Their Role in Inflammation. *Nutrients*, 5(3), 771-787. doi:10.3390/nu5030771

[257] Carr, A. (2012, November 23). Depressed mood associated with gluten sensitivity—resolution of symptoms with a gluten-free diet. *Department of Pathology, University of Otago | Journal of the New Zealand Medical Association*. Vol 125 No 1366

[258] Carrasco, A. (2012, November 28). Why You Might Have a Gluten Sensitivity and Not Even Know It. *MindBodyGreen*. Retrieved October 22, 2015, from http://www.mindbodygreen.com/0-6950/Why-You-Might-Have-a-Gluten-Sensitivity-and-Not-Even-Know-It.html

[259] Lionetti, E., Leonardi, S., Franzonello, C., Mancardi, M., Ruggieri, M., & Catassi, C. (2015). Gluten Psychosis: Confirmation of a New Clinical Entity. *Nutrients*, 7(7), 5532-5539. doi:10.3390/nu7075235

[260] Punder, K. D., & Pruimboom, L. (2013). The Dietary Intake of Wheat and other Cereal Grains and Their Role in Inflammation. *Nutrients*, 5(3), 771-787. doi:10.3390/nu5030771

[261] Myers, A. (2013, November 14). 5 Reasons to Avoid the Gluten-Free Aisle. *Primal Docs*. Retrieved October 22, 2015, from http://primaldocs.com/opinion/5-reasons-to-avoid-the-gluten-free-aisle/

[262] FDA. (2015, August 30). What is Gluten-Free? FDA Has an Answer. *FDA U.S. Food and Drug Administration | U.S. Department of Health and Human Services*. Retrieved October 22, 2015, from http://www.fda.gov/ForConsumers/ConsumerUpdates/ucm363069.htm

[263] Myers, A. (2013, November 14). 5 Reasons to Avoid the Gluten-Free Aisle. *Primal Docs*. Retrieved October 22, 2015, from http://primaldocs.com/opinion/5-reasons-to-avoid-the-gluten-free-aisle/

[264] HSPH. (2013, January 10). Foods identified as 'whole grain' not always healthy. *HSPH | Harvard School of Public Health | HSPH News*. Retrieved October 22, 2015, from http://www.hsph.harvard.edu/news/press-releases/foods-identified-as-whole-grain-not-always-healthy/

[265] Ibid

[266] Lew, J. (2013, October 1). Catalytic Hydrogenation of Alkenes. *USDAVIS Chemwiki*. Retrieved October 23, 2015, from http://chemwiki.ucdavis.edu/Organic_Chemistry/Hydrocarbons/Alkenes/Reactivity_of_Alkenes/Catalytic_Hydrogenation

[267] Freeman, I. P. (2000). Margarines and Shortenings. *Ullmanns Encyclopedia of Industrial Chemistry*. doi:10.1002/14356007.a16_145

[268] Marchand, V. (2010). Trans fats: What physicians should know. Canadian Pediatric Society, Nutrition and Gastroenterology Committee. *Pediatrics and Child Health*. doi:10.1093/pch/15.6.373

[269] Mozaffarian, D., Pischon, T., Hankinson, S., Rifai, N., Joshipura, K., Willett, W., et al. (2004, April). Dietary intake of trans fatty acids and systemic inflammation in women. *The American Journal of Clinical Nutrition*. 79(4):606-12

[270] Micha, R., & Mozaffarian, D. (2008). Trans fatty acids: Effects on cardiometabolic health and implications for policy. *Prostaglandins, Leukotrienes and Essential Fatty Acids, 79*(3-5), 147-152. doi:10.1016/j.plefa.2008.09.008

[271] Ibid

[272] Risérus, U. (2006). Trans fatty acids and insulin resistance. *Atherosclerosis Supplements, 7*(2), 37-39. doi:10.1016/j.atherosclerosissup.2006.04.008

[273] Reuters. (2008, April 11). Trans-fats linked to breast cancer risk in study | Reuters. *Reuters.com | Business & Financial News, Breaking US & International News*. Retrieved October 23, 2015, from http://www.reuters.com/article/2008/04/11/us-cancer-breast-fats-idUSN1122758320080411

[274] Ibid

[275] ABC News. (2011, March 10). Trans Fat and Depression | Video - ABC News. ABCNews.com - Breaking News, *ABC News*. Retrieved October 23, 2015, from http://abcnews.go.com/Health/video/trans-fat-depression-heart-disease-mental-illness-diet-13107625

[276] Ibid

[277] Ibid

[278] Ibid

[279] Stender, S., Dyerberg, J., & Astrup, A. (2006). High Levels Of Industrially Produced Trans Fat In Popular Fast Foods. *New England Journal of Medicine, 354*(15), 1650-1652.

[280] CDC. (2010, December 15). Trans Fat. *Centers for Disease Control and Prevention | Nutrition for Everyone | CDC.gov*. Retrieved October 23, 2015, from www.cdc.gov/nutrition/downloads/trans_fat_final.pdf
http://www.cdc.gov/nutrition/everyone/basics/fat/transfat.html

[281] Fulkerson, L. (Director). (2011). *Forks over knives* [Documentary]. Dr. T. Colin Campbell, Ph.D.. United States : Monica Beach Media.

[282] Feskanich, D., Willett, W. C., Stampfer, M. J., & Colditz, G. A. (1997). Milk, dietary calcium, and bone fractures in women: a 12-year prospective study. *American Journal of Public Health, 87*(6), 992-997. doi:10.2105/ajph.87.6.992

[283] National Center for Biotechnology Information, U.S. National Library of Medicine. (2012, February 24). Osteoporosis. National Library of Medicine - PubMed Health. Retrieved March 20, 2017, from https://www.ncbi.nlm.nih.gov/pubmedhealth/PMHT0024680/

[284] Feskanich, D., Willett, W. C., Stampfer, M. J., & Colditz, G. A. (1997). *Milk, dietary calcium, and bone fractures in women: a 12-year prospective study*. American Journal of Public Health, 87(6), 992-997.

[285] Ibid

[286] Fulkerson, L. (Director). (2011). *Forks over knives* [Documentary]. Dr. T. Colin Campbell, Ph.D.. United States : Monica Beach Media.

[287] Campbell, T. C., & Campbell, T. M. (2005). The China study: the most comprehensive study of nutrition ever conducted and the startling implications for diet, weight loss and long-term health. Dallas, Tex.: BenBella Books.

[288] Abelow, B. J., Holford, T. R., & Insogna, K. L. (1992). Cross-cultural association between dietary animal protein and hip fracture: A hypothesis. *Calcified Tissue International, 50*(1), 14-18. doi:10.1007/bf00297291

[289] Ochoa, M. S., MD. (2016, March 21). 7 Ways Milk and Dairy Products Are Making You Sick. Retrieved March 21, 2017, from https://www.forksoverknives.com/7-ways-milk-and-dairy-products-are-making-you-sick/

[290] Ibid

[291] Abelow, B. J., Holford, T. R., & Insogna, K. L. (1992). Cross-cultural association between dietary animal protein and hip fracture: A hypothesis. *Calcified Tissue International, 50*(1), 14-18. doi:10.1007/bf00297291

[292] Campbell, T. C., & Campbell, T. M. (2005). The China study: the most comprehensive study of nutrition ever conducted and the startling implications for diet, weight loss and long-term health. Dallas, Tex.: BenBella Books.

[293] Ibid

[294] Cumming, R. G., & Klineberg, R. J. (1994). Case-Control Study of Risk Factors for Hip Fractures in the Elderly. *American Journal of Epidemiology, 139*(5), 493-503. doi:10.1093/oxfordjournals.aje.a117032

[295] Dairy Australia. (2010, August 13). Use of hormones in milk production. *Dairy Australia*. Retrieved October 30, 2013, from http://www.dairyaustralia.com.au/Standard-Items/News/Dairy-News/Use-of-hormones-in-milk-production.aspx

[296] Dhanwal, D., Dennison, E., Harvey, N., & Cooper, C. (2011). Epidemiology of hip fracture: Worldwide geographic variation. *Indian Journal of Orthopaedics, 45*(1), 15. doi:10.4103/0019-5413.73656

[297] Encyclopedia Britannica. (2001, February 1). Casein (protein). *Encyclopedia Britannica Online*. Retrieved October 26, 2015, from http://www.britannica.com/EBchecked/topic/97854/Casein

[298] Ibid

299 Hyman, M. (2013, July 25). Got Proof? Lack of Evidence for Milk's Benefits. *Dr Mark Hyman*. Retrieved October 26, 2015, from http://drhyman.com/blog/2013/07/05/got-proof-lack-of-evidence-for-milks-benefits/#close

300 American Cancer Society. (2014, September 10). Recombinant Bovine Growth Hormone. *American Cancer Society - Cancer.org.* Retrieved October 26, 2015, from http://www.cancer.org/cancer/cancercauses/othercarcinogens/athome/recombinant-bovine-growth-hormone

301 FDA. (2014, July 28). Product Safety Information - Report on the Food and Drug Administration's Review of the Safety of Recombinant Bovine Somatotropin. *U. S. Food and Drug Administration*. Retrieved July 03, 2017, from https://www.fda.gov/animalveterinary/safetyhealth/productsafetyinformation/ucm130321.htm#top

302 Larsson, S., Bergkvist, L., & Wolk, A. (2004, November). Milk and lactose intakes and ovarian cancer risk in the Swedish Mammography Cohort. *The American Journal of Clinical Nutrition.* 80(5):1353-7 PMID: 15531686

303 Ibid

304 Ibid

305 Ibid

306 Campbell, T. C., & Campbell, T. M. (2005). The China study: the most comprehensive study of nutrition ever conducted and the startling implications for diet, weight loss and long-term health. Dallas, Tex.: BenBella Books.

307 Park, S., Kim, J., Kim, Y., Lee, S. J., Lee, S. D., & Chung, M. K. (2014). A Milk Protein, Casein, as a Proliferation Promoting Factor in Prostate Cancer Cells. *The World Journal of Men's Health*, 32(2), 76. doi:10.5534/wjmh.2014.32.2.76

308 Campbell, T. C., & Campbell, T. M. (2005). The China study: the most comprehensive study of nutrition ever conducted and the startling implications for diet, weight loss and long-term health. Dallas, Tex.: BenBella Books.

309 Appleton, B. S., & Campbell, T. C. (1983, May). Effect of high and low dietary protein on the dosing and postdosing periods of aflatoxin B1-induced hepatic preneoplastic lesion development in the rat. *Cancer Research.* 43(5):2150-4 PMID: 6131741

310 Campbell, T. C., & Campbell, T. M. (2005). The China study: the most comprehensive study of nutrition ever conducted and the startling implications for diet, weight loss and long-term health. Dallas, Tex.: BenBella Books.

311 Maruyama, K., Oshima, T., & Ohyama, K. (2010). Exposure to exogenous estrogen through intake of commercial milk produced from pregnant cows. *Pediatrics International*, 52(1), 33-38. doi:10.1111/j.1442-200x.2009.02890.x

312 Ireland, C. (2006, December 7). Hormones in milk can be dangerous - Ganmaa Davaasambuu, a Ph.D.. *Harvard University Gazette*. Retrieved from http://news.harvard.edu/gazette/2006/12.07/11-dairy.html

313 Ibid

314 Shaw, J. (2016, December 22). Modern Milk. *Harvard Magazine*. Retrieved June 22, 2017, from http://harvardmagazine.com/2007/05/modern-milk.html

315 MALEKINEJAD, H., & REZABAKHSH, A. (2015). Hormones in Dairy Foods and Their Impact on Public Health - A Narrative Review Article. *Iranian Journal of Public Health*, 44(6), 742–758.

316 Newmark, H. L., & Heaney, R. P. (2010). Dairy Products and Prostate Cancer Risk. *Nutrition and Cancer*, 62(3), 297-299. doi:10.1080/01635580903407221

317 Davies, T. W., Palmer, C. R., Ruja, E., & Lipscombe, J. M. (1996). Adolescent milk, dairy product and fruit consumption and testicular cancer. *British Journal of Cancer*, 74(4), 657–660.

318 Ireland, C. (2006, December 7). Hormones in milk can be dangerous - Ganmaa Davaasambuu, a Ph.D.. *Harvard University Gazette*. Retrieved from http://news.harvard.edu/gazette/2006/12.07/11-dairy.html

319 Shaw, J. (2016, December 22). Modern Milk. *Harvard Magazine*. Retrieved June 22, 2017, from http://harvardmagazine.com/2007/05/modern-milk.html

320 Zang, J., Shen, M., Du, S., Chen, T., & Zou, S. (2015). The Association between Dairy Intake and Breast Cancer in Western and Asian Populations: A Systematic Review and Meta-Analysis. *Journal of Breast Cancer*, 18(4), 313. doi:10.4048/jbc.2015.18.4.313

321 Shaw, J. (2016, December 22). Modern Milk. *Harvard Magazine*. Retrieved June 22, 2017, from http://harvardmagazine.com/2007/05/modern-milk.html

322 Maruyama, K., Oshima, T., & Ohyama, K. (2010). Exposure to exogenous estrogen through intake of commercial milk produced from pregnant cows. *Pediatrics International*, 52(1), 33-38. doi:10.1111/j.1442-200x.2009.02890.x

323 Ibid

324 Ibid

325 Shaw, J. (2016, December 22). Modern Milk. *Harvard Magazine*. Retrieved June 22, 2017, from http://harvardmagazine.com/2007/05/modern-milk.html

326 Silverstone, A., & Pearson, V. (2011). *The kind diet: a simple guide to feeling great, losing weight, and saving the planet*. Emmaus, PA: Rodale.

327 Ibid

328 Davies, T. W., Palmer, C. R., Ruja, E., & Lipscombe, J. M. (1996). Adolescent milk, dairy product and fruit consumption and testicular cancer. *British Journal of Cancer*, 74(4), 657–660.

329 MALEKINEJAD, H., & REZABAKHSH, A. (2015). Hormones in Dairy Foods and Their Impact on Public Health - A Narrative Review Article. *Iranian Journal of Public Health*, 44(6), 742–758.

[330] NDDIC. (n.d.). National Digestive Diseases - U.S. DEPARTMENT OF HEALTH AND HUMAN SERVICES Information Clearinghouse (NDDIC). *Lactose Intolerance - A service of the National Institute of Diabetes and Digestive and Kidney Diseases*. Retrieved October 26, 2015, from http://digestive.niddk.nih.gov/ddiseases/pubs/lactoseintolerance/#what

[331] Docena, G. H., Fernandez, R., Chirdo, F. G., & Fossati, C. A. (1996). Identification of Casein as the major allergenic and antigenic protein of cow's milk. *Allergy*, 51(6), 412-416. doi:10.1111/j.1398-9995.1996.tb00151.x

[332] Mayo Clinic. (2011, August 11). Casein Allergy Overview. *Mayo Clinic*. Retrieved October 26, 2015, from http://www.mayoclinic.com/health/milk-allergy/DS01008/DSECTION=causes

[333] Masoodi, T. A., & Shafi, G. (2010). Analysis of Casein alpha S1 & S2 proteins from different mammalian species. Bioinformation, 4(9), 430-435. doi:10.6026/97320630004430

[334] American Diabetes Association. (n.d.). Type 1 Diabetes - Diabetes Basics. *American Diabetes Association*. Retrieved October 26, 2015, from http://www.diabetes.org/diabetes-basics/type-1/

[335] Luopajärvi, K., Savilahti, E., Virtanen, S. M., Ilonen, J., Knip, M., Åkerblom, H. K., & Vaarala, O. (2008). Enhanced levels of cow's milk antibodies in infancy in children who develop type 1 diabetes later in childhood. *Pediatric Diabetes*, 9(5), 434-441. doi:10.1111/j.1399-5448.2008.00413.x

[336] Ibid

[337] Ibid

[338] Wendel, B. (Director). (2012). Forks over knives - the extended interviews [Documentary].Dr. Neal Barnard, MD., Clinical Researcher. United States: Virgil Films.

[339] Knip, M., Veijola, R., Virtanen, S. M., Hyoty, H., Vaarala, O., & Akerblom, H. K. (2005). Environmental Triggers and Determinants of Type 1 Diabetes. *Diabetes, 54*(Supplement 2). doi:10.2337/diabetes.54.suppl_2.s125

[340] Luopajärvi, K., Savilahti, E., Virtanen, S. M., Ilonen, J., Knip, M., Åkerblom, H. K., & Vaarala, O. (2008). Enhanced levels of cow's milk antibodies in infancy in children who develop type 1 diabetes later in childhood. *Pediatric Diabetes*, 9(5), 434-441. doi:10.1111/j.1399-5448.2008.00413.x

[341] Ibid

[342] Jenness, R. (1979, July). The composition of human milk. *Seminars in Perinatology*. 3(3):225-39 PMID: 392766

[343] Goldes, M. (1989, September 25). Studies Confirm Cholesterol-Heart Attack Link; The Fault in the Milk. *The New York Times*. Retrieved April 05, 2017, from http://www.nytimes.com/1989/09/26/opinion/l-studies-confirm-cholesterol-heart-attack-link-the-fault-in-the-milk-466689.html

[344] Enig, P. M., PhD. (2003, December 13). Milk Homogenization & Heart Disease. The *Weston A. Price Foundation* . Retrieved April 05, 2017, from https://www.westonaprice.org/health-topics/know-your-fats/milk-homogenization-heart-disease/

[345] Grant, W. B. (1998, August). Milk and other dietary influences on coronary heart disease. *Alternative Medicine Review: A Journal of Clinical Therapeutic*. 3(4):281-94 PMID: 9727089

[346] Motarjemi, Y., & Lelieveld, H. (2014). *Food safety management: a practical guide for the food industry*. Amsterdam: Elsevier.

[347] Ibid

[348] Ibid

[349] Ibid

[350] CDC. (2016, December 19). Raw Milk Questions and Answers. *Centers for Disease Control and Prevention*. Retrieved April 06, 2017, from https://www.cdc.gov/foodsafety/rawmilk/raw-milk-questions-and-answers.html#past

[351] Alkanhal, H. A., Al-Othman, A. A., & Hewedi, F. M. (2001). Changes in protein nutritional quality in fresh and recombined ultra high temperature treated milk during storage. *International Journal of Food Sciences and Nutrition*, 52(6), 509-514. doi:10.1080/713671811

[352] Roth-Walter, F., Berin, M. C., Arnaboldi, P., Escalante, C. R., Dahan, S., Rauch, J., . . . Mayer, L. (2008). Pasteurization of milk proteins promotes allergic sensitization by enhancing uptake through Peyer's patches. *Allergy*, 63(7), 882-890. doi:10.1111/j.1398-9995.2008.01673.x

[353] Baldwin, H. B. (1916). Some Observations On Homogenized Milk And Cream. *American Journal of Public Health*, 6(8), 862-864. doi:10.2105/ajph.6.8.862

[354] Editors - Encyclopedia Britannica. (1998, July 20). Homogenization. *Encyclopedia Britannica*. Retrieved April 06, 2017, from https://www.britannica.com/topic/homogenization

[355] Augustin (Marcus), S. A. (2015). *The hungry brain: the nutrition/cognition connection*. New York, NY: Skyhorse Publishing.

[356] Oster, K. A., Ross, D. J., Dawkins, H. H., Sampsidis, N., & Morrison, M. D. (1983). *The XO factor: Homogenized Milk May Cause Your Heart Attack*. New York: Park City Press.

[357] Ibid

[358] Ibid

[359] Doehner, W. (2005). Xanthine oxidase inhibition for chronic heart failure: is allopurinol the next therapeutic advance in heart failure? *Heart*, 91(6), 707-709. doi:10.1136/hrt.2004.057190

[360] Cabot, S., Ronald, R., & Jasinska, M. (2009). *Cholesterol: the real truth ; are the drugs you take making you sick*. Auckland, N.Z.: Royal New Zealand Foundation of the Blind.

[361] Ibid

[362] IARC Working Group on the Evaluation of Carcinogenic Risk to Humans. (1970, January 01). Ingested Nitrate and Nitrite, and Cyanobacterial Peptide Toxins. *International Agency for Research on Cancer; 2010. (IARC Monographs on the Evaluation of Carcinogenic Risks to Humans*, No. 94.)

[363] Ibid

[364] Morton Salt. (2001, February 1). MORTON® TENDER QUICK® Product Overview. *Morton Salt*. Retrieved October 26, 2015, from http://www.mortonsalt.com/for-your-home/culinary-salts/meat-curing-and-pickling-salts/178/morton-tender-quick/

[365] Hardin, A. (2011, August 26). Myth or Fact: Hot Dogs Cause Cancer. *DukeHealth.org*. Retrieved January 17, 2014, from http://www.dukehealth.org/health_library/health_articles/myth-or-fact-hot-dogs-cause-cancer

[366] HSPH News. (2010, May 17). Eating processed meats, but not unprocessed red meats, may raise risk of heart disease and diabetes. *HSPH News - Harvard School of Public Health*. Retrieved October 26, 2015, from http://www.hsph.harvard.edu/news/press-releases/processed-meats-unprocessed-heart-disease-diabetes/

[367] Ibid

[368] Micha, R., Wallace, S. K., & Mozaffarian, D. (2010). Red and Processed Meat Consumption and Risk of Incident Coronary Heart Disease, Stroke, and Diabetes Mellitus: A Systematic Review and Meta-Analysis. *Circulation, 121*(21), 2271-2283. doi:10.1161/circulationaha.109.924977

[369] Ibid

[370] Glade, M. (2008). World Cancer Research Fund/American Institute For Cancer Research, Food, Nutrition, Physical Activity And The Prevention Of Cancer: A Global Perspective , American Institute For Cancer Research, Washington, D.C (2007) ISBN: 978-0-9722522-2-5.. *Nutrition, 24*(4), 393-398.

[371] Ibid

[372] Monte, S. M., Neusner, A., Chu, J., & Lawton, M. (2009). Epidemiological Trends Strongly Suggest Exposures as Etiologic Agents in the Pathogenesis of Sporadic Alzheimers Disease, Diabetes Mellitus, and Non-Alcoholic Steatohepatitis. *Journal of Alzheimers Disease, 17*(3), 519-529. doi:10.3233/jad-2009-1070

[373] Sindelar, J. J., Ph.D.. (2012, March 1). What's the Deal with Nitrates and Nitrites Used in Meat Products?. *University of Wisconsin Meat Science & Muscle Biology Lab | University of Wisconsin Meat Laboratory*. Retrieved June 26, 2017, from http://fyi.uwex.edu/meats/files/2012/02/Nitrate-and-nitrite-in-cured-meat_10-18-2012.pdf

[374] Hardin, A. (2011, August 26). Myth or Fact: Hot Dogs Cause Cancer. *DukeHealth.org*. Retrieved January 17, 2014, from http://www.dukehealth.org/health_library/health_articles/myth-or-fact-hot-dogs-cause-cancer

[375] Ibid

[376] Monte, S. M., Neusner, A., Chu, J., & Lawton, M. (2009). Epidemiological Trends Strongly Suggest Exposures as Etiologic Agents in the Pathogenesis of Sporadic Alzheimers Disease, Diabetes Mellitus, and Non-Alcoholic Steatohepatitis. *Journal of Alzheimers Disease, 17*(3), 519-529. doi:10.3233/jad-2009-1070

[377] Glade, M. (2008). World Cancer Research Fund/American Institute For Cancer Research, Food, Nutrition, Physical Activity And The Prevention Of Cancer: A Global Perspective , American Institute For Cancer Research, Washington, D.C (2007) ISBN: 978-0-9722522-2-5.. *Nutrition, 24*(4), 393-398.

[378] Ibid

[379] Ibid

[380] Tricker, A., & Preussmann, R. (1991). Carcinogenic N-nitrosamines in the diet: occurrence, formation, mechanisms and carcinogenic potential. *Mutation Research/Genetic Toxicology, 259*(3-4), 277-289. doi:10.1016/0165-1218(91)90123-4

[381] Cancer.org. (2011, June 29). Known and Probable Human Carcinogens. *American Cancer Society - Cancer.org*. Retrieved October 26, 2015, from http://www.cancer.org/cancer/cancercauses/othercarcinogens/generalinformationaboutcarcinogens/known-and-probable-human-carcinogens

[382] Weldon, G., & Campbell, S. (2007, October 31). Landmark Report: Excess Body Fat Causes Cancer Panel Also Implicates Red Meat, Processed Meat and Alcohol. *American Institute for Cancer Research*. Retrieved June 22, 2017, from http://preventcancer.aicr.org/site/News2?page=NewsArticle&id=12898&news_iv_ctrl=0&abbr=pr

[383] Barnard, N., MD. (2011, August 10). Could Processed Meat Give You Cancer?. *The Huffington Post*. Retrieved January 17, 2014, from http://www.huffingtonpost.com/neal-barnard-md/processed-meat-cancer_b_919034.html

[384] Santarelli, R., Pierre, F., & Corpet, D. (2008). Processed Meat and Colorectal Cancer: A Review of Epidemiologic and Experimental Evidence. *Nutrition and Cancer, 60*(2), 131-144. doi:10.1080/01635580701684872

[385] Ibid

[386] Weldon, G., & Campbell, S. (2007, October 31). Landmark Report: Excess Body Fat Causes Cancer Panel Also Implicates Red Meat, Processed Meat and Alcohol. *American Institute for Cancer Research*. Retrieved June 22, 2017, from http://preventcancer.aicr.org/site/News2?page=NewsArticle&id=12898&news_iv_ctrl=0&abbr=pr

[387] American Cancer Society. (2016, February 10). What Are the Risk Factors for Stomach Cancer?. *American Cancer Society*. Retrieved June 26, 2017, from https://www.cancer.org/cancer/stomach-cancer/causes-risks-prevention/risk-factors.html

[388] Barnard, N., MD. (2011, August 10). Could Processed Meat Give You Cancer?. *The Huffington Post*. Retrieved October 26, 2015, from http://www.huffingtonpost.com/neal-barnard-md/processed-meat-cancer_b_919034.html

[389] Rohrmann, S., Overvad, K., Bueno-de-Mesquita, H. B., Jakobsen, M. U., Egeberg, R., Tjønneland, A., et al. (2013, March 7). Meat consumption and mortality - results from the European Prospective Investigation into Cancer and Nutrition. *BMC Medicine*. BioMed Central Ltd. Volume 11. DOI: 10.1186/1741-7015-11-63.

[390] Ibid

[391] Ibid

[392] Ibid

[393] Ibid

[394] Calorie Counter. (2013, March 26). Calories in Bologna. *The Calorie Counter*. Retrieved October 26, 2015, from http://thecaloriecounter.com/Foods/700/42161/1/Food.aspx

[395] NCI. (2014, May 22). Childhood Cancers. *National Cancer Institute - NCI*. Retrieved October 26, 2015, from http://www.cancer.gov/cancertopics/factsheet/Sites-Types/childhood

[396] Liu, C., Hsu, Y., Wu, M., Pan, P., Ho, C., Su, L., . . . Christiani, D. C. (2009). Cured meat, vegetables, and bean-curd foods in relation to childhood acute leukemia risk: A population based case-control study. *BMC Cancer*, 9(1). doi:10.1186/1471-2407-9-15

[397] Ibid

[398] Ibid

[399] JAD. (2009, July 1). Researchers find possible environmental causes for Alzheimer's, diabetes. *JAD - Press Releases | Journal of Alzheimer's Disease*. Retrieved October 26, 2015, from http://www.j-alz.com/press/2009/20090706.html

[400] DeLaMonte, S. M., Neusner, A., Chu, J., & Lawton, M. (2009). Epidemiological Trends Strongly Suggest Exposures as Etiologic Agents in the Pathogenesis of Sporadic Alzheimers Disease, Diabetes Mellitus, and Non-Alcoholic Steatohepatitis. *Journal of Alzheimers Disease, 17*(3), 519-529. doi:10.3233/jad-2009-1070

[401] Ibid

[402] Rhode Island Hospital. (2011, November 2). Diet and Dementia: Toxic Preservatives Contribute to Alzheimer's Disease. *The Alzheimer's Disease and Memory Disorders Center - Rhode Island Hospital*. Retrieved October 26, 2015, from http://www.rhodeislandhospital.org/services/alzheimers/memory-disorders/diet-and-dementia-toxic-preservatives-contribute-to-alzheimers-disease.html

[403] Mergenthaler, P., Lindauer, U., Dienel, G. A., & Meisel, A. (2013). Sugar for the brain: the role of glucose in physiological and pathological brain function. *Trends in Neurosciences, 36*(10), 587-597. doi:10.1016/j.tins.2013.07.001

[404] DeLaMonte, S. M., & Wands, J. R. (2008, November). Alzheimer's Disease Is Type 3 Diabetes–Evidence Reviewed. *Journal of Diabetes Science and Technology*, 2(6), 1101–1113. PMCID: PMC2769828. doi: 10.1177/193229680800200619

[405] DeLaMonte, S. (2011, June 4). Alzheimer's: Diabetes of the Brain?. *The Dr. Oz Show*. Retrieved June 27, 2017, from http://www.doctoroz.com/article/alzheimers-diabetes-brain?page=3

[406] Scanlan, R. A., Ph.D. (n.d.). Nitrosamines and Cancer. *Oregonstate.edu - The Linus Pauling Institute*. Retrieved January 20, 2014, from http://lpi.oregonstate.edu/search/osu/Nitrosamines%20and%20Cancer/0/1/

[407] DeLaMonte, S. M., Neusner, A., Chu, J., & Lawton, M. (2009). Epidemiological Trends Strongly Suggest Exposures as Etiologic Agents in the Pathogenesis of Sporadic Alzheimers Disease, Diabetes Mellitus, and Non-Alcoholic Steatohepatitis. *Journal of Alzheimers Disease, 17*(3), 519-529. doi:10.3233/jad-2009-1070

[408] DeLaMonte, S. (2011, June 4). Alzheimer's: Diabetes of the Brain?. *The Dr. Oz Show*. Retrieved June 27, 2017, from http://www.doctoroz.com/article/alzheimers-diabetes-brain?page=3

[409] Ibid

[410] Ibid

[411] Rhode Island Hospital. (2011, November 2). Diet and Dementia: Toxic Preservatives Contribute to Alzheimer's Disease. *The Alzheimer's Disease and Memory Disorders Center - Rhode Island Hospital*. Retrieved October 26, 2015, from http://www.rhodeislandhospital.org/services/alzheimers/memory-disorders/diet-and-dementia-toxic-preservatives-contribute-to-alzheimers-disease.html

[412] DeLaMonte, S. M., Neusner, A., Chu, J., & Lawton, M. (2009). Epidemiological Trends Strongly Suggest Exposures as Etiologic Agents in the Pathogenesis of Sporadic Alzheimers Disease, Diabetes Mellitus, and Non-Alcoholic Steatohepatitis. *Journal of Alzheimers Disease, 17*(3), 519-529. doi:10.3233/jad-2009-1070

[413] Rhode Island Hospital. (2011, November 2). Diet and Dementia: Toxic Preservatives Contribute to Alzheimer's Disease. *The Alzheimer's Disease and Memory Disorders Center - Rhode Island Hospital*. Retrieved October 26, 2015, from http://www.rhodeislandhospital.org/services/alzheimers/memory-disorders/diet-and-dementia-toxic-preservatives-contribute-to-alzheimers-disease.html

[414] Eubank, W., Carpenter, J. D., & Maltsberger, B. A. (1998). Nitrate in Drinking Water. *UNIVERSITY OF MISSOURI Extension - The Ohio State University*. Retrieved October 27, 2015, from http://extension.missouri.edu/p/WQ103

[415] Ibid

[416] EPA. (2009, July 3). Basic Information about Nitrate in Drinking Water. *EPA United States Protection Agency*. Retrieved October 27, 2015, from http://water.epa.gov/drink/contaminants/basicinformation/nitrate.cfm

[417] Eubank, W., Carpenter, J. D., & Maltsberger, B. A. (1998). Nitrate in Drinking Water. *UNIVERSITY OF MISSOURI Extension - The Ohio State University*. Retrieved October 27, 2015, from http://extension.missouri.edu/p/WQ103

[418] Ibid

[419] Helmenstine, Ph.D., A. M. (n.d.). Reverse Osmosis | What Is Reverse Osmosis and How Does It Work?. *About.com Chemistry*. Retrieved October 27, 2015, from http://chemistry.about.com/od/waterchemistry/a/reverseosmosis.htm

[420] Lewis, G. M., & Wang, L. (2007, August). Arsenic Removal From Drinking Water by Point-of-Use Reverse Osmosis (POU RO), U.S. EPA Demonstration Project at Sunset Ranch Development in Homedale, ID, Final Performance Evaluation Report. *EPA*. EPA/600/R-07/082

[421] EPA. (2006, January 9). Arsenic in Drinking Water Arsenic Virtual Trade Show. *EPA - United States Environmental Protection Agency*. Retrieved October 27, 2015, from http://cfpub.epa.gov/safewater/arsenic/arsenictradeshow/arsenic.cfm?action=Ion%20Exchange

[422] Ibid

[423] USBR. (2010, September 20). Electrodialysis (ED) and Electrodialysis Reversal (EDR) . *United States Department of Interior Bureau of Reclamation*. Retrieved October 27, 2015, from http://www.usbr.gov/pmts/water/publications/reportpdfs/Primer%20Files/07%20-%20Electrodialysis.pdf

[424] EPA. (2009, April 17). Radionuclides in Drinking Water Electrodialysis/Electrodialysis Reversal. *EPA - United States Environmental Protection Agency*. Retrieved October 27, 2015, from http://cfpub.epa.gov/safewater/radionuclides/radionuclides.cfm?action=Rad_Electrodialysis

[425] EPA. (2005, September). Water Health Series | Bottled Water Basics. *EPA - United States Environmental Protection Agency*. Retrieved January 26, 2014, from http://www.epa.gov/ogwdw000/faq/pdfs/fs_healthseries_bottlewater.pdf

[426] Burros, M. (1981, December 23). THE NITRITE QUESTION: WHAT CAN YOU EAT?. *The New York Times*. Retrieved October 27, 2015, from http://www.nytimes.com/1981/12/23/garden/the-nitrite-question-what-can-you-eat.html

[427] The Health Effects of Nitrate, Nitrite, and N-Nitroso Compounds. (1981). doi:10.17226/19738

[428] Katan, M. B. (2009). Nitrate in foods: harmful or healthy?. *The American Journal of Clinical Nutrition*. Retrieved October 27, 2015, from http://ajcn.nutrition.org/content/90/1/11.full

[429] JAD. (2009, July 1). Researchers find possible environmental causes for Alzheimer's, diabetes. *JAD - Press Releases | Journal of Alzheimer's Disease*. Retrieved October 27, 2015, from http://www.j-alz.com/press/2009/20090706.html

[430] Schmähl, D., & Eisenbrand, G. (1982). Influence of ascorbic acid on the endogenous (intragastral) formation of N-nitroso compounds. *International journal for vitamin and nutrition research Supplement = Internationale Zeitschrift für Vitamin- und Ernährungsforschung. Supplement.* 23:91-102 PMID: 6811491

[431] Fields, Ph.D, R. D. (2011, April 1). The New Brain How your brain—and our understanding of it—are constantly changing | Why We Prefer Certain Colors Colors influence object preference in many situations. *Psychology Today*. Retrieved October 27, 2015, from http://www.psychologytoday.com/blog/the-new-brain/201104/why-we-prefer-certain-colors

[432] Smythe, C. (2008, October 6). Salmon-Labeling Suit Lands On Solicitor Gen.'s Desk. *Law360 A LexisNexis Company*. Retrieved October 27, 2015, from https://www.law360.com/articles/71711

[433] KSU. (2003, June 5). Why is a colouring additive used in salmon and poultry feed?. Kansas State University. Retrieved January 28, 2014, from http://www.foodsafety.ksu.edu/articles/533/canthaxanthin_factsheet.pdf

[434] Gogoi, P. (2006, October 01). An Insider's Guide to Food Labels. *Bloomberg*. Retrieved July 03, 2017, from https://www.bloomberg.com/news/articles/2006-09-30/an-insiders-guide-to-food-labelsbusinessweek-business-news-stock-market-and-financial-advice

[435] IPCS Inchem. (2003, March 1). 635. Canthaxanthin (WHO Food Additives Series 22). *IPCS INCHEM*. Retrieved November 6, 2015, from http://www.inchem.org/documents/jecfa/jecmono/v22je09.htm

[436] Beaulieu, R. A., Warwar, R. E., & Buerk, B. M. (2013). Canthaxanthin Retinopathy with Visual Loss: A Case Report and Review. *Case Reports in Ophthalmological Medicine*, 2013, 1-4. doi:10.1155/2013/140901

[437] Center for Food Safety. (2011, February 8). IN THE SUPREME COURT OF CALIFORNIA FARM RAISED SALMON CASES. *Center for Food Safety*. Retrieved January 28, 2014, from http://www.centerforfoodsafety.org/files/ca_salmon_label_opinion_2-11-08.pdf

[438] FDA. (2009, December). For Industry | Color Additive Status List. *U.S. Food and Drug Administration*. Retrieved November 4, 2015, from http://www.fda.gov/ForIndustry/ColorAdditives/ColorAdditiveInventories/ucm106626.htm

[439] Associated Press. (1990, January 30). F.D.A. Limits Red Dye No. 3. *The New York Times*. Retrieved November 4, 2015, from http://www.nytimes.com/1990/01/30/science/fda-limits-red-dye-no-3.html

[440] FDA. (2009, December). For Industry | Color Additive Status List. *U.S. Food and Drug Administration*. Retrieved November 4, 2015, from http://www.fda.gov/ForIndustry/ColorAdditives/ColorAdditiveInventories/ucm106626.htm

[441] Associated Press. (1990, January 29). FDA Bans Some Uses of Red No. 3 Additive. *Los Angeles Times*. Retrieved November 4, 2015, from http://articles.latimes.com/1990-01-29/business/fi-917_1_fda-bans

[442] Ibid

[443] Kim, S. (2013, June 26). 11 Food Ingredients Banned Outside the U.S. That We Eat. *ABC News*. Retrieved November 4, 2015, from http://abcnews.go.com/Lifestyle/Food/11-foods-banned-us/story?id=19457237

[444] Säätelä, E. (2013, October 23). Foods Americans eat that are banned around the world. *Fox News*. Retrieved March 23, 2017, from http://www.foxnews.com/food-drink/2013/10/23/foods-americans-eat-that-are-banned-around-world.html

[445] Columbia Psychiatry. (2010, September 22). How bad is Red 40 and more synthetic dyes?. *Columbia University Medical Center | Columbia Psychiatry*. Retrieved November 4, 2015, from http://columbiapsychiatry.org/http%3A/%252Fwww.eatingwell.com/food_news_origins/food_news/the_hidden_health_risks_of_food_dyes%3Fpage%3D2

[446] Prival, M.D., M., Peiperl, M.D., & Bell, S.J.. (1993, October). Determination of combined benzidine in FD & C yellow no. 5 (tartrazine), using a highly sensitive analytical method. *Science Direct | also published Food and Chemical Toxicology* Volume 31, Issue 10, October 1993, Pages 751–758. Retrieved November 4, 2015, from http://www.sciencedirect.com/science/article/pii/027869159390147Q

[447] EPA. (2000, January). 4-Aminobiphenyl Hazard Summary-Created in April 1992; Revised in January 2000. *EPA-United States Environmental Protection Agency*. Retrieved November 4, 2015, from http://www.epa.gov/ttn/atw/hlthef/aminobip.html

[448] EPA. (2014, January 15). Benzidine Dyes Action Plan Summary | Existing Chemicals . *EPA - EPA-United States Environmental Protection Agency*. Retrieved November 4, 2015, from http://www.epa.gov/oppt/existingchemicals/pubs/actionplans/benzidine.html http://www2.epa.gov/assessing-and-managing-chemicals-under-tsca/benzidine-dyes-action-plan

[449] EPA. (2000, January). 4-Aminobiphenyl Hazard Summary-Created in April 1992; Revised in January 2000. *EPA-United States Environmental Protection Agency*. Retrieved November 4, 2015, from http://www.epa.gov/ttn/atw/hlthef/aminobip.html

[450] EPA. (2005, March). Supplemental Guidance for Assessing Susceptibility from Early Life Exposure to Carcinogens. *EPA 630/R-03/003F*. Also, http://www2.epa.gov/risk/supplemental-guidance-assessing-susceptibility-early-life-exposure-carcinogens

[451] Kim, S. (2013, June 26). 11 Food Ingredients Banned Outside the U.S. That We Eat. *ABC News*. Retrieved November 4, 2015, from http://abcnews.go.com/Lifestyle/Food/11-foods-banned-us/story?id=19457237#1

[452] FDA. (2003, September 29). FDA Public Health Advisory: Subject: Reports of Blue Discoloration and Death in Patients Receiving Enteral Feedings Tinted With The Dye, FD&C Blue No. 1. *FDA - United States Food and Drug Administration*. Retrieved November 4, 2015, from http://www.fda.gov/ForIndustry/ColorAdditives/ColorAdditivesinSpecificProducts/InMedicalDevices/ucm142395.htm

[453] Kim, S. (2013, June 26). 11 Food Ingredients Banned Outside the U.S. That We Eat. *ABC News*. Retrieved November 4, 2015, from http://abcnews.go.com/Lifestyle/Food/11-foods-banned-us/story?id=19457237#2

[454] Sciencelab.com, Inc.. (2013, May 21). Material Safety Data Sheet FD&C Blue #2, Catalog Codes: SLF2182, CAS#: 860-22-0. *Sciencelab.com, Inc.*. Retrieved November 4, 2015, from http://www.sciencelab.com/msds.php?msdsId=9924015

[455] Drugs.com. (2011, October 19). FD&C Green No. 3 Excipient (pharmacologically inactive substance). *Drugs.com - Drug Information Online*. Retrieved November 4, 2015, from http://www.drugs.com/inactive/fd-c-green-no-3-252.html#ref1

[456] Ibid

[457] Gavigan, C. (2013, September 23). Food Dyes: Red Does Not Mean GO. *The Huffington Post*. Retrieved November 4, 2015, from http://www.huffingtonpost.com/christopher-gavigan/food-dye_b_3792860.html

[458] FDA. (2009, December). For Industry | Color Additive Status List. *U.S. Food and Drug Administration*. Retrieved November 4, 2015, from http://www.fda.gov/ForIndustry/ColorAdditives/ColorAdditiveInventories/ucm106626.htm

[459] Columbia Psychiatry. (2010, September 22). How bad is Red 40 and more synthetic dyes?. *Columbia University Medical Center | Columbia Psychiatry*. Retrieved November 4, 2015, from http://columbiapsychiatry.org/http%3A/%252Fwww.eatingwell.com/food_news_origins/food_news/the_hidden_health_risks_of_food_dyes%3Fpage%3D2

[460] Bhat, R. (2017). *Sustainability challenges in the agrofood sector*. Hoboken, NJ: John Wiley & Sons.

[461] McCann, D., Barrett, A., Cooper, A., Crumpler, D., Dalen, L., Grimshaw, K., et al. (2007, November 3). Food additives and hyperactive behaviour in 3-year-old and 8/9-year-old children in the community: a randomised, double-blinded, placebo-controlled trial. *Yearbook of Pediatrics*, 2009, 94-95. doi:10.1016/s0084-3954(08)79206-6 | *The Lancet*, Volume 370, Issue 9598, 1560 - 1567

[462] Ibid

[463] Columbia Psychiatry. (2010, September 22). How bad is Red 40 and more synthetic dyes?. *Columbia University Medical Center | Columbia Psychiatry*. Retrieved November 4, 2015, from http://columbiapsychiatry.org/http%3A/%252Fwww.eatingwell.com/food_news_origins/food_news/the_hidden_health_risks_of_food_dyes%3Fpage%3D2

[464] FDA. (2009, December). For Industry | Color Additive Status List. *U.S. Food and Drug Administration*. Retrieved November 4, 2015, from http://www.fda.gov/ForIndustry/ColorAdditives/ColorAdditiveInventories/ucm106626.htm

[465] Hennessey, R. (2012, August 27). Living in Color: The Potential Dangers of Artificial Dyes. *Forbes Magazine*. Retrieved November 4, 2015, from http://www.forbes.com/sites/rachelhennessey/2012/08/27/living-in-color-the-potential-dangers-of-artificial-dyes/

[466] Layton, L. (2011, April 3). FDA panel rejects need for warnings on food coloring. *The Washington Post*. Retrieved November 4, 2015, from http://www.washingtonpost.com/politics/fda-panel-rejects-need-for-warnings-on-food-coloring/2011/03/31/AF0AaxBC_story.html

[467] Hudson, W. (2014, January 7). American mom wants European M&Ms. *CNN Health - Cable News Network*. Retrieved November 4, 2015, from http://www.cnn.com/2014/01/07/health/mms-candy-artificial-dyes/index.html

[468] Donahue, W. (2011, April 6). Artificial food dyes | FDA takes another look at artificial food dyes, consider possible links to behavior disorders. *Chicago Tribune*. Retrieved November 4, 2015, from http://articles.chicagotribune.com/2011-04-06/features/sc-food-0401-kids-dyes-20110406_1_artificial-food-dyes-fd-c-natural-colorants

[469] Columbia Psychiatry. (2010, September 22). How bad is Red 40 and more synthetic dyes?. *Columbia University Medical Center | Columbia Psychiatry*. Retrieved November 4, 2015, from http://columbiapsychiatry.org/http%3A/%252Fwww.eatingwell.com/food_news_origins/food_news/the_hidden_health_risks_of_food_dyes%3Fpage%3D2

[470] Dartmouth College. (n.d.). Arsenic: A Murderous History. - *Dartmouth Toxic Metals Superfund Research Program*. Retrieved November 4, 2015, from http://www.dartmouth.edu/~toxmetal/arsenic/history.html

[471] EPA. (2013, September 12). Arsenic in Drinking Water. *EPA United States Environmental Protection Agency*. Retrieved November 4, 2015, from http://water.epa.gov/lawsregs/rulesregs/sdwa/arsenic/index.cfm

[472] Dartmouth College. (2013, August 13). Arsenic: A Murderous History. - *Dartmouth Toxic Metals Superfund Research Program*. Retrieved November 4, 2015, from http://www.dartmouth.edu/~toxmetal/arsenic/history.html

[473] Ibid

[474] Johns Hopkins Bloomberg School of Public Health. (2013, May 11). Poultry Drug Increases Levels of Toxic Arsenic in Chicken Meat. *Johns Hopkins Bloomberg School of Public Health*. Retrieved November 4, 2015, from http://www.jhsph.edu/news/news-releases/2013/nachman_arsenic_chicken.html

[475] Nachman, K. E., Baron, P. A., Raber, G., Francesconi, K. A., Navas-Acien, A., & Love, D. C. (2013). Roxarsone, Inorganic Arsenic, and Other Arsenic Species in Chicken: A U.S.-Based Market Basket Sample. *Environmental Health Perspectives, 121*(7), 818-824. doi:10.1289/ehp.1206245

[476] USDA. (2012, April). Poultry - Production and Value. *United States Department of Agriculture National Agricultural Statistics Service*. Retrieved November 4, 2015, from http://usda01.library.cornell.edu/usda/nass/PoulProdVa//2010s/2012/PoulProdVa-04-26-2012.txt Also, http://search.usa.gov/search?utf8=%E2%9C%93&affiliate=usda-nass&query=Poultry+-+Production+and+Value

[477] Nachman, K. E., Baron, P. A., Raber, G., Francesconi, K. A., Navas-Acien, A., & Love, D. C. (2013). Roxarsone, Inorganic Arsenic, and Other Arsenic Species in Chicken: A U.S.-Based Market Basket Sample. *Environmental Health Perspectives, 121*(7), 818-824. doi:10.1289/ehp.1206245

[478] Johns Hopkins Bloomberg School of Public Health. (2013, May 11). Poultry Drug Increases Levels of Toxic Arsenic in Chicken Meat. *Johns Hopkins Bloomberg School of Public Health*. Retrieved November 5, 2015, from http://www.jhsph.edu/news/news-releases/2013/nachman_arsenic_chicken.html

[479] Nachman, K. E., Baron, P. A., Raber, G., Francesconi, K. A., Navas-Acien, A., & Love, D. C. (2013). Roxarsone, Inorganic Arsenic, and Other Arsenic Species in Chicken: A U.S.-Based Market Basket Sample. *Environmental Health Perspectives, 121*(7), 818-824. doi:10.1289/ehp.1206245

[480] EPA. (2013, September 12). Arsenic in Drinking Water. *EPA United States Environmental Protection Agency*. Retrieved November 5, 2015, from http://water.epa.gov/lawsregs/rulesregs/sdwa/arsenic/index.cfm

[481] Ibid

[482] Johns Hopkins Bloomberg School of Public Health. (2013, May 11). Poultry Drug Increases Levels of Toxic Arsenic in Chicken Meat. *Johns Hopkins Bloomberg School of Public Health*. Retrieved November 5, 2015, from http://www.jhsph.edu/news/news-releases/2013/nachman_arsenic_chicken.html

[483] Strom, S. (2013, October 1). F.D.A. Bans Three Arsenic Drugs Used in Poultry and Pig Feeds. *The New York Times*. Retrieved November 5, 2015, from http://www.nytimes.com/2013/10/02/business/fda-bans-three-arsenic-drugs-used-in-poultry-and-pig-feeds.html?_r=0

[484] Ibid

[485] EPA. (2013, September 12). Arsenic in Drinking Water. *EPA United States Environmental Protection Agency*. Retrieved November 5, 2015, from http://water.epa.gov/lawsregs/rulesregs/sdwa/arsenic/index.cfm

[486] Strom, S. (2013, October 1). F.D.A. Bans Three Arsenic Drugs Used in Poultry and Pig Feeds. *The New York Times*. Retrieved November 5, 2015, from http://www.nytimes.com/2013/10/02/business/fda-bans-three-arsenic-drugs-used-in-poultry-and-pig-feeds.html?_r=0

[487] Consumer Reports Magazine. (2012, November 1). Arsenic in Your Food |Our findings show a real need for federal standards for this toxin. *Consumer Reports magazine | Consumer Reports Investigation*. Retrieved November 5, 2015, from http://www.consumerreports.org/cro/magazine/2012/11/arsenic-in-your-food/index.htm

[488] EPA. (2012, March 6). Basic Information about the Arsenic Rule. *United States Environmental Protection Agency*. Retrieved November 5, 2015, from http://water.epa.gov/lawsregs/rulesregs/sdwa/arsenic/Basic-Information.cfm

[489] American Chemical Society. (1999, April 1). New Hampshire Study Shows Well Water Has Higher Arsenic Levels Than Municipal. *ScienceDaily*. Retrieved November 5, 2015, from www.sciencedaily.com/releases/1999/04/990401061229.htm

[490] NRDC.org. (1999, April 29). Summary Findings of NRDC's 1999 Bottled Water Report. *NRDC: Natural Resources Defense Council*. Retrieved November 5, 2015, from http://www.nrdc.org/water/drinking/nbw.asp

[491] NRDC.org. (2009, February 12). Arsenic in Drinking Water. *Natural Resources Defense Council*. Retrieved November 5, 2015, from http://www.nrdc.org/water/drinking/qarsenic.asp#bottled

[492] HHS.gov. (2009, July 8). Regulation of Bottled Water. *U.S. Department of Health and Human Services*. Retrieved November 5, 2015, from http://www.hhs.gov/asl/testify/2009/07/t20090708a.html

[493] NRDC.org. (1999, April 29). Summary Findings of NRDC's 1999 Bottled Water Report. *NRDC: Natural Resources Defense Council*. Retrieved November 5, 2015, from http://www.nrdc.org/water/drinking/nbw.asp

[494] CDC.gov. (2010, May 3). Arsenic and Drinking Water from Private Wells. *Centers for Disease Control and Prevention*. Retrieved November 5, 2015, from http://www.cdc.gov/healthywater/drinking/private/wells/disease/arsenic.html

[495] Ibid

[496] EPA. (2006, January 9). Arsenic in Drinking Water Arsenic Virtual Trade Show. *EPA - United States Environmental Protection Agency*. Retrieved from http://cfpub.epa.gov/safewater/arsenic/arsenictradeshow/arsenic.cfm?action=Ion%20Exchange

[497] CDC.gov. (2010, May 3). Arsenic and Drinking Water from Private Wells. *Centers for Disease Control and Prevention*. Retrieved from http://www.cdc.gov/healthywater/drinking/private/wells/disease/arsenic.html

[498] Consumer Reports Magazine. (2012, November 1). Arsenic in Your Food |Our findings show a real need for federal standards for this toxin. *Consumer Reports magazine | Consumer Reports Investigation*. Retrieved November 5, 2015, from http://www.consumerreports.org/cro/magazine/2012/11/arsenic-in-your-food/index.htm

[499] FDA. (2013, September 27). Questions & Answers: Arsenic in Rice and Rice Products. *U.S. Food and Drug Administration*. Retrieved November 5, 2015, from http://www.fda.gov/Food/FoodborneIllnessContaminants/Metals/ucm319948.htm

[500] Consumer Reports Magazine. (2012, November 1). Arsenic in Your Food |Our findings show a real need for federal standards for this toxin. *Consumer Reports magazine | Consumer Reports Investigation*. Retrieved November 5, 2015, from http://www.consumerreports.org/cro/magazine/2012/11/arsenic-in-your-food/index.htm

[501] Goodman, B., MA. (2011, December 5). Reviewed by Louise Chang, MD. Eating Rice May Raise Arsenic Levels. *WebMD*. Retrieved November 5, 2015, from http://www.webmd.com/baby/news/20111204/eating-rice-may-raise-arsenic-levels?page=2

[502] EPA. (2013, September 12). Arsenic in Drinking Water. *EPA United States Environmental Protection Agency*. Retrieved November 5, 2015, from http://water.epa.gov/lawsregs/rulesregs/sdwa/arsenic/index.cfm

[503] American Cancer Society. (2011, February 17). Arsenic. *American Cancer Society*. Retrieved November 5, 2015, from http://www.cancer.org/cancer/cancercauses/othercarcinogens/intheworkplace/arsenic

[504] Goodman, B., MA. (2011, December 5). Reviewed by Louise Chang, MD. Eating Rice May Raise Arsenic Levels. *WebMD*. Retrieved November 5, 2015, from http://www.webmd.com/baby/news/20111204/eating-rice-may-raise-arsenic-levels?page=2

[505] Ibid

[506] Wu, H., Grandjean, P., Hu, F. B., & Sun, Q. (2015). Consumption of White Rice and Brown Rice and Urinary Inorganic Arsenic Concentration. *Epidemiology*, 26(6). doi:10.1097/ede.0000000000000369

[507] Goodman, B., MA. (2011, December 5). Reviewed by Louise Chang, MD. Eating Rice May Raise Arsenic Levels. *WebMD*. Retrieved November 5, 2015, from http://www.webmd.com/baby/news/20111204/eating-rice-may-raise-arsenic-levels?page=2

[508] Gilbert-Diamond, D., Cottingham, K. L., Gruber, J. F., Punshon, T., Sayarath, V., Gandolfi, A. J., . . . Karagas, M. R. (2011). Rice consumption contributes to arsenic exposure in US women. *Proceedings of the National Academy of Sciences*, 108(51), 20656-20660. doi:10.1073/pnas.1109127108

[509] Goodman, B., MA. (2011, December 5). Reviewed by Louise Chang, MD. Eating Rice May Raise Arsenic Levels. *WebMD*. Retrieved November 5, 2015, from http://www.webmd.com/baby/news/20111204/eating-rice-may-raise-arsenic-levels?page=2

[510] Ibid

[511] Dr. Oz Show. (2011, September 12). Dr. Oz Investigates: Arsenic in Apple Juice. *The Dr. Oz Show*. Retrieved November 5, 2015, from http://www.doctoroz.com/videos/dr-oz-investigates-arsenic-apple-juice

[512] Ibid

[513] Ibid

[514] Ibid

[515] Ibid

[516] Dr. Oz Show. (2011, September 9). Arsenic in Apple Juice. *The Dr. Oz Show*. Retrieved November 5, 2015, from http://www.doctoroz.com/videos/arsenic-apple-juice

[517] Ibid

[518] Dr. Oz Show. (2011, September 14). Statement on Behalf of Juicy Juice. *The Dr. Oz Show*. Retrieved November 5, 2015, from http://www.doctoroz.com/videos/statement-behalf-juicy-juice

[519] Dr. Oz Show. (2011, September 12). Statement on Behalf of Gerber. *The Dr. Oz Show*. Retrieved November 5, 2015, from http://www.doctoroz.com/videos/gerber-statement

[520] Dr. Oz Show. (2011, September 14). Statement on Behalf of Juicy Juice. *The Dr. Oz Show*. Retrieved November 5, 2015, from http://www.doctoroz.com/videos/statement-behalf-juicy-juice

521 Consumer Reports Magazine. (2012, January). Arsenic in your juice | How much is too much? Federal limits don't exist. *Consumer Reports Magazine*. Retrieved November 5, 2015, from http://www.consumerreports.org/cro/magazine/2012/01/arsenic-in-your-juice/index.htm

522 FDA. (2014, October 14). Steroid Hormone Implants Used for Growth in Food-Producing Animals. FDA, *U.S. Food and Drug Administration*. Retrieved November 6, 2015, from http://www.fda.gov/AnimalVeterinary/SafetyHealth/ProductSafetyInformation/ucm055436.htm

523 FDA Veterinarian Newsletter. (2002). THE USE OF STEROID HORMONES FOR GROWTH PROMOTION IN FOOD-PRODUCING ANIMALS. *U.S. Food and Drug Administration FDA Veterinarian Newsletter Volume XVI, No V*. Retrieved April 29, 2014 from http://www.fda.gov/AnimalVeterinary/NewsEvents/FDAVeterinarianNewsletter/ucm110712.htm

524 Al-Husseini, W., Gondro, C., Quinn, K., Cafe, L. M., Herd, R. M., Gibson, J. P., . . . Chen, Y. (2014). Hormonal growth implants affect feed efficiency and expression of residual feed intake-associated genes in beef cattle. *Animal Production Science, 54*(5), 550. doi:10.1071/an12398

525 FDA. (2014, October 14). Steroid Hormone Implants Used for Growth in Food-Producing Animals. FDA, *U.S. Food and Drug Administration*. Retrieved November 6, 2015, from http://www.fda.gov/AnimalVeterinary/SafetyHealth/ProductSafetyInformation/ucm055436.htm

526 Gandhi, R., Ph.D., & Snedeker, S. M., Ph.D. (2003, May 2). Consumer Concerns About Hormones in Food. *Cornell University Archival Website*. Retrieved November 6, 2015, from http://envirocancer.cornell.edu/Factsheet/Diet/fs37.hormones.cfm

527 Johnson, R. (2014, April 22). The U.S.-EU Beef Hormone Dispute. *UNT Digital Library*. Retrieved November 6, 2015, from http://digital.library.unt.edu/ark:/67531/metadc287939/ and fas.org/sgp/crs/row/R40449.pdf

528 European Commission. (2017, June 23). Hormones in Meat - Food Safety - European Commission. Retrieved July 04, 2017, from https://ec.europa.eu/food/safety/chemical_safety/meat_hormones_en

529 Smith, M., Ph.D., J.D. (2005, November/December). Beef Hormone Trade Dispute | FDA Veterinarian Newsletter . *U.S. Food and Drug Administration*. Retrieved April 29, 2014 from http://www.fda.gov/AnimalVeterinary/NewsEvents/FDAVeterinarianNewsletter/ucm092839.htm

530 FDA Veterinarian Newsletter. (2002). THE USE OF STEROID HORMONES FOR GROWTH PROMOTION IN FOOD-PRODUCING ANIMALS. *U.S. Food and Drug Administration FDA Veterinarian Newsletter Volume XVI, No V*. Retrieved April 29, 2014 from http://www.fda.gov/AnimalVeterinary/NewsEvents/FDAVeterinarianNewsletter/ucm110712.htm

531 FDA. (2014, October 14). Steroid Hormone Implants Used for Growth in Food-Producing Animals. FDA, *U.S. Food and Drug Administration*. Retrieved November 6, 2015, from http://www.fda.gov/AnimalVeterinary/SafetyHealth/ProductSafetyInformation/ucm055436.htm

532 Al-Husseini, W., Gondro, C., Quinn, K., Cafe, L. M., Herd, R. M., Gibson, J. P., . . . Chen, Y. (2014). Hormonal growth implants affect feed efficiency and expression of residual feed intake-associated genes in beef cattle. *Animal Production Science, 54*(5), 550. doi:10.1071/an12398

533 Weil, A., MD. (2006, October 31). Avoiding Hormones in Meat and Poultry?. *WEIL Q & A LIBRARY*. Retrieved November 6, 2015, from http://www.drweil.com/drw/u/id/QAA400066

534 Rodriguez, C. A., Bongiovanni, A. M., & Borrego, L. C. (1985). An epidemic of precocious development in Puerto Rican children. *The Journal of Pediatrics, 107*(3), 393-396. doi:10.1016/s0022-3476(85)80513-8

535 Ibid

536 Johns Hopkins Children's Center. (2008, March 10). Precocious Puberty - What is Precocious Puberty?. *Johns Hopkins Children's Center*. Retrieved November 6, 2015, from http://www.hopkinschildrens.org/precocious-puberty.aspx

537 Rodriguez, C. A., Bongiovanni, A. M., & Borrego, L. C. (1985). An epidemic of precocious development in Puerto Rican children. *The Journal of Pediatrics,* 107(3), 393-396. doi:10.1016/s0022-3476(85)80513-8

538 Ibid

539 FDA. (2015, October 22). Bovine Somatotropin (BST). *U.S. Food and Drug Administration*. Retrieved November 6, 2015, from http://www.fda.gov/AnimalVeterinary/SafetyHealth/ProductSafetyInformation/ucm055435.htm

540 Brinckman, D. (1999, December 16). AgBioForum 3(2&3): The Regulation Of rBST: The European Case. *AgBioForum The Journal of Agrobiotechnology Management & Economics*. Retrieved November 6, 2015, from http://www.agbioforum.org/v3n23/v3n23a15-brinckman.htm

541 American Cancer Society. (2014, September 10). Recombinant Bovine Growth Hormone. *American Cancer Society - Cancer.org*. Retrieved November 6, 2015, from http://www.cancer.org/cancer/cancercauses/othercarcinogens/athome/recombinant-bovine-growth-hormone

542 Hyman, M. (2013, July 25). Got Proof? Lack of Evidence for Milk's Benefits. *Dr Mark Hyman*. Retrieved from http://drhyman.com/blog/2013/07/05/got-proof-lack-of-evidence-for-milks-benefits/#close

543 American Cancer Society. (2014, September 10). Recombinant Bovine Growth Hormone. *American Cancer Society - Cancer.org*. Retrieved November 6, 2015, from http://www.cancer.org/cancer/cancercauses/othercarcinogens/athome/recombinant-bovine-growth-hormone

544 Roizen, M. (2013, January 22). Why should I be concerned about antibiotics in meat and fish?. *Sharecare - Food Production & Health*. Retrieved November 9, 2015, from http://www.sharecare.com/health/food-production-and-health/why-concerned-antibiotics-meat-fish

545 Johns Hopkins Bloomberg School of Public Health. (2011, November 9). Testing of Seafood Imported into the U.S. Is Inadequate. *Johns Hopkins Bloomberg School of Public Health*. Retrieved November 9, 2015, from http://www.jhsph.edu/news/news-releases/2011/love-seafood.html

[546] PEW. (2013, February 6). Record-High Antibiotic Sales for Meat and Poultry Production | Project: Pew Campaign on Human Health and Industrial Farming. *The PEW Charitable Trusts Health Initiatives*. Retrieved November 9, 2015, from http://www.pewhealth.org/other-resource/record-high-antibiotic-sales-for-meat-and-poultry-production-85899449119

[547] Ibid

[548] Bren, L. (2006, January-February). About FDA | FDA Consumer magazine| Animal Health and Consumer Protection. *U.S. Food and Drug Administration*. Retrieved November 9, 2015, from http://www.fda.gov/AboutFDA/WhatWeDo/History/ProductRegulation/AnimalHealthandConsumerProtection/

[549] FDA. (2013, December 11). Phasing Out Certain Antibiotic Use in Farm Animals. *U.S. Food and Drug Administration*. Retrieved November 9, 2015, from http://www.fda.gov/ForConsumers/ConsumerUpdates/ucm378100.htm

[550] UCDavis. (2008, January 23). Prohibited Antimicrobial Agents in Seafood. *University of California, Davis*. Retrieved November 9, 2015, from http://safeseafood.ucdavis.edu/background.htm

[551] U.S. GAO. (2011, April 14). U.S. GAO - Seafood Safety: FDA Needs to Improve Oversight of Imported Seafood and Better Leverage Limited Resources Report to Congressional Requesters. *United States Government Accountability Office - GAO* . Retrieved November 9, 2015, from http://www.gao.gov/products/GAO-11-286
http://www.gao.gov/assets/320/317734.pdf

[552] Ibid

[553] FDA. (2013, August 5). Import Alert 16-131 "Detention Without Physical Examination of Aquacultured Catfish, Basa, Shrimp, Dace, and Eel from China- Presence of New Animal Drugs and/or Unsafe Food Additives". *FDA - United States Food and Drug Administration*. Retrieved November 9, 2015, from http://www.accessdata.fda.gov/cms_ia/importalert_33.html

[554] Ibid

[555] Ibid

[556] Johns Hopkins Bloomberg School of Public Health. (2011, November 9). Testing of Seafood Imported into the U.S. Is Inadequate. *Johns Hopkins Bloomberg School of Public Health*. Retrieved November 9, 2015, from http://www.jhsph.edu/news/news-releases/2011/love-seafood.html

[557] Ibid

[558] Ibid

[559] Ibid

[560] FDA. (2013, August 5). Import Alert 16-131 "Detention Without Physical Examination of Aquacultured Catfish, Basa, Shrimp, Dace, and Eel from China- Presence of New Animal Drugs and/or Unsafe Food Additives". *FDA - United States Food and Drug Administration*. Retrieved November 9, 2015, from http://www.accessdata.fda.gov/cms_ia/importalert_33.html

[561] Roizen, M. (2013, January 22). Why should I be concerned about antibiotics in meat and fish?. *Sharecare - Food Production & Health*. Retrieved November 9, 2015, from http://www.sharecare.com/health/food-production-and-health/why-concerned-antibiotics-meat-fish

[562] FDA. (2013, December 11). Phasing Out Certain Antibiotic Use in Farm Animals . *U.S. Food and Drug Administration*. Retrieved November 9, 2015, from http://www.fda.gov/ForConsumers/ConsumerUpdates/ucm378100.htm

[563] Lupkin, S. (2013, December 24). Your Christmas Ham's Vet May Be the Gatekeeper to Antibiotics. *ABC News*. Retrieved November 9, 2015, from http://abcnews.go.com/Health/livestock-vets-prescribe-low-dose-antibiotics/story?id=21312309

[564] FDA. (2013, December 11). Phasing Out Certain Antibiotic Use in Farm Animals . *U.S. Food and Drug Administration*. Retrieved November 9, 2015, from http://www.fda.gov/ForConsumers/ConsumerUpdates/ucm378100.htm

[565] Marshall, B. M., & Levy, S. B. (2011). Food Animals and Antimicrobials: Impacts on Human Health. *Clinical Microbiology Reviews*, 24(4), 718-733. doi:10.1128/cmr.00002-11

[566] Spellberg, B., Bartlett, J. G., & Gilbert, D. N. (2013). The Future of Antibiotics and Resistance. *New England Journal of Medicine*, 368(4), 299-302. doi:10.1056/nejmp1215093

[567] Davies, J., & Davies, D. (2010). Origins and Evolution of Antibiotic Resistance. *Microbiology and Molecular Biology Reviews*, 74(3), 417-433. doi:10.1128/mmbr.00016-10

[568] FDA. (2013, December 11). Phasing Out Certain Antibiotic Use in Farm Animals . *U.S. Food and Drug Administration*. Retrieved November 9, 2015, from http://www.fda.gov/ForConsumers/ConsumerUpdates/ucm378100.htm

[569] Roizen, M. (2013, January 22). Why should I be concerned about antibiotics in meat and fish?. *Sharecare - Food Production & Health*. Retrieved November 9, 2015, from http://www.sharecare.com/health/food-production-and-health/why-concerned-antibiotics-meat-fish

[570] FDA. (2012, November 19). Questions and Answers on Monosodium Glutamate (MSG). *U.S. Food and Drug Administration*. Retrieved November 9, 2015, from http://www.fda.gov/Food/IngredientsPackagingLabeling/FoodAdditivesIngredients/ucm328728.htm

[571] Fulton, A. (2011, July 22). Got Enhanced Meat? USDA Rule May Make It Easier To Tell. *NPR*. Retrieved November 9, 2015, from http://www.npr.org/blogs/health/2011/07/22/138606851/got-enhanced-meat-usda-rule-may-make-it-easier-to-tell

[572] USDA. (2013, August 6). Water in Meat and Poultry. *United States Department of Agriculture - Food Safety and Inspection Service*. Retrieved November 10, 2015, from http://www.fsis.usda.gov/wps/portal/fsis/topics/food-safety-education/get-answers/food-safety-fact-sheets/meat-preparation/water-in-meat-and-poultry/ct_index

[573] Ibid

574 Hull, J. (2008, September). Cooking Down Maltodextrin. *Dr. Janet Hull | Alternative Health and Nutrition*. Retrieved November 10, 2015, from http://www.janethull.com/newsletter/0908/cooking_down_maltodextrin.php

575 FDA. (2013, April 1). CFR - Code of Federal Regulations Sec. 184.1444 Maltodextrin. *U.S. Food and Drug Administration*. Retrieved November 10, 2015, from http://www.accessdata.fda.gov/scripts/cdrh/cfdocs/cfcfr/CFRSearch.cfm?fr=184.1444

576 Hull, J. (2008, September). Cooking Down Maltodextrin. *Dr. Janet Hull | Alternative Health and Nutrition*. Retrieved November 10, 2015, from http://www.janethull.com/newsletter/0908/cooking_down_maltodextrin.php

577 FDA. (2013, April 1). Sec. 184.1639 Potassium lactate | CFR - Code of Federal Regulations Title 21 . *U.S. Food and Drug Administration*. Retrieved November 10, 2015, from http://www.accessdata.fda.gov/scripts/cdrh/cfdocs/cfcfr/CFRSearch.cfm?fr=184.1639

578 Ibid

579 Ibid

580 Med-Health. (2015, November 12). Sodium Phosphate. *Med-Health.net | Health News Written by Medical Doctors*. Retrieved November 10, 2015, from http://www.med-health.net/Sodium-Phosphate.html

581 Robinson, A. (2013, September 6). Food Additives: What is Sodium Phosphate?. *Livestrong.com*. Retrieved November 10, 2015, from http://www.livestrong.com/article/40858-sodium-phosphate-label/

582 Med-Health. (2015, November 12). Sodium Phosphate. *Med-Health.net | Health News Written by Medical Doctors*. Retrieved November 10, 2015, from http://www.med-health.net/Sodium-Phosphate.html

583 Robinson, A. (2013, September 6). Food Additives: What is Sodium Phosphate?. *Livestrong.com*. Retrieved November 10, 2015, from http://www.livestrong.com/article/40858-sodium-phosphate-label/

584 NutritionData. (2003, August 30). Food Additives | Individual Food Additives (alphabetical listing). *NutritionData*. Retrieved November 10, 2015, from http://nutritiondata.self.com/topics/food-additives

585 FDA. (2014, January 13). FDA warns of possible harm from exceeding recommended dose of over-the-counter sodium phosphate products to treat constipation. *U.S. Food and Drug Administration*. Retrieved November 10, 2015, from http://www.fda.gov/Drugs/DrugSafety/ucm380757.htm

586 NIH. (2014, April 15). Sodium Phosphate: MedlinePlus Drug Information. *U.S National Library of Medicine | National Institutes of Health*. Retrieved November 10, 2015, from http://www.nlm.nih.gov/medlineplus/druginfo/meds/a609019.html

587 FDA. (2014, January 13). FDA warns of possible harm from exceeding recommended dose of over-the-counter sodium phosphate products to treat constipation. *U.S. Food and Drug Administration*. Retrieved November 10, 2015, from http://www.fda.gov/Drugs/DrugSafety/ucm380757.htm

588 NIH. (2014, April 15). Sodium Phosphate: MedlinePlus Drug Information. *U.S National Library of Medicine | National Institutes of Health*. Retrieved November 10, 2015, from http://www.nlm.nih.gov/medlineplus/druginfo/meds/a609019.html

589 Ibid

590 Ehrlich, S. D. (2011, June 17). Phosphorus. *University of Maryland Medical Center*. Retrieved November 10, 2015, from http://umm.edu/health/medical/altmed/supplement/phosphorus

591 USDA. (1995, March 17). Labeling and Consumer Protection Propietary Mixture Suppliers and Manufacturers. *United States Department of Agriculture*. Retrieved November 10, 2015, from http://www.fsis.usda.gov/OPPDE/larc/Ingredients/PMC_QA.htm

592 Siegel-Itzkovich, J. (2005). Health committee warns of potential dangers of soya. *Bmj, 331*(7511), 254-0. doi:10.1136/bmj.331.7511.254-a

593 Ibid

594 Ibid

595 Warren, B. S., BCERF & Devine, C. , Ph.D., R.D. (2002, July 1). PhytoEstrogens and Breast Cancer Fact Sheet #01. *Cornell University Program on Breast Cancer and Environmental Risk Factors*. Retrieved November 10, 2015, from http://envirocancer.cornell.edu/FactSheet/Diet/fs1.phyto.cfm

596 Ireland, C. (2006, December 7). Hormones in milk can be dangerous - Ganmaa Davaasambuu, a Ph.D.. *Harvard University Gazette*. Retrieved November 10, 2015, from http://news.harvard.edu/gazette/2006/12.07/11-dairy.html

597 Clark, R. A., M.S., Snedeker, S., Ph.D., & Devine, C. Ph.D. (2002, July 2). Cornell University Program on Breast Cancer and Environmental Risk Factors. Estrogen and Breast Cancer Risk: part 1. Retrieved November 10, 2015, from http://envirocancer.cornell.edu/FactSheet/General/fs10.Estrogen.cfm

598 Travis, R. C., & Key, T. J. (2003). OEstrogen exposure and breast cancer risk. *Breast Cancer Research,5*(5). doi:10.1186/bcr628

599 Harvard School of Public Health. (2014, February 12). Straight talk about soy. *Harvard School of Public Health | The Nutrition Source*. Retrieved November 10, 2015, from http://www.hsph.harvard.edu/nutritionsource/2014/02/12/straight-talk-about-soy/#ref31

600 Ibid

601 Ibid

602 USDA ERS -Adoption of Genetically Engineered Crops in the U.S.: Recent Trends in GE Adoption. (2015, July 9). *USDA ERS - Economic Research Service*. Retrieved November 12, 2015, from http://www.ers.usda.gov/data-products/adoption-of-genetically-engineered-crops-in-the-us/recent-trends-in-ge-adoption.aspx#.UwUmbmJdWdI

603 WebMD. (2015, June 10). Genetically Modified Foods (Biotech Foods) Pros and Cons | Are Biotech Foods Safe to Eat?. *WebMD*. Retrieved November 12, 2015, from http://www.webmd.com/food-recipes/features/are-biotech-foods-safe-to-eat

604 Ibid

[605] Wilkerson, J. (2015, August 10). Why Roundup Ready Crops Have Lost their Allure - Science in the News. *Harvard University The Graduate School of Arts and Sciences*. Retrieved May 25, 2016, from http://sitn.hms.harvard.edu/flash/2015/roundup-ready-crops/

[606] Myers, J. P., Antoniou, M. N., Blumberg, B., Carroll, L., Colborn, T., Everett, L. G., . . . Benbrook, C. M. (2016). Concerns over use of glyphosate-based herbicides and risks associated with exposures: a consensus statement. *Environmental Health, 15*(1). doi:10.1186/s12940-016-0117-0

[607] Mercola, J. (2013, October 6). Toxicology Expert Speaks Out About Roundup and GMOs | Dr. Huber: Things You Need to Know About GMO and Roundup. *Mercola.com*. Retrieved May 26, 2016, from http://articles.mercola.com/sites/articles/archive/2013/10/06/dr-huber-gmo-foods.aspx

[608] Ibid

[609] Samsel, A., & Seneff, S. (2013). Glyphosate's Suppression of Cytochrome P450 Enzymes and Amino Acid Biosynthesis by the Gut Microbiome: Pathways to Modern Diseases. *Entropy, 15*(4), 1416-1463. doi:10.3390/e15041416

[610] Myers, J. P., Antoniou, M. N., Blumberg, B., Carroll, L., Colborn, T., Everett, L. G., . . . Benbrook, C. M. (2016). Concerns over use of glyphosate-based herbicides and risks associated with exposures: a consensus statement. *Environmental Health, 15*(1). doi:10.1186/s12940-016-0117-0

[611] Mercola, J. (2013, October 6). Toxicology Expert Speaks Out About Roundup and GMOs | Dr. Huber: Things You Need to Know About GMO and Roundup. *Mercola.com*. Retrieved May 26, 2016, from http://articles.mercola.com/sites/articles/archive/2013/10/06/dr-huber-gmo-foods.aspx

[612] Ibid

[613] Weitz & Luxenberg. (2017). Roundup Weed Killer Could Cause Cancer. *Weitz & Luxenberg*. Retrieved August 10, 2017, from http://www.weedkillercancer.com/?utm_source=google&utm_medium=paid-search&utm_campaign=roundup&gclid=CIjYgdONzdUCFU-BswodMzcKUg

[614] Baum Hedlund Law. (2017). Monsanto Roundup Lawsuit. *Baum, Hedlund, Aristei, Goldman*. Retrieved August 10, 2017, from https://www.baumhedlundlaw.com/toxic-tort-law/monsanto-roundup-lawsuit/?gclid=EAIaIQobChMIh7fezY3N1QIVCIlpCh0C0wpVEAAYAiAAEgJjdvD_BwE

[615] Chlanger, Z. (2016, February 19). THE FDA WILL BEGIN TESTING FOOD FOR GLYPHOSATE, THE MOST HEAVILY USED FARM CHEMICAL EVER. *Newsweek*. Retrieved May 26, 2016, from http://www.newsweek.com/fda-will-begin-testing-food-glyphosate-most-heavily-used-farm-chemical-ever-428790

[616] Liener, I. E. (1994). Implications of antinutritional components in soybean foods. *Critical Reviews in Food Science and Nutrition, 34*(1), 31-67. doi:10.1080/10408399409527649

[617] Dictionary. (2007, February 10). Anti-nutrients. *Dictionary.com*. Retrieved November 12, 2015, from http://dictionary.reference.com/browse/anti-nutrients

[618] Fallon, S., & Enig, M. G.,Ph.D.. (n.d.). Newest Research On Why You Should Avoid Soy. *Mercola.com*. Retrieved November 12, 2015, from http://www.mercola.com/article/soy/avoid_soy.htm

[619] Doerge, D. R., & Sheehan, D. M. (2002). Goitrogenic and Estrogenic Activity of Soy Isoflavones. Environmental Health Perspectives, 110(S3), 349-353. doi:10.1289/ehp.02110s3349

[620] Fallon, S., & Enig, M. G.,Ph.D.. (1999, October 25). Newest Research On Why You Should Avoid Soy. *Mercola.com*. Retrieved November 12, 2015, from http://www.mercola.com/article/soy/avoid_soy.htm

[621] Ibid

[622] Daniel, K. T., PhD, CCN. (2005). *The whole soy story: the dark side of America's favorite health food*. Washington, DC: New Trends Publishing.

[623] Ibid

[624] Ibid

[625] Ibid

[626] Ibid

[627] Ibid

[628] Ibid

[629] Ibid

[630] Ibid

[631] Ibid

[632] Fallon, S., & Enig, M. G.,Ph.D.. (1999, October 25). Newest Research On Why You Should Avoid Soy. *Mercola.com*. Retrieved November 12, 2015, from http://www.mercola.com/article/soy/avoid_soy.htm

[633] Reddy, N., & Pierson, M. (1994). Reduction in antinutritional and toxic components in plant foods by fermentation. *Food Research International, 27*(3), 281-290. doi:10.1016/0963-9969(94)90096-5

[634] Mercola, J. (2012, August 23). The Health Dangers of Soy. *The Huffington Post Healthy Living*. Retrieved November 12, 2015, from http://www.huffingtonpost.com/dr-mercola/soy-health_b_1822466.html

[635] Ibid

[636] Direct Publishing Ltd. (2010, July 8). The Atkins Diet and Alcohol Consumption. *Atkins Diet Advisor*. Retrieved November 12, 2015, from http://www.atkins-diet-advisor.com/atkins-diet-and-alcohol.html

[637] Columbia University. (2014, February 20). Do drinking and weight loss mix?. *Go Ask Alice! | Columbia University*. Retrieved November 12, 2015, from http://goaskalice.columbia.edu/do-drinking-and-weight-loss-mix

[638] Ibid

[639] About, Inc. (2014, January 20). Calories in Orange Juice fresh pressed. *Calorie Count*. Retrieved November 12, 2015, from http://caloriecount.about.com/calories-orange-juice-i9206

[640] USDA. (2008, July 9). Chapter 9 Alcoholic Beverages. *USDA Health.gov*. Retrieved November 12, 2015, from http://www.health.gov/dietaryguidelines/dga2005/document/html/chapter9.htm

[641] Samuel Adams®. (n.d.). Samuel Adams® - Boston Lager - Our Flagship Craft Beer. *samueladams*. Retrieved July 10, 2017, from https://www.samueladams.com/craft-beers/boston-lager

[642] USDA. (2008, July 9). Chapter 9 Alcoholic Beverages. *USDA Health.gov*. Retrieved November 12, 2015, from http://www.health.gov/dietaryguidelines/dga2005/document/html/chapter9.htm

[643] Ibid

[644] Ibid

[645] American Cancer Society. (2014, February 12). Alcohol Use and Cancer. *American Cancer Society*. Retrieved November 12, 2015, from http://www.cancer.org/cancer/cancercauses/dietandphysicalactivity/alcohol-use-and-cancer

[646] Ibid

[647] Ibid

[648] Hanson, D. J., Ph.D.(n.d.). Drinking Alcohol, Weight & Obesity. *Potsdam State University of New York | Sociology Department*. Retrieved November 12, 2015, from http://www2.potsdam.edu/alcohol/InTheNews/MedicalReports/index-Weight.html#.U5pHgP4U88w

[649] Maia, R. D. (2014). Risks and Forms of Cancer Associated with Alcohol Consumption. *Cancer Research Journal*, 2(6), 30. doi:10.11648/j.crj.s.2014020601.13

[650] Rehm, J., Shield, K.(2014). Alcohol consumption. World Cancer Report 2014. *International Agency for Research on Cancer*, Lyon, France

[651] Ibid

[652] Shuman, T. C. (2005, October 1). Reviewed by Elizabeth Klodas, MD, FACC on February 19, 2014. The Link Between Drinking Alcohol and Heart Disease?. *WebMD*. Retrieved from http://www.webmd.com/heart-disease/guide/heart-disease-alcohol-your-heart

[653] Baum-Baicker, C. (1985). The health benefits of moderate alcohol consumption: A review of the literature. *Drug and Alcohol Dependence*, 15(3), 207-227. doi:10.1016/0376-8716(85)90001-8

[654] MacMath, T.(1990, November). Alcohol and gastrointestinal bleeding. *Emergency medicine clinics of North America*, Department of Surgery, University of Florida Health Science Center/Jaksonville. 8(4):859-72. PMID: 2226291

[655] USDA. (2008, July 9). Chapter 9 Alcoholic Beverages. *USDA Health.gov*. Retrieved November 12, 2015, from http://www.health.gov/dietaryguidelines/dga2005/document/html/chapter9.htm

[656] Hanson, D. J., Ph.D.(n.d.). Drinking Alcohol, Weight & Obesity. *Potsdam State University of New York | Sociology Department*. Retrieved November 12, 2015, from http://www2.potsdam.edu/alcohol/InTheNews/MedicalReports/index-Weight.html#.U5pHgP4U88w

[657] Otaka, M., Konishi, N., Odashima, M., Jin, M., Wada, I., Matsuhashi, T., . . . Watanabe, S. (2007). Effect of Alcohol Consumption on Leptin Level in Serum, Adipose Tissue, and Gastric Mucosa. *Digestive Diseases and Sciences*, 52(11), 3066-3069. doi:10.1007/s10620-006-9635-x

[658] Cabot, S., MD. (2013, October 24). Alcohol can mess with your appetite hormones and make it impossible to lose weight. *Liver Doctor*. Retrieved November 12, 2015, from http://www.liverdoctor.com/alcohol-can-mess-appetite-hormones-make-impossible-lose-weight/

[659] Ibid

[660] Ibid

[661] Ibid

[662] Purohit, V., Bode, J. C., Bode, C., Brenner, D. A., Choudhry, M. A., Hamilton, F., . . . Turner, J. R. (2008). Alcohol, intestinal bacterial growth, intestinal permeability to endotoxin, and medical consequences: Summary of a symposium. *Alcohol*, 42(5), 349-361. doi:10.1016/j.alcohol.2008.03.131

[663] Hartmann, P., Seebauer, C. T., & Schnabl, B. (2015). Alcoholic Liver Disease: The Gut Microbiome and Liver Cross Talk. *Alcoholism: Clinical and Experimental Research*, 39(5), 763-775. doi:10.1111/acer.12704

[664] Copeland, S., Warren, H. S., Lowry, S. F., Calvano, S. E., & Remick, D. (2005). Acute Inflammatory Response to Endotoxin in Mice and Humans. *Clinical and Vaccine Immunology*, 12(1), 60-67. doi:10.1128/cdli.12.1.60-67.2005

[665] Liang, H., Hussey, S. E., Sanchez-Avila, A., Tantiwong, P., & Musi, N. (2013). Effect of Lipopolysaccharide on Inflammation and Insulin Action in Human Muscle. *PLoS ONE*, 8(5). doi:10.1371/journal.pone.0063983

[666] The Pennsylvania State University. (2014, April 26). Exotoxins and Endotoxins. *MICRB 106 | Eberly College of Science*. Retrieved August 23, 2017, from https://online.science.psu.edu/micrb106_wd/node/6029

[667] Purohit, V., Bode, J. C., Bode, C., Brenner, D. A., Choudhry, M. A., Hamilton, F., . . . Turner, J. R. (2008). Alcohol, intestinal bacterial growth, intestinal permeability to endotoxin, and medical consequences: Summary of a symposium. *Alcohol*, 42(5), 349-361. doi:10.1016/j.alcohol.2008.03.131

[668] Ibid

[669] Salaspuro, M. (1997). Microbial metabolism of ethanol and acetaldehyde and clinical consequences. *Addiction Biology, 2*(1), 35-46. doi:10.1080/13556219772840

[670] Lachenmeier, D. W., Kanteres, F., & Rehm, J. (2009). Carcinogenicity of acetaldehyde in alcoholic beverages: risk assessment outside Ethanol metabolism. *Addiction, 104*(4), 533-550. doi:10.1111/j.1360-0443.2009.02516.x

[671] Purohit, V., Bode, J. C., Bode, C., Brenner, D. A., Choudhry, M. A., Hamilton, F., . . . Turner, J. R. (2008). Alcohol, intestinal bacterial growth, intestinal permeability to endotoxin, and medical consequences: Summary of a symposium. *Alcohol, 42*(5), 349-361. doi:10.1016/j.alcohol.2008.03.131

[672] Engen, P. A., Green, S. J., Voigt, R. M., Forsyth, C. B., & Keshavarzian, A. (2015). The Gastrointestinal Microbiome: Alcohol Effects on the Composition of Intestinal Microbiota. *Alcohol Research: current reviews.* 37(2):223-36

[673] Ibid

[674] Ibid

[675] Ibid

[676] Ibid

[677] Ibid

[678] Brent, G. A. (2012). Mechanisms of Thyroid hormone action. *Journal of Clinical Investigation, 122*(9), 3035-3043. doi:10.1172/jci60047

[679] Balhara, Y. S., & Deb, K. (2013). Impact of alcohol use on Thyroid function. *Indian Journal of Endocrinology and Metabolism, 17*(4), 580. doi:10.4103/2230-8210.113724

[680] Rachdaoui, N., & Sarkar, D. K. (2013). Effects of Alcohol on the Endocrine System. *Endocrinology and Metabolism Clinics of North America, 42*(3), 593-615. doi:10.1016/j.ecl.2013.05.008

[681] Balhara, Y. S., & Deb, K. (2013). Impact of alcohol use on Thyroid function. *Indian Journal of Endocrinology and Metabolism, 17*(4), 580. doi:10.4103/2230-8210.113724

[682] Rachdaoui, N., & Sarkar, D. K. (2013). Effects of Alcohol on the Endocrine System. *Endocrinology and Metabolism Clinics of North America, 42*(3), 593-615. doi:10.1016/j.ecl.2013.05.008

[683] Hage, M. P., & Azar, S. T. (2012). The Link between Thyroid Function and Depression. *Journal of Thyroid Research, 2012*, 1-8. doi:10.1155/2012/590648

[684] Gavaler, J. Ph.D., (1998). Alcoholic beverages as a source of Estrogens. *Alcohol Health and Research World.* 22(3):220-7.

[685] Warren, B. S., BCERF & Devine, C. , Ph.D., R.D. (2002, July 1). PhytoEstrogens and Breast Cancer Fact Sheet #01. *Cornell University Program on Breast Cancer and Environmental Risk Factors.* Retrieved November 10, 2015, from http://envirocancer.cornell.edu/FactSheet/Diet/fs1.phyto.cfm

[686] Milligan, S. R., Kalita, J. C., Heyerick, A., Rong, H., Cooman, L. D., & Keukeleire, D. D. (1999). Identification of a Potent PhytoEstrogen in Hops (Humulus lupulus L.) and Beer. *The Journal of Clinical Endocrinology & Metabolism, 84*(6), 2249-2249. doi:10.1210/jcem.84.6.5887

[687] Ibid

[688] Couwenbergs, C.J. (1988, October). Acute effects of drinking beer or wine on the steroid hormones of healthy men. *Journal of Steroid Biochemistry.* 31(4A):467-73. PMID: 3172777

[689] Ibid

[690] Johnson, R. E., & Murad, M. H. (2009). Gynecomastia: Pathophysiology, Evaluation, and Management. *Mayo Clinic Proceedings, 84*(11), 1010-1015. doi:10.1016/s0025-6196(11)60671-x

[691] Grossmann, M., Fui, M. T., & Dupuis, P. (2014). Lowered Testosterone in male obesity: Mechanisms, morbidity and management. *Asian Journal of Andrology, 16*(2), 223. doi:10.4103/1008-682x.122365

[692] Ramasamy, R., Schulster, M., & Bernie, A. (2016). The role of estradiol in male reproductive function. *Asian Journal of Andrology, 18*(3), 435. doi:10.4103/1008-682x.173932

[693] Benegal, V., & Arackal, B. (2007). Prevalence of sexual dysfunction in male subjects with alcohol dependence. *Indian Journal of Psychiatry, 49*(2), 109. doi:10.4103/0019-5545.33257

[694] Key, T. J., Appleby, P. N., Reeves, G. K., Roddam, A. W., Helzlsouer, K. J., Alberg, A. J., . . . Strickler, H. D. (2011). Circulating sex hormones and breast cancer risk factors in postmenopausal women: reanalysis of 13 studies. *British Journal of Cancer, 105*(5), 709-722. doi:10.1038/bjc.2011.254

[695] Bradley, K. A., Badrinath, S., Bush, K., Boyd-Wickizer, J., & Anawalt, B. (1998). Medical risks for women who drink alcohol. *Journal of General Internal Medicine, 13*(9), 627-639. doi:10.1046/j.1525-1497.1998.cr187.x

[696] Chakraborty, S., Ganti, A. K., Marr, A., & Batra, S. K. (2010). Lung cancer in women: role of Estrogens. *Expert Review of Respiratory Medicine, 4*(4), 509-518. doi:10.1586/ers.10.50

[697] Travis, R. C., & Key, T. J. (2003). OEstrogen exposure and breast cancer risk. *Breast Cancer Research, 5*(5). doi:10.1186/bcr628

[698] Hamajima, N, Hirose K, Tajima, K, Rohan, T, Calle, E, Heath, CW Jr, Coates, RJ, Liff, JM, Talamini, R, Chantarakul, N, Koetsawang, S, Rachawat, D, Morabia, A, Schuman, L,... Meirik, O. (2002). Alcohol, tobacco and breast cancer--collaborative reanalysis of individual data from 53 epidemiological studies, including 58,515 women with breast cancer and 95,067 women without the disease. *British Journal of Cancer, 87*(11), 1234-1245. doi:10.1038/sj.bjc.6600596

[699] Allen, N. E., Beral, V., Casabonne, D., Kan, S. W., Reeves, G. K., Brown, A., & Green, J. (2009). Moderate Alcohol Intake and Cancer Incidence in Women. *JNCI Journal of the National Cancer Institute, 101*(5), 296-305. doi:10.1093/jnci/djn514

700 Ibid

701 Gavaler, J. Ph.D., (1998). Alcoholic beverages as a source of Estrogens. *Alcohol Health and Research World*. 22(3):220-7.

702 Rohsenow, D., & Howland, J. (2010, June). The role of beverage congeners in hangover and other residual effects of alcohol intoxication: a review. *Current Drug Abuse Review*. 3(2):76-9. PMID: 20712591

703 Gude, D. (2012). Alcohol and fertility. *Journal of Human Reproductive Sciences*, 5(2), 226. doi:10.4103/0974-1208.101030

704 Vignera, S. L., Condorelli, R. A., Balercia, G., Vicari, E., & Calogero, A. E. (2012). Does alcohol have any effect on male reproductive function? A review of literature. *Asian Journal of Andrology*, 15(2), 221-225. doi:10.1038/aja.2012.118

705 Emanuele, M., & Emanuele, N. (2001). Alcohol and the male reproductive system. *Alcohol Research and Health: The journal of the National Institute on Alcohol Abuse and Alcoholism*. 25(4):282-7. PMID: 11910706

706 Grotheer, P., Marshall, M., & Simonne, A. (2013). Sulfites: Separating Fact from Fiction. EDIS *New Publications RSS: Publication #FCS8787 | University of Florida*. Retrieved November 12, 2015, from http://edis.ifas.ufl.edu/fy731

707 Vally, H., & Misso, N. L. (2012). Adverse reactions to the sulphite additives. *Gastroenterology and Hepatology From Bed to Bench*, 5(1), 16–23. PMCID: PMC4017440

708 Yang, W. H., & Purchase, E. C. R. (1985). Adverse reactions to sulfites. *Canadian Medical Association Journal*, 133(9), 865–880. PMCID: PMC1346296

709 Ibid

710 Ibid

711 Vally, H., & Misso, N. L. (2012). Adverse reactions to the sulphite additives. *Gastroenterology and Hepatology From Bed to Bench*, 5(1), 16–23. PMCID: PMC4017440

712 Grotheer, P., Marshall, M., & Simonne, A. (2013). Sulfites: Separating Fact from Fiction. EDIS *New Publications RSS: Publication #FCS8787 | University of Florida*. Retrieved November 12, 2015, from http://edis.ifas.ufl.edu/fy731

713 Lester, M. R. (1995). Sulfite sensitivity: significance in human health. *Journal of the American College of Nutrition*, 14(3), 229-232. doi:10.1080/07315724.1995.10718500

714 Grotheer, P., Marshall, M., & Simonne, A. (2013). Sulfites: Separating Fact from Fiction. EDIS *New Publications RSS: Publication #FCS8787 | University of Florida*. Retrieved November 12, 2015, from http://edis.ifas.ufl.edu/fy731

715 Ibid

716 Ibid

717 Ibid

718 Vally, H., & Misso, N. L. (2012). Adverse reactions to the sulphite additives. *Gastroenterology and Hepatology From Bed to Bench*, 5(1), 16–23. PMCID: PMC4017440

719 Ibid

720 WebMD. (2012, April 26). Reviewed by Brunilda Nazario, MD. Tyramine-Rich Foods: Do They Trigger Migraines?. *WebMD*. Retrieved November 12, 2015, from http://www.webmd.com/migraines-headaches/guide/tyramine-and-migraines

721 Moffett, A., Swash, M., & Scott, D. F. (1972). Effect of tyramine in migraine: a double-blind study. *Journal of Neurology, Neurosurgery & Psychiatry*, 35(4), 496-499. doi:10.1136/jnnp.35.4.496

722 Ibid

723 Clugston, R. D., & Blaner, W. S. (2012). The Adverse Effects of Alcohol on Vitamin A Metabolism. *Nutrients*, 4(12), 356-371. doi:10.3390/nu4050356

724 Laufer, E. M., Hartman, T. J., Baer, D. J., Gunter, E. W., Dorgan, J. F., Campbell, W. S., . . . Taylor, P. R. (2004). Effects of moderate alcohol consumption on folate and vitamin B12 status in postmenopausal women. *European Journal of Clinical Nutrition*, 58(11), 1518-1524. doi:10.1038/sj.ejcn.1602002

725 Hoyumpa, A. M. (1986). Mechanisms of Vitamin Deficiencies in Alcoholism. *Alcoholism: Clinical and Experimental Research*, 10(6), 573-581. doi:10.1111/j.1530-0277.1986.tb05147.x

726 Ibid

727 ATSDR. (2011, March 3). Toxic Substances Portal - Propylene Glycol. *ATSDR - Agency for Toxic Substances and Disease Registry*. Retrieved November 12, 2015, from http://www.atsdr.cdc.gov/substances/toxsubstance.asp?toxid=240

728 Zitomer, D., Ferguson, N., Mcgrady, K., & Schilling, J. (2001). Anaerobic Co-Digestion of Aircraft Deicing Fluid and Municipal Wastewater Sludge. *Water Environment Research*, 73(6), 645-654. doi:10.2175/106143001x143376

729 EPA. (2012, November 19). Antifreeze, Common Wastes & Materials. *EPA*. Retrieved November 12, 2015, from http://www.epa.gov/epawaste/conserve/materials/antifree.htm

730 DOW. (2013). Pure Flavor Solutions Dow Propylene Glycol USP/EP for the Food-Processing Industry. *The Dow Chemical Company*. Retrieved November 12, 2015, from http://msdssearch.dow.com/PublishedLiteratureDOWCOM/dh_064f/0901b8038064fc36.pdf?filepath=propyleneglycol/pdfs/noreg/117-01632.pdf&fromPage=GetDoc

731 Ibid

732 Ibid

733 Ibid

734 ATSDR. (2011, March 3). Toxic Substances Portal - Propylene Glycol. *ATSDR - Agency for Toxic Substances and Disease Registry*. Retrieved November 12, 2015, from http://www.atsdr.cdc.gov/substances/toxsubstance.asp?toxid=240

735 FDA. (2013, April 1). CFR - Code of Federal Regulations Title 21 Sec. 184.1666 Propylene glycol. *U.S. Food and Drug Administration*. Retrieved November 12, 2015, from http://www.accessdata.fda.gov/scripts/cdrh/cfdocs/cfcfr/CFRSearch.cfm?fr=184.1666

736 Ibid

737 Ibid

738 Ibid

739 Ibid

740 Ibid

741 Ibid

742 ATSDR. (2011, March 3). Toxic Substances Portal - Propylene Glycol. *ATSDR Agency for Toxic Substances and Disease Registry*. Retrieved November 12, 2015, from http://www.atsdr.cdc.gov/PHS/PHS.asp?id=1120&tid=240

743 FDA. (2013, April 1). CFR - Code of Federal Regulations Title 21 Sec. 184.1666 Propylene glycol. *U.S. Food and Drug Administration*. Retrieved November 12, 2015, from http://www.accessdata.fda.gov/scripts/cdrh/cfdocs/cfcfr/CFRSearch.cfm?fr=184.1666

744 ATSDR. (2011, March 3). Toxic Substances Portal - Propylene Glycol. *ATSDR - Agency for Toxic Substances and Disease Registry*. Retrieved November 12, 2015, from http://www.atsdr.cdc.gov/substances/toxsubstance.asp?toxid=240

745 Ibid

746 Ibid

747 Szajewski, J., MD. (1991, July). Propylene glycol | Main risks and target organs. *IPCS INCHEM Chemical Safety Information from Intergovernmental Organizations*. Retrieved November 12, 2015, from http://www.inchem.org/documents/pims/chemical/pim443.htm#SectionTitle:2.1 Main risks and target organs

748 Medical-Dictionary. (2009, January 1). Stupor. *Medical-Dictionary | The FreeDictionary.com*. Retrieved November 12, 2015, from http://medical-dictionary.thefreedictionary.com/stupor

749 Medical-Dictionary. (2009). Hyperaemia. *Medical-Dictionary | The FreeDictionary.com*. Retrieved November 12, 2015, from http://medical-dictionary.thefreedictionary.com/hyperaemia

750 MedlinePlus. (2012, October 14). Lactic acidosis. *MedlinePlus Medical Encyclopedia U.S National Library of Medicine*. Retrieved November 13, 2015, from http://www.nlm.nih.gov/medlineplus/ency/article/000391.htm

751 Szajewski, J., MD. (1991, July). Propylene glycol | Main risks and target organs. *IPCS INCHEM Chemical Safety Information from Intergovernmental Organizations*. Retrieved November 12, 2015, from http://www.inchem.org/documents/pims/chemical/pim443.htm

752 Mercola.com. (2010, July 29). Do You Know What's in Your Shampoo? Retrieved December November 12, 2015, from http://articles.mercola.com/sites/articles/archive/2010/07/29/do-you-know-whats-in-your-shampoo.aspx#!

753 ATSDR. (2011, March 3). Toxic Substances Portal - Propylene Glycol. *ATSDR - Agency for Toxic Substances and Disease Registry*. Retrieved November 12, 2015, from http://www.atsdr.cdc.gov/substances/toxsubstance.asp?toxid=240

754 Collins, MD, R., & Buckley, RDN, CDE, S. (2015, April 29). The Latest Research on Fats and Cholesterol. *South Denver Cardiology*. Retrieved March 27, 2017, from https://www.southdenver.com/wp-content/uploads/2012/09/The-Latest-Research-on-Fats-and-Cholesterol-for-web.pdf

755 Dr. Oz Show. (2012, February 24). 5 Diet Myths Making You Gain Weight. *The Dr. Oz Show*. Retrieved November 13, 2015, from http://www.doctoroz.com/videos/5-diet-myths-making-you-gain-weight?page=3

756 Ibid

757 Glassman, K., & Mahoney, S. (2012). *The new you (and improved!) diet: 8 rules to lose weight and change your life forever*. New York: Rodale.

758 Ibid

759 Fox News. (2013, June 6). 5 low-fat foods that are making you fat. *Fox News Network*. Retrieved November 13, 2015, from http://www.foxnews.com/health/2013/06/06/5-low-fat-foods-that-are-making-fat/

760 Glassman, K., & Mahoney, S. (2012). *The new you (and improved!) diet: 8 rules to lose weight and change your life forever*. New York: Rodale.

761 USDA. (2005). Dietary Guidelines for Americans - Chapter 6 Fats. *USDA Health.gov*. Retrieved November 13, 2015, from http://www.health.gov/dietaryguidelines/dga2005/document/html/chapter6.htm

762 HSPH. (2002, July 7). Fats and Cholesterol: Out with the Bad, In with the Good. *Harvard School of Public Health - The Nutrition Source*. Retrieved July 5, 2014, from https://www.hsph.harvard.edu/nutritionsource/cholesterol/

763 Berg, J. M., Tymoczko JL, Stryer L. (2002). Section 26.4 Important Derivatives of Cholesterol Include Bile Salts and Steroid Hormones. *Biochemistry. 5th edition*. New York: W H Freeman

764 USDA. (2010). Dietary guidelines for Americans, 2010. *U.S. Department of Agriculture. U.S. Department of Health and Human Services | www.dietaryguidelines.gov*. Retrieved September 23, 2016, from http://www.cnpp.usda.gov/sites/default/files/dietary_guidelines_for_americans/PolicyDoc.pdf

765 Millen, B. DrPH, RD, Chair. Lichtenstein, A, DSc, Vice Chair (2015). Scientific Report of the 2015 Dietary Guidelines Advisory Committee. *US Departments of Agriculture and Health and Human Services*. Retrieved September 28, 2016, from https://health.gov/dietaryguidelines/2015-scientific-report/pdfs/scientific-report-of-the-2015-dietary-guidelines-advisory-committee.pdf

766 LoGiudice, P., Bleakney, S., & Bongiorno, P. (2012, October 29). The Surprising Health Benefits of Coconut Oil. *The Dr. Oz Show.* Retrieved November 13, 2015, from http://www.doctoroz.com/videos/surprising-health-benefits-coconut-oil

767 Mccarty, M. F., & Dinicolantonio, J. J. (2016). Lauric acid-rich medium-chain triglycerides can substitute for other oils in cooking applications and may have limited pathogenicity. *Open Heart, 3*(2). doi:10.1136/openhrt-2016-000467

768 Cardoso, D. A., Moreira, A. S., De, G. M., Raggio, R., & Rosa, G. (2015, November 01). A COCONUT EXTRA VIRGIN OIL-RICH DIET INCREASES HDL CHOLESTEROL AND DECREASES WAIST CIRCUMFERENCE AND BODY MASS IN CORONARY ARTERY DISEASE PATIENTS. *Nutrición hospitalaria, Spain.* 32(5):2144-52. doi: 10.3305/nh.2015.32.5.9642

769 Brown, M. J., RD. (2017, June 03). MCT Oil 101 - A Review of Medium-Chain Triglycerides. *Authority Nutrition.* Retrieved July 11, 2017, from https://authoritynutrition.com/mct-oil-101/

770 Pereira, R. A., Sevá-Pereira, A., & De, A. F. (1988, April-June). Absorption of medium chain triglycerides in patients with blind loop syndrome. *Instituto Brasileiro de Estudos e Pesquisas de Gastroenterologia, Brazil.* 25(2):75-81 PMID: 3255274

771 Faber, J., Goldstein, R., Blondheim, O., Stankiewicz, H., Darwashi, A., Bar-Maor, J. A., . . . Freier, S. (1988). Absorption of Medium Chain Triglycerides in the Stomach of the Human Infant. *Journal of Pediatric Gastroenterology and Nutrition, 7*(2), 189-195. doi:10.1097/00005176-198803000-00006

772 Wolinsky, I., & Driskell, J. A. (2004). *Nutritional ergogenic Aids.* Boca Raton (Fla.): CRC Press.

773 Cardoso, D. A., Moreira, A. S., De, G. M., Raggio, R., & Rosa, G. (2015, November 01). A COCONUT EXTRA VIRGIN OIL-RICH DIET INCREASES HDL CHOLESTEROL AND DECREASES WAIST CIRCUMFERENCE AND BODY MASS IN CORONARY ARTERY DISEASE PATIENTS. *Nutrición hospitalaria, Spain.* 32(5):2144-52. doi: 10.3305/nh.2015.32.5.9642

774 Ibid

775 Assunção, M. L., Ferreira, H. S., Santos, A. F., Cabral, C. R., & Florêncio, T. M. (2009). Effects of Dietary Coconut Oil on the Biochemical and Anthropometric Profiles of Women Presenting Abdominal Obesity. *Lipids, 44*(7), 593-601. doi:10.1007/s11745-009-3306-6

776 St-Onge, M.-P., & Bosarge, A. (2008). Weight-loss diet that includes consumption of medium-chain triacylglycerol oil leads to a greater rate of weight and fat mass loss than does olive oil. *The American Journal of Clinical Nutrition, 87*(3), 621–626.

777 Ibid

778 Drummond, J. C., Golding, J., Zilva, S. S., & Coward, K. H. (1920). The Nutritive Value of Lard. *Biochemical Journal, 14*(6), 742–753.

779 Odia, O. J., Ofori, S., & Maduka, O. (2015). Palm oil and the heart: A review. *World Journal of Cardiology, 7*(3), 144–149. doi: 10.4330/wjc.v7.i3.144.

780 American Egg Board. (2013). Eggs Facts | Fat. *Incredible Edible Egg.* Retrieved November 13, 2015, from http://www.incredibleegg.org/egg-facts/eggcyclopedia/f/fat

781 Filipiak-Florkiewicz A., Deren K., Florkiewicz A., Topolska K., Juszczak L., Cieslik E. (2017). The quality of eggs (organic and nutraceutical vs. conventional) and their technological properties. *Poultry Science.* (7):2480-2490. doi: 10.3382/ps/pew488.

782 Karsten, H., Patterson, P., Stout, R., & Crews, G. (2010). Vitamins A, E and fatty acid composition of the eggs of caged hens and pastured hens. *Renewable Agriculture and Food Systems*, 25(01), 45-54. doi:10.1017/s1742170509990214

783 Ginter, E., & Simko, V. (2016). New data on harmful effects of trans-fatty acids. *Bratislava Medical Journal, 117*(05), 251-253. doi:10.4149/bll_2016_048

784 USDA. (2010). Dietary guidelines for Americans, 2010. U.S. *Department of Agriculture. U.S. Department of Health and Human Services | www.dietaryguidelines.gov.* Retrieved September 23, 2016, from http://www.cnpp.usda.gov/sites/default/files/dietary_guidelines_for_americans/PolicyDoc.pdf

785 Millen, B. DrPH, RD, Chair. Lichtenstein, A, DSc, Vice Chair (2015). Scientific Report of the 2015 Dietary Guidelines Advisory Committee. *US Departments of Agriculture and Health and Human Services.* Retrieved September 28, 2016, from https://health.gov/dietaryguidelines/2015-scientific-report/pdfs/scientific-report-of-the-2015-dietary-guidelines-advisory-committee.pdf

786 NIH. (2011, June 24). Vitamin B12 Dietary Supplement Fact Sheet . *National Institutes of Health NIH.* Retrieved November 13, 2015, from http://ods.od.nih.gov/factsheets/VitaminB12-HealthProfessional/#h6

787 MedlinePlus. (2013, February 18). Vitamin B12: MedlinePlus Medical Encyclopedia. *U.S National Library of Medicine.* Retrieved November 14, 2015, from http://www.nlm.nih.gov/medlineplus/ency/article/002403.htm

788 Liem, I. T., Steinkraus, K. H., & Cronk, T. C. (1977). Production of vitamin B-12 in tempeh, a fermented soybean food. *Applied and Environmental Microbiology*, 34(6), 773–776

789 MedlinePlus. (2013, February 18). Vitamin B12: MedlinePlus Medical Encyclopedia. *U.S National Library of Medicine.* Retrieved November 14, 2015, from http://www.nlm.nih.gov/medlineplus/ency/article/002403.htm

790 Maresz, K., PhD. (2015, February). Proper Calcium Use: Vitamin K2 as a Promoter of Bone and Cardiovascular Health. *Integrative Medicine: A Clinician's Journal.* 14(1): 34–39. PMCID: PMC4566462

791 Hirano, J., & Ishii, Y. (2002). Effects of vitamin K2, vitamin D, and calcium on the bone metabolism of rats in the growth phase. *Journal of Orthopedic Science*, 7(3), 364-369. doi:10.1007/s007760200061

792 Maresz, K., PhD. (2015, February). Proper Calcium Use: Vitamin K2 as a Promoter of Bone and Cardiovascular Health. *Integrative Medicine: A Clinician's Journal.* 14(1): 34–39. PMCID: PMC4566462

[793] Ibid

[794] Ibid

[795] Bellows, L., Moore, R., & Gross, A. (2013, September). Dietary Supplements: Vitamins and Minerals. *Colorado State University*. Retrieved November 14, 2015, from http://www.ext.colostate.edu/pubs/foodnut/09338.html

[796] HSPH. (2014, June 9). Fats and Cholesterol: Out with the Bad, In with the Good. *Harvard School of Public Health - The Nutrition Source*. Retrieved Retrieved July 5, 2014, from https://www.hsph.harvard.edu/nutritionsource/types-of-fat/

[797] American Heart Association. (2015, October 7). Monounsaturated Fats. *The American Heart Association*. Retrieved November 14, 2015, from http://www.heart.org/HEARTORG/GettingHealthy/FatsAndOils/Fats101/Monounsaturated-Fats_UCM_301460_Article.jsp

[798] Ibid

[799] American Heart Association. (2015, October 7). Polyunsaturated Fats. *The American Heart Association*. Retrieved November 14, 2015, from http://www.heart.org/HEARTORG/GettingHealthy/FatsAndOils/Fats101/Polyunsaturated-Fats_UCM_301461_Article.jsp

[800] Zelman, K. M., MPH, RD, LD. (2007, November 1). Reviewed by Louise Chang, MD. Good Fats vs. Bad Fats: Get the Skinny on Fat. *WebMD*. Retrieved November 14, 2015, from http://www.webmd.com/diet/features/skinny-fat-good-fats-bad-fats?page=2

[801] Ibid

[802] Zivkovic, A. M., Telis, N., German, J. B., & Hammock, B. D. (2011). Dietary omega-3 fatty acids aid in the modulation of inflammation and metabolic health. *California Agriculture, 65*(3), 106-111. doi:10.3733/ca.v065n03p106

[803] Mozaffarian, D., & Rimm, E. B. (2006). Fish Intake, Contaminants, and Human Health. *Jama, 296*(15), 1885. doi:10.1001/jama.296.15.1885

[804] USDA. (2005). Dietary Guidelines for Americans - Chapter 6 Fats. *USDA Health.gov*. Retrieved November 14, 2015, from http://www.health.gov/dietaryguidelines/dga2005/document/html/chapter6.htm

[805] Ibid

[806] Patterson, E., Wall, R., Fitzgerald, G. F., Ross, R. P., & Stanton, C. (2012). Health Implications of High Dietary Omega-6 Polyunsaturated Fatty Acids. *Journal of Nutrition and Metabolism, 2012*, 1-16. doi:10.1155/2012/539426

[807] Simopoulos, A. (2002). The importance of the ratio of omega-6/omega-3 essential fatty acids. *Biomedicine & Pharmacotherapy, 56*(8), 365-379. doi:10.1016/s0753-3322(02)00253-6

[808] Ibid

[809] MacLean, P. S., Bergouignan, A., Cornier, M.-A., & Jackman, M. R. (2011). Biology's response to dieting: the impetus for weight regain. *American Journal of Physiology - Regulatory, Integrative and Comparative Physiology, 301*(3), R581–R600. doi: 10.1152/ajpregu.00755.2010

[810] Blomain, E. S., Dirhan, D. A., Valentino, M. A., Kim, G. W., & Waldman, S. A. (2013). Mechanisms of Weight Regain following Weight Loss. *ISRN Obesity, 2013*, 210524. doi: 10.1155/2013/210524

[811] WIN. (2014, October 15). Weight-loss and Nutrition Myths. *U.S. Department of Health and Human Services | NIH*. Retrieved November 14, 2015, from http://win.niddk.nih.gov/publications/myths.htm

[812] Paintal, A. S. (1954). A study of gastric stretch receptors. Their role in the peripheral mechanism of satiation of hunger and thirst. *The Journal of Physiology, 126*(2), 255-270. doi:10.1113/jphysiol.1954.sp005207

[813] DeNoon, D. (2007, April 11). Reviewed by Louise Chang, MD.. Diets Don't Work Long-Term. *WebMD*. Retrieved November 16, 2015, from http://www.webmd.com/diet/news/20070411/diets-dont-work-long-term

[814] University of MD Medical Center. (2010, November 17). Weight loss and age. *Baltimore Washington Medical Center*. Retrieved November 16, 2015, from http://www.mybwmc.org/library/1/001962

[815] Bulik, C., Ph.D. & Taylor, N., M.S., R.D. (2005, January 9). Are All Diets Unhealthy?.*About Health*. Retrieved November 16, 2015, December from http://seniorhealth.about.com/od/arthritis/a/diet_unhealthy.htm

[816] DeNoon, D. (2007, April 11). Reviewed by Louise Chang, MD.. Diets Don't Work Long-Term. *WebMD*. Retrieved November 16, 2015, from http://www.webmd.com/diet/news/20070411/diets-dont-work-long-term

[817] Fuchs, D., & Strasser, B. (2016). Diet Versus Exercise in Weight Loss and Maintenance: Focus on Tryptophan. *International Journal of Tryptophan Research, 9*. doi:10.4137/ijtr.s33385

[818] McIntosh, J. (2014, September 1). What is serotonin? What does serotonin do?. *Medical News Today*. Retrieved November 16, 2015, from http://www.medicalnewstoday.com/articles/232248.php

[819] McDonald, L. (2009, June 12). Carbohydrate Intake and Depression – Q&A | Dieting and Depression. *Body Recomposition*. Retrieved November 16, 2015, from http://www.bodyrecomposition.com/nutrition/carbohydrate-intake-and-depression-qa.html/

[820] Bulik, C., Ph.D. & Taylor, N., M.S., R.D. (2005, January 9). Are All Diets Unhealthy?.*About Health*. Retrieved November 16, 2015, from http://seniorhealth.about.com/od/arthritis/a/diet_unhealthy.htm

[821] DeNoon, D. (2007, April 11). Reviewed by Louise Chang, MD.. Diets Don't Work Long-Term. *WebMD*. Retrieved November 16, 2015, from http://www.webmd.com/diet/news/20070411/diets-dont-work-long-term

[822] Quotegarden. (2013, September 6). Ayurveda Quotes, Sayings Supporting Ayurvedic Nutrition. *quotegarden.com*. Retrieved November 17, 2015, from http://www.quotegarden.com/ayurveda.html

[823] FDA. (2017, May 4). Consumer Updates - Sometimes Drugs and the Liver Don't Mix. *US Food and Drug Administration*. Retrieved July 12, 2017, from https://www.fda.gov/ForConsumers/ConsumerUpdates/ucm398855.htm

824 MerckManuals. (2014, June).Revision by Steven K. Herrine, MD. Liver Injury Caused by Drugs | Drugs and the Liver: Merck Manual Professional. *The Merck Manual for Healthcare Professionals*. Retrieved November 16, 2015, from http://www.merckmanuals.com/professional/hepatic_and_biliary_disorders/drugs_and_the_liver/liver_injury_caused_by_drugs.html?qt=&sc=&alt=

825 Björnsson, E., Jacobsen, E. I., & Kalaitzakis, E. (2012). Hepatotoxicity associated with statins: Reports of idiosyncratic liver injury post-marketing. *Journal of Hepatology, 56*(2), 374-380. doi:10.1016/j.jhep.2011.07.023

826 Suk, K. T., & Kim, D. J. (2012). Drug-induced liver injury: present and future. *Clinical and Molecular Hepatology, 18*(3), 249. doi:10.3350/cmh.2012.18.3.249

827 Dean, C. (2005, October 9). Dr. Carolyn Dean, author of The Magnesium Miracle. *The Magnesium Miracle*. Retrieved September 05, 2017, from http://drcarolyndean.com/magnesium_miracle/

828 AboutLawsuits. (2010, February 23). Lipitor, Zocor and Other Cholesterol Drugs May Raise Diabetes Risk: Study - AboutLawsuits.com. *AboutLawsuitscom RSS*. Retrieved November 16, 2015, from http://www.aboutlawsuits.com/lipitor-zocor-statins-raise-diabetes-risk-8459/

829 Kohn, L. T., Corrigan, J., & Donaldson, M. S. (2000). *To err is human building a safer health system*. Washington, D.C.: National Academy Press.

830 Merck & Co., Inc. (Revised 2016, October). PRINIVIL® (lisinopril) tablets, for oral use. *U.S. Food and Drug Administration*. Retrieved November 8, 2016, from http://www.accessdata.fda.gov/drugsatfda_docs/label/2016/019558s060lbl.pdf

831 WebMD. (2017, March 15). High Blood Pressure and Erectile Dysfunction (ED). *WebMD*. Retrieved January 19, 2018, from https://www.webmd.com/erectile-dysfunction/guide/blood-pressure-medication-and-ed#1

832 Rosen, R. C., Kostis, J. B., & Jekelis, A. W. (1988). Beta-blocker effects on sexual function in normal males. *Archives of Sexual Behavior, 17*(3), 241-255. doi:10.1007/bf01541742

833 AstraZeneca. (Revised 2012, October). TENORMIN® (atenolol) Tablets. *U.S. Food and Drug Administration*. Retrieved November 8, 2016, from http://www.accessdata.fda.gov/drugsatfda_docs/label/2012/018240s032lbl.pdf

834 Ogbru, O. (2013, October 21). Beta Blockers: Drug Facts, Side Effects and Dosing. *MedicineNet*. Retrieved November 16, 2015, from http://www.medicinenet.com/beta_blockers/article.htm

835 Ogbru, O. (2012, May 22). Statins Symptoms, Causes, Treatment - What are the side effects of statins? - MedicineNet. *MedicineNet*. Retrieved November 16, 2015, from http://www.medicinenet.com/statins/page3.htm

836 Helfand, M., Carson, S., & Kelley, C. (2004). *Drug class review on HMG-CoA reductase inhibitors (statins)*. Portland, Or.: Oregon Evidence-based Practice Center, Oregon Health & Science University.

837 Björnsson, E., Jacobsen, E. I., & Kalaitzakis, E. (2012). Hepatotoxicity associated with statins: Reports of idiosyncratic liver injury post-marketing. *Journal of Hepatology, 56*(2), 374-380. doi:10.1016/j.jhep.2011.07.023

838 Pfizer Ireland Pharmaceuticals. (Revised 2007, March). Lipitor® (Atorvastatin Calcium) Tablets. *U.S. Food and Drug Administration*. Retrieved November 9, 2016, from http://www.accessdata.fda.gov/drugsatfda_docs/label/2007/020702s047lbl.pdf

839 Deichmann, R., Lavie, C., & Andrews, S. (2010). Coenzyme Q10 and Statin-Induced Mitochondrial Dysfunction. *The Ochsner Journal, 10*(1), 16–21.

840 Saini, R. (2011). Coenzyme Q10: The essential nutrient. *Journal of Pharmacy and Bioallied Sciences,3*(3), 466. doi:10.4103/0975-7406.84471

841 Madmani, M. E., Solaiman, A. Y., Agha, K. T., Madmani, Y., Shahrour, Y., Essali, A., & Kadro, W. (2014). Coenzyme Q10 for heart failure. *Cochrane Database of Systematic Reviews*. doi:10.1002/14651858.cd008684.pub2

842 Quinzii, C. M., Dimauro, S., & Hirano, M. (2006). Human Coenzyme Q10 Deficiency. *Neurochemical Research, 32*(4-5), 723-727. doi:10.1007/s11064-006-9190-z

843 Garrido-Maraver, J., Cordero, M. D., Oropesa-Ávila, M., Vega, A. F., Mata, M. D., Pavón, A. D., . . . Sánchez-Alcázar, J. A. (2014). Coenzyme Q10 Therapy. *Molecular Syndromology, 5*(3-4), 187-197. doi:10.1159/000360101

844 Rubinstein, J., Aloka, F., & Abela, G. S. (2009). Statin Therapy Decreases Myocardial Function as Evaluated Via Strain Imaging. *Clinical Cardiology, 32*(12), 684-689. doi:10.1002/clc.20644

845 Ibid

846 Pfizer Ireland Pharmaceuticals. (Revised 2007, March). Lipitor® (Atorvastatin Calcium) Tablets. *U.S. Food and Drug Administration*. Retrieved November 9, 2016, from http://www.accessdata.fda.gov/drugsatfda_docs/label/2007/020702s047lbl.pdf

847 ConsumerMedSafety.org. (2012, March 26). FDA Expands Advice on Statin Risks | FDA Alert Posted: February 27, 2011. *Prevent Medication Errors - Consumer Med Safety*. Retrieved July 13, 2017, from http://www.consumermedsafety.org/latest-fda-medication-alerts/special-alerts/item/532-fda-expands-advice-on-statin-risks

848 FDA-Center for Drug Evaluation and Research. (2016, January 19). Drug Safety and Availability - FDA Drug Safety Communication: Important safety label changes to cholesterol-lowering statin drugs. *US Food & Drug Administration*. Retrieved July 13, 2017, from https://www.fda.gov/Drugs/DrugSafety/ucm293101.htm

849 Deichmann, R., Lavie, C., & Andrews, S. (2010). Coenzyme Q10 and Statin-Induced Mitochondrial Dysfunction. *The Ochsner Journal, 10*(1), 16–21.

850 Quinzii, C. M., Dimauro, S., & Hirano, M. (2006). Human Coenzyme Q10 Deficiency. *Neurochemical Research, 32*(4-5), 723-727. doi:10.1007/s11064-006-9190-z

[851] Reinolds, G. (2013, May 22). Can Statins Cut the Benefits of Exercise?. *The New York Times*. Retrieved January 14, 2018, from https://mobile.nytimes.com/blogs/well/2013/05/22/can-statins-curb-the-benefits-of-exercise/?referer=

[852] Mikus, C. R., Boyle, L. J., Borengasser, S. J., Oberlin, D. J., Naples, S. P., Fletcher, J., . . . Thyfault, J. P. (2013). Simvastatin Impairs Exercise Training Adaptations. *Journal of the American College of Cardiology*, 62(8), 709-714. doi:10.1016/j.jacc.2013.02.074

[853] FDA-Center for Drug Evaluation and Research. (2016, January 19). Drug Safety and Availability - FDA Drug Safety Communication: Important safety label changes to cholesterol-lowering statin drugs. *US Food & Drug Administration*. Retrieved July 13, 2017, from https://www.fda.gov/Drugs/DrugSafety/ucm293101.htm

[854] Sattar, N., Preiss, D., Murray, H. M., Welsh, P., Buckley, B. M., Craen, A. J., . . . Ford, I. (2010). Statins and risk of incident diabetes: a collaborative meta-analysis of randomised statin trials. *The Lancet*,375(9716), 735-742. doi:10.1016/s0140-6736(09)61965-6

[855] FDA-Center for Drug Evaluation and Research. (2016, January 19). Drug Safety and Availability - FDA Drug Safety Communication: Important safety label changes to cholesterol-lowering statin drugs. *US Food & Drug Administration*. Retrieved July 13, 2017, from https://www.fda.gov/Drugs/DrugSafety/ucm293101.htm

[856] Sukhija, R., Prayaga, S., Marashdeh, M., Bursac, Z., Kakar, P., Bansal, D., . . . Mehta, J. L. (2009). Effect of Statins on Fasting Plasma Glucose in Diabetic and Nondiabetic Patients. *Journal of Investigative Medicine*, 57(3), 495-499. doi:10.2310/jim.0b013e318197ec8b

[857] Carter, A. A., Gomes, T., Camacho, X., Juurlink, D. N., Shah, B. R., & Mamdani, M. M. (2013). Risk of incident diabetes among patients treated with statins: population based study. *Bmj*, 346(May23 4). doi:10.1136/bmj.f2610

[858] Aiman, U., Najmi, A., & Khan, R. (2014). Statin induced diabetes and its clinical implications. *Journal of Pharmacology and Pharmacotherapeutics*, 5(3), 181. doi:10.4103/0976-500x.136097

[859] Topol, E. (2012, March 4). The Diabetes Dilemma for Statin Users. *The New York Times*. Retrieved November 16, 2015, from http://www.nytimes.com/2012/03/05/opinion/the-diabetes-dilemma-for-statin-users.html

[860] Sattar, N., Preiss, D., Murray, H. M., Welsh, P., Buckley, B. M., Craen, A. J., . . . Ford, I. (2010). Statins and risk of incident diabetes: a collaborative meta-analysis of randomised statin trials. *The Lancet*,375(9716), 735-742. doi:10.1016/s0140-6736(09)61965-6

[861] Koh, K. K., Quon, M. J., Han, S. H., Lee, Y., Kim, S. J., & Shin, E. K. (2010). Atorvastatin Causes Insulin Resistance and Increases Ambient Glycemia in Hypercholesterolemic Patients. *Journal of the American College of Cardiology*, 55(12), 1209-1216. doi:10.1016/j.jacc.2009.10.053

[862] Saiontz & Kirk, P.A.. (2014). Lipitor Lawsuit - Lawyers Reviewing Lipitor Diabetes Lawsuits. *Saiontz Kirk PA YouHaveALawyercom Lipitor Lawsuit Comments*. Retrieved November 16, 2015, from http://www.youhavealawyer.com/lipitor/

[863] Brunetti, L., & Kalabalik, J. (2012). Management of Type-2 Diabetes Mellitus in Adults: Focus on Individualizing Non-Insulin Therapies. *Pharmacy and Therapeutics*, 37(12), 687–696.

[864] Nasri, H., & Rafieian-Kopaei, M. (2014). Metformin: Current knowledge. *Journal of Research in Medical Sciences : The Official Journal of Isfahan University of Medical Sciences*, 19(7), 658–664.

[865] Ko, S., Ko, S., Ahn, Y., Song, K., Han, K., Park, Y., . . . Kim, H. (2014). Association of Vitamin B12Deficiency and Metformin Use in Patients with Type 2 Diabetes. *Journal of Korean Medical Science*,29(7), 965. doi:10.3346/jkms.2014.29.7.965

[866] Svare, A. (2009). A patient presenting with symptomatic hypomagnesemia caused by metformin-induced diarrhoea: a case report. *Cases Journal*, 2(1), 156. doi:10.1186/1757-1626-2-156

[867] U.S. National Library of Medicine. (2017, February 6). DRUG RECORD Metformin. *Clinical and Research Information of Drug-Induced Liver Injury | National Institutes of Health, U.S. Department of Health & Human Services*. Retrieved July 14, 2017, from https://livertox.nih.gov/Metformin.htm

[868] Mayo Clinic/Micromedex. (2017, March 01). Metformin (Oral Route) Side Effects. *Mayo Clinic*. Retrieved July 14, 2017, from http://www.mayoclinic.org/drugs-supplements/metformin-oral-route/side-effects/drg-20067074

[869] FDA. (2011, June 15). FDA Drug Safety Communication: Update to ongoing safety review of Actos (pioglitazone) and increased risk of bladder cancer | Safety Announcement. *U.S. Food and Drug Administration | FDA Drug Safety Communication*. Retrieved November 16, 2015, from http://www.fda.gov/Drugs/DrugSafety/ucm259150.htm

[870] Ibid

[871] NHLBI. (2011, July 1). How Are Arrhythmias Treated?. *NHLBI - National Heart, Lung, and Blood Institute - NIH - National Institutes of Health*. Retrieved November 16, 2015, from http://www.nhlbi.nih.gov/health/health-topics/topics/arr/treatment.html

[872] Ibid

[873] Ibid

[874] Do, C., Huyghe, E., Lapeyre-Mestre, M., Montastruc, J. L., & Bagheri, H. (2009). Statins and Erectile Dysfunction. *Drug Safety*, 32(7), 591-597. doi:10.2165/00002018-200932070-00005

[875] Rizvi, K., Hapmson, J., & Harvey, J. (2002). Do lipid-lowering drugs cause erectile dysfunction? A systematic review. *Family Practice*, 19(1), 95-98.

[876] Ibid

[877] Martinez, J., & Samadi, Dr. (2014, April 16). Erectile dysfunction drugs linked to skin cancer?. *Fox News*. Retrieved August 6, 2014, from http://www.foxnews.com/health/2014/04/16/erectile-dysfunction-drugs-linked-to-skin-cancer/

[878] Sokolove Law. (n.d.). Viagra and Revatio Linked to Melanoma Skin Cancer. *Sokolove Law*. Retrieved November 16, 2015, from http://web.sokolovelaw.com/viagrabing?utm_source=Bing&utm_medium=PPC&utm_campaign=ViagraSC4-21-

14&utm_Adgroup=Brand%20Side%20Effects&utm_keyword=+Viagra%20+melanoma&utm_Match=Broad&cvosrc=ppc.bing.=+Viagra%20+
melanoma&mm_campaign=4BDE9E745715A26B2D575451D9DB3393&keyword=%2BViagra%20%2Bmelanoma

[879] Firger, J. (2014, June 4). Viagra may increase melanoma risk, study finds. *CBS News.* Retrieved November 16, 2015, from
http://www.cbsnews.com/news/viagra-may-increase-melanoma-risk/

[880] Aleccia, J. (2014, April 7). Viagra May Boost Risk of Deadly Skin Cancer, Study Finds. *NBC News.* Retrieved November 16, 2015, from
http://www.nbcnews.com/health/health-news/viagra-may-boost-risk-deadly-skin-cancer-study-finds-n73976

[881] Litster Frost Injury Lawyers. (2014, April 15). Viagra® Melanoma Skin Cancer Lawsuit. *Litster Frost Injury Lawyers.* Retrieved November 16, 2015, from http://melanomaedlawyer.com/

[882] Li, W., Qureshi, A. A., Robinson, K. C., & Han, J. (2014). Sildenafil Use and Increased Risk of Incident Melanoma in US Men A Prospective Cohort Study. *JAMA Internal Medicine, 174*(6), 964. doi:10.1001/jamainternmed.2014.594

[883] Grissinger, M. (2013). Multiple Brand Names for the Same Generic Drug Can Cause Confusion. Pharmacy and Therapeutics, 38(6), 305.

[884] Pfizer Labs. (2010, January). VIAGRA® (sildenafil citrate) Tablets. *U.S. Food and Drug Administration.* Retrieved November 10, 2016, from
http://www.accessdata.fda.gov/drugsatfda_docs/label/2011/020895s036lbl.pdf

[885] Pfizer. (2015, October). Potential Side Effects. *VIAGRA Side Effects* . Retrieved November 16, 2015, from
https://www.viagra.com/learning/what-are-possible-side-effects

[886] You, H., Lu, W., Zhao, S., Hu, Z., & Zhang, J. (2013). The relationship between statins and depression: a review of the literature. *Expert Opinion on Pharmacotherapy, 14*(11), 1467-1476. doi:10.1517/14656566.2013.803067

[887] Bakalar, N. (2012, March 5). Mental Health: Use of Statins May Lower Depression Risk. *The New York Times.* Retrieved November 16, 2015, from http://www.nytimes.com/2012/03/06/health/research/possible-link-between-statin-use-and-lower-depression-risk.html

[888] Borland, S. (2011, January 19). Statins 'may cause loss of memory and depression'. *Mail Online.* Retrieved November 16, 2015, from
http://www.dailymail.co.uk/health/article-1348435/Statins-cause-loss-memory-depression.html

[889] Cham, S., Koslik, H. J., & Golomb, B. A. (2015). Mood, Personality, and Behavior Changes During Treatment with Statins: A Case Series. *Drug Safety - Case Reports, 3*(1). doi:10.1007/s40800-015-0024-2

[890] Ibid

[891] FDA. (2007, May 3). FDA Proposes New Warnings About Suicidal Thinking, Behavior in Young Adults Who Take Antidepressant Medications. *U.S. Food and Drug Administration.* Retrieved July 15, 2017, from
https://www.fda.gov/ForConsumers/ConsumerUpdates/ucm048950.htm

[892] Ibid

[893] Laugren, T. (2011, August 23). XANAX® alprazolam tablets, USP. *U.S. Food and Drug Administration.* Retrieved November 11, 2016, from
http://www.accessdata.fda.gov/drugsatfda_docs/label/2011/018276s045lbl.pdf

[894] Ibid

[895] Higgins, A., Nash, M., & Lynch, A. M. (2010). Antidepressant-associated sexual dysfunction: impact, effects, and treatment. *Drug, Healthcare and Patient Safety, 2,* 141–150. http://doi.org/10.2147/DHPS.S7634

[896] Alprazolam.org. (2014). Alprazolam Sexual Effects. *Alprazolam.org Reviews, Ratings and Information.* Retrieved November 16, 2015, from
http://www.alprazolam.org/sexual-effects.html

[897] Laugren, T. (2011, August 23). XANAX® alprazolam tablets, USP. *U.S. Food and Drug Administration.* Retrieved November 11, 2016, from
http://www.accessdata.fda.gov/drugsatfda_docs/label/2011/018276s045lbl.pdf

[898] Alprazolam.org. (2014). Alprazolam Sexual Effects. *Alprazolam.org Reviews, Ratings and Information.* Retrieved November 16, 2015, from
http://www.alprazolam.org/sexual-effects.html

[899] Laugren, T. (2011, August 23). XANAX® alprazolam tablets, USP. *U.S. Food and Drug Administration.* Retrieved November 11, 2016, from
http://www.accessdata.fda.gov/drugsatfda_docs/label/2011/018276s045lbl.pdf

[900] Colten, H. R., & Altevogt, B. M. (2006). *Sleep disorders and sleep deprivation: an unmet public health problem | 3 Extent and Health Consequences of Chronic Sleep Loss and Sleep Disorders.* Washington, DC: Institute of Medicine.

[901] Sanofi-aventis. (2014, October). AMBIEN® (zolpidem tartrate) tablets, for oral use, C-IV Reference ID: 4022123 *U.S. Food and Drug Administration.* Retrieved July 15, 2017, from https://www.accessdata.fda.gov/drugsatfda_docs/label/2016/019908s037lbl.pdf

[902] Ibid

[903] FDA. (2013, May 14). FDA Drug Safety Communication: Risk of next-morning impairment after use of insomnia drugs; FDA requires lower recommended doses for certain drugs containing zolpidem (Ambien, Ambien CR, Edluar, and Zolpimist). *U.S. Food and Drug Adminstration.* Retrieved November 16, 2015, from http://www.fda.gov/Drugs/DrugSafety/ucm334033.htm

[904] Drugs.com. (2017). Ambien CR Side Effects in Detail. *Drugs.com.* Retrieved July 15, 2017, from https://www.drugs.com/sfx/ambien-cr-side-effects.html

[905] Sanofi-aventis. (2014, October). AMBIEN® (zolpidem tartrate) tablets, for oral use, C-IV Reference ID: 4022123 *U.S. Food and Drug Administration.* Retrieved July 15, 2017, from https://www.accessdata.fda.gov/drugsatfda_docs/label/2016/019908s037lbl.pdf

[906] CDC. (2011, February 23). Vitamins and Minerals. *Centers for Disease Control and Prevention.* Retrieved November 16, 2015, from
http://www.cdc.gov/nutrition/everyone/basics/Vitamins/
https://ods.od.nih.gov/factsheets/list-VitaminsMinerals/

[907] Ibid

[908] Ibid

[909] Nierenberg, C. (2014, April 2). Reviewed by Maryann Tomovich Jacobsen, MS, RD. Taking Too Many Vitamins? Side Effects of Vitamin Overdosing. *WebMD*. Retrieved November 16, 2015, from http://www.webmd.com/food-recipes/features/effects-of-taking-too-many-Vitamins

[910] De Lourdes Samaniego-Vaesken, M., Alonso-Aperte, E., & Varela-Moreiras, G. (2012). Vitamin food fortification today. *Food & Nutrition Research*, 56. doi: 10.3402/fnr.v56i0.5459

[911] MedlinePlus. (2011, December 15). Updated by: Eric Perez, MD, St. Luke's / Roosevelt Hospital Center, NY. Multiple Vitamin overdose: MedlinePlus Medical Encyclopedia. *U.S National Library of Medicine*. Retrieved June 17, 2014, from http://www.nlm.nih.gov/medlineplus/ency/article/002596.htm

[912] Johnson, L. E., MD, PhD. (2012, December). Vitamin C - Vitamin Deficiency, Dependency, and Toxicity. *Merck Manual for Health Care Professionals*. Retrieved November 16, 2015, from http://www.merckmanuals.com/professional/nutritional_disorders/Vitamin_deficiency_dependency_and_toxicity/Vitamin_c.html?qt=&sc=&alt=

[913] Zhou, S. (2014). Excess vitamin intake: An unrecognized risk factor for obesity. *World Journal of Diabetes*, 5(1), 1. doi:10.4239/wjd.v5.i1.1

[914] Ibid

[915] Bellows, L., Moore, R., & Gross, A. (2013, September). Dietary Supplements: Vitamins and Minerals. *Colorado State University*. Retrieved June 17, 2014, from http://www.ext.colostate.edu/pubs/foodnut/09338.html

[916] Saul, A. (2012). *Doctor yourself: Natural healing that works* (2nd ed.). Laguna Beach, CA: Basic Health Publications.

[917] Bellows, L., Moore, R., & Gross, A. (2013, September). Dietary Supplements: Vitamins and Minerals. *Colorado State University*. Retrieved June 17, 2014, from http://www.ext.colostate.edu/pubs/foodnut/09338.html

[918] NIH. (2013, November 21). Calcium - Dietary Supplement Fact Sheet: — Health Professional Fact Sheet. *National Institutes of Health*. Retrieved November 17, 2015, from http://ods.od.nih.gov/factsheets/Calcium-HealthProfessional/

[919] Ibid

[920] MerckManuals. (2014, June).Revision by Steven K. Herrine, MD. Liver Injury Caused by Drugs | Drugs and the Liver: Merck Manual Professional. *The Merck Manual for Healthcare Professionals*. Retrieved November 17, 2015, from http://www.merckmanuals.com/professional/hepatic_and_biliary_disorders/drugs_and_the_liver/liver_injury_caused_by_drugs.html?qt=&sc=&alt=

[921] Björnsson, E. (2016). Hepatotoxicity by Drugs: The Most Common Implicated Agents. *International Journal of Molecular Sciences*, 17(2), 224. doi:10.3390/ijms17020224

[922] Suk, K. T., & Kim, D. J. (2012). Drug-induced liver injury: present and future. *Clinical and Molecular Hepatology*, 18(3), 249. doi:10.3350/cmh.2012.18.3.249

[923] Zijp, I. M., Korver, O., & Tijburg, L. B. (2000). Effect of Tea and Other Dietary Factors on Iron Absorption. Critical Reviews in Food Science and Nutrition, 40(5), 371-398. doi:10.1080/10408690091189194

[924] Ibid

[925] MedlinePlus. (2013, April 29). Iron. *U.S National Library of Medicine*. Retrieved November 17, 2015, from http://www.nlm.nih.gov/medlineplus/druginfo/natural/912.html

[926] Zijp, I. M., Korver, O., & Tijburg, L. B. (2000). Effect of Tea and Other Dietary Factors on Iron Absorption. Critical Reviews in Food Science and Nutrition, 40(5), 371-398. doi:10.1080/10408690091189194

[927] Morck T.A., Lynch S.R., Cook J.D. (1983, March). Inhibition of food iron absorption by coffee. *American Journal of Clinical Nutrition*. 37(3):416-20. PMID: 6402915

[928] Ibid

[929] Ibid

[930] Chung, H. R. (2014). Iodine and thyroid function. *Annals of Pediatric Endocrinology & Metabolism*, 19(1), 8. doi:10.6065/apem.2014.19.1.8

[931] Dean, C. (2017). *Magnesium miracle*. New York, NY: Ballantine.

[932] Ibid

[933] Al-Hakeim, H. (2009). Serum levels of lipids, calcium and magnesium in women with hypothyroidism and cardiovascular diseases. *Journal of Laboratory Physicians*, 1(2), 49. doi:10.4103/0974-2727.59698

[934] Jahnen-Dechent, W., & Ketteler, M. (2012). Magnesium basics. *Clinical Kidney Journal*, 5(Suppl 1), I3-I14. doi:10.1093/ndtplus/sfr163

[935] Killilea, D. W., & Maier, J. A. (2008, June). A connection between magnesium deficiency and aging: new insights from cellular studies. *Nutrition and Metabolism Center, Children's Hospital Oakland Research Institute*. 21(2): 77–82. DOI: 10.1684/mrh.2008.0134

[936] Douban S, Brodsky M, Whang D. (1996, September). Significance of magnesium in congestive heart failure. *American Heart Journal*. 132(3):664-71. PMID: 8800040

[937] Rosanoff, A. (2005, February). [Magnesium and hypertension]. *Clinical Calcium*. 15(2):255-60. PMID: 15692166

[938] Abbasi, B., Kimiagar, M., Sadeghniiat, K., Shirazi, M. M., Hedayati, M., & Rashidkhani, B. (2012). The effect of magnesium supplementation on primary insomnia in elderly: A double-blind placebo-controlled clinical trial. *Journal of Research in Medical Sciences*. 17(12), 1161–1169. PMC3703169

939 Galland, L. (1988). Magnesium and inflammatory bowel disease.
Magnesium. 7(2):78-83. PMID: 3294519

940 Swaminathan, R. (2003). Magnesium Metabolism and its Disorders. *The Clinical Biochemist Reviews*, 24(2), 47–66. PMC1855626

941 Jahnen-Dechent, W., & Ketteler, M. (2012). Magnesium basics. *Clinical Kidney Journal*, 5(Suppl 1), I3-I14. doi:10.1093/ndtplus/sfr163

942 MedlinePlus. (2013, February 18). Vitamins: MedlinePlus Medical Encyclopedia. *U.S National Library of Medicine | National Institutes of Health*. Retrieved November 17, 2015, from http://www.nlm.nih.gov/medlineplus/ency/article/002399.htm

943 MedicineNet. (2007, January 17). Ask the Experts: Fat- and Water-Soluble Vitamins. *MedicineNet.com | Ask the Experts*. Retrieved June 18, 2014, from http://www.medicinenet.com/script/main/art.asp?articlekey=79102

944 National Research Council (US) Subcommittee on the Tenth Edition of the Recommended Dietary Allowances. (1999). *Recommended dietary allowances: 10th Edition*. Washington: National Academy Press. ISBN-10: 0-309-04633-5 ISBN-10: 0-309-04041-8

945 FDA. (2016, September 20). Fortify Your Knowledge About Vitamins. *U.S. Food and Drug Administration*. Retrieved November 18, 2016, from http://www.fda.gov/ForConsumers/ConsumerUpdates/ucm118079.htm#water

946 Ibid

947 MedlinePlus. (2013, February 18). Vitamins: MedlinePlus Medical Encyclopedia. *U.S National Library of Medicine | National Institutes of Health*. Retrieved November 17, 2015, from http://www.nlm.nih.gov/medlineplus/ency/article/002399.htm

948 NIH. (2011, September 20). Zinc. *NIH - National Institutes of Health | U.S. Department of Health and Human Services*. Retrieved November 17, 2015, from http://ods.od.nih.gov/factsheets/Zinc-QuickFacts/

949 Singh, M., & Das, R. R. (2013). Zinc for the common cold. *Cochrane Database of Systematic Reviews*. doi:10.1002/14651858.cd001364.pub4, PMID: 23775705

950 Hemilä, H., & Chalker, E. (2015). The effectiveness of high dose zinc acetate lozenges on various common cold symptoms: a meta-analysis. *BMC Family Practice*, 16(1). doi:10.1186/s12875-015-0237-6

951 NIH. (2011, September 20). Zinc. *NIH - National Institutes of Health | U.S. Department of Health and Human Services*. Retrieved November 17, 2015, from http://ods.od.nih.gov/factsheets/Zinc-QuickFacts/

952 NIH. (2014, February 3). Magnesium. *NIH - National Institutes of Health | U.S. Department of Health and Human Services*. Retrieved November 17, 2015, from http://ods.od.nih.gov/factsheets/Magnesium-QuickFacts/#h3

953 Ibid

954 NIH. (2011, June 24). Iodine. *NIH - National Institutes of Health | U.S. Department of Health and Human Services*. Retrieved November 17, 2015, from http://ods.od.nih.gov/factsheets/Iodine-QuickFacts/#h3

955 Ibid

956 NIH. (2013, November 4). Dietary Supplement Fact Sheet: Chromium — Health Professional Fact Sheet. *U.S National Library of Medicine | U.S. Department of Health & Human Services*. Retrieved November 18, 2016, from https://ods.od.nih.gov/factsheets/Chromium-HealthProfessional/

957 Ibid

958 MedlinePlus. (2013, February 18). Copper in diet: MedlinePlus Medical Encyclopedia. *U.S National Library of Medicine*. Retrieved November 17, 2015, from http://www.nlm.nih.gov/medlineplus/ency/article/002419.htm

959 Ibid

960 Ehrlich, S. (2013, May 31). Manganese. *University of Maryland Medical Center*. Retrieved November 18, 2016, from http://umm.edu/health/medical/altmed/supplement/manganese

961 Ibid

962 MedlinePlus. (2013, February 18). Iron in diet: MedlinePlus Medical Encyclopedia. *U.S National Library of Medicine*. Retrieved November 17, 2015, from http://www.nlm.nih.gov/medlineplus/ency/article/002422.htm

963 Zelman, K. M. (2004, August 2). Top 10 Iron-Rich Foods: Foods High in Iron. *WebMD*. Retrieved November 17, 2015, from http://www.webmd.com/diet/features/top-10-iron-rich-foods

964 MedlinePlus. (2012, June 23). Potassium in diet: MedlinePlus Medical Encyclopedia. *U.S National Library of Medicine*. Retrieved November 17, 2015, from http://www.nlm.nih.gov/medlineplus/ency/article/002413.htm

965 Ibid

966 MedlinePlus. (2013, February 18). Selenium in diet: MedlinePlus Medical Encyclopedia. *U.S National Library of Medicine*. Retrieved November 17, 2015, from http://www.nlm.nih.gov/medlineplus/ency/article/002414.htm

967 Ibid

968 NIH. (2013, June 2). Selenium. *NIH - National Institutes of Health | U.S. Department of Health and Human Services*. Retrieved November 17, 2015, from http://ods.od.nih.gov/factsheets/Selenium-HealthProfessional/

969 University of Maryland Medical Center. (2013, May 7). Sulfur. *University of Maryland Medical Center*. Retrieved November 17, 2015, from http://umm.edu/health/medical/altmed/supplement/sulfur

970 Harvard Health Publications. (n.d.). Listing of Vitamins. *Harvard School of Public Health - Harvard Health Publications*. Retrieved November 17, 2015, from http://www.health.harvard.edu/newsweek/Listing_of_Vitamins.htm

971 University of Maryland Medical Center. (2013, May 7). Sulfur. *University of Maryland Medical Center*. Retrieved November 17, 2015, from http://umm.edu/health/medical/altmed/supplement/sulfur

[972] NIH. (2011, June 24). Vitamin D Fact Sheet for Consumers . *National Institutes of Health NIH*. Retrieved November 17, 2015, from http://ods.od.nih.gov/factsheets/VitaminD-QuickFacts/

[973] NIH. (2013, November 21). Calcium - Dietary Supplement Fact Sheet: — Health Professional Fact Sheet. *National Institutes of Health*. Retrieved November 17, 2015, from http://ods.od.nih.gov/factsheets/Calcium-HealthProfessional/

[974] Ehrlich, S. D. (2011, May 10). Omega-3 fatty acids. *University of Maryland Medical Center*. Retrieved November 17, 2015, from http://umm.edu/health/medical/altmed/supplement/omega3-fatty-acids

[975] NIH MedlinePlus. (2009). Orthopedic Health: Joint Health and Care: Prevention, Symptoms, Diagnosis & Treatment. *U.S National Library of Medicine | National Institutes of Health*. Retrieved November 17, 2015, from http://www.nlm.nih.gov/medlineplus/magazine/issues/spring09/articles/spring09pg14.html

[976] Ibid

[977] Jerosch, J. (2011). Effects of Glucosamine and Chondroitin Sulfate on Cartilage Metabolism in OA: Outlook on Other Nutrient Partners Especially Omega-3 Fatty Acids. *International Journal of Rheumatology*. doi: 10.1155/2011/969012. PMCID: PMC3150191

[978] Christiansen, B. A., Bhatti, S., Goudarzi, R., & Emami, S. (2015). Management of Osteoarthritis with Avocado/Soybean Unsaponifiables. *Cartilage*, 6(1), 30–44. doi: 10.1177/1947603514554992

[979] Consumer Reports Developed in cooperation with the American Academy of Orthopaedic Surgeons. (2014, March 11). Osteoarthritis of the Knee | Popular supplements don't work. *Choosing Wisely An initiative of the ABIM Foundation*. Retrieved June 09, 2016, from http://www.choosingwisely.org/patient-resources/osteoarthritis-of-the-knee/

[980] CDC.gov. (2012, October 10). Water: Meeting Your Daily Fluid Needs. *Centers for Disease Control and Prevention*. Retrieved June 18, 2014, from http://www.cdc.gov/nutrition/everyone/basics/water.html

[981] Missouri Department of Health & Senior Services. (n.d.). Water: An Important Nutrient | **[PDF]** 20131015_12345 flyers-Partners.indd. *Missouri Department of Health & Senior Services*. Retrieved November 17, 2015, from http://search.mo.gov/search?as_sitesearch=health.mo.gov/living/families/wic&q=Water:+An+Important+Nutrient&site=dhss&output=xml_no_dtd&client=dhss&num=10&proxystylesheet=dhss&x=0&y=0&ie=UTF-8&ulang=en&ip=69.255.250.121&access=p&sort=date:D:L:d1&entqr=3&entqrm=0&wc=200&wc_mc=1&oe=UTF-8&ud=1

[982] Vorvick, L. J. (2013, August 19). Water in die. *U.S National Library of Medicine | MedlinePlus Medical Encyclopedia*. Retrieved November 17, 2015, from http://www.nlm.nih.gov/medlineplus/ency/article/002471.htm

[983] Ornish, D. (1990). *Dr. Dean Ornish's program for reversing heart disease: the only system scientifically proven to reverse heart disease without drugs or surgery*. New York: Random House.

[984] PMRI. (2011, Novermber 16). Bio - Dean Ornish, MD. *PMRI - Preventive Medicine Research Institute*. Retrieved November 17, 2015, from http://www.pmri.org/dean_ornish.html

[985] Cochran, A. (2014, March 4). Does your doctor have ties to big pharma? How you'll be able to find out. *CBS NEWS*. Retrieved January 12, 2016, from http://www.cbsnews.com/news/does-your-doc-have-ties-to-big-pharma-how-youll-be-able-to-find-out/

[986] Ornish, D. (2007). *The spectrum: how to customize a way of eating and living just right for you and your family*. New York: Ballantine Books.

[987] Ornish, D. (1990). *Dr. Dean Ornish's program for reversing heart disease: the only system scientifically proven to reverse heart disease without drugs or surgery*. New York: Random House.

[988] Huffington Post. (2011, May 13). Caldwell B. Esselstyn, Jr., MD. *The Huffington Post*. Retrieved November 17, 2015, from http://www.huffingtonpost.com/caldwell-b-esselstyn-jr-md

[989] Ibid

[990] Esselstyn, C. B. (2007). *Prevent and reverse heart disease: the revolutionary, scientifically proven, nutrition-based cure*. New York: Avery.

[991] Ibid

[992] Tousoulis, D., Kampoli, A., Papageorgiou, C. T., & Stefanadis, C. (2012). The Role of Nitric Oxide on Endothelial Function. *Current Vascular Pharmacology*, 10(1), 4-18. doi:10.2174/157016112798829760

[993] Ibid

[994] Tuso, P., Stroll, S., & Li, W. (2015). A Plant-Based Diet, Atherogenesis, and Coronary Artery Disease Prevention. *The Permanente Journal*, 62-67. doi:10.7812/tpp/14-036

[995] Ibid

[996] Hong, Y. M. (2010). Atherosclerotic Cardiovascular Disease Beginning in Childhood. *Korean Circulation Journal*, 40(1), 1. doi:10.4070/kcj.2010.40.1.1

[997] Abraham, D., & Distler, O. (2007). How does endothelial cell injury start? The role of endothelin in systemic sclerosis. *Arthritis Research & Therapy*, 9(Suppl 2). doi:10.1186/ar2186

[998] Tuso, P., Stroll, S., & Li, W. (2015). A Plant-Based Diet, Atherogenesis, and Coronary Artery Disease Prevention. *The Permanente Journal*, 62-67. doi:10.7812/tpp/14-036

[999] NIH. (2016, April 6). What Is Cholesterol? | Atherosclerosis. *U.S. Department of Health & Human Services*. Retrieved April 10, 2017, from https://www.nhlbi.nih.gov/health/health-topics/topics/hbc

[1000] Ibid

[1001] Ibid

[1002] Maresz, K., PhD. (2015, February). Proper Calcium Use: Vitamin K2 as a Promoter of Bone and Cardiovascular Health. *Integrative Medicine: A Clinician's Journal*. 14(1): 34–39.
PMCID: PMC4566462

[1003] Hirano, J., & Ishii, Y. (2002). Effects of vitamin K2, vitamin D, and calcium on the bone metabolism of rats in the growth phase. *Journal of Orthopaedic Science*, 7(3), 364-369. doi:10.1007/s007760200061

[1004] Maresz, K., PhD. (2015, February). Proper Calcium Use: Vitamin K2 as a Promoter of Bone and Cardiovascular Health. *Integrative Medicine: A Clinician's Journal*. 14(1): 34–39.
PMCID: PMC4566462

[1005] Ibid

[1006] Ibid

[1007] Ibid

[1008] Harvard Medical School. (2010, August). Stress and the sensitive gut. *Harvard Health Publication | Harvard Medical School*. Retrieved November 17, 2015, from http://www.health.harvard.edu/newsletters/Harvard_Mental_Health_Letter/2010/August/stress-and-the-sensitive-gut?utm_source=mental&utm_medium=pressrelease&utm_campaign=mental0810

[1009] Sasselli, V., Pachnis, V., & Burns, A. J. (2012). The enteric nervous system. *Developmental Biology*,366(1), 64-73. doi:10.1016/j.ydbio.2012.01.012

[1010] King, R. M. (2013, February). The Enteric Nervous System: The Brain in the Gut. *King's Psychology Network*. Retrieved November 18, 2015, from http://www.psyking.net/id36.htm

[1011] Nezami, B. G., & Srinivasan, S. (2010). Enteric Nervous System in the Small Intestine: Pathophysiology and Clinical Implications. *Current Gastroenterology Reports*, 12(5), 358-365. doi:10.1007/s11894-010-0129-9

[1012] Harvard Medical School. (2010, August). Stress and the sensitive gut. *Harvard Health Publication | Harvard Medical School*. Retrieved November 18, 2015, from http://www.health.harvard.edu/newsletters/Harvard_Mental_Health_Letter/2010/August/stress-and-the-sensitive-gut?utm_source=mental&utm_medium=pressrelease&utm_campaign=mental0810

[1013] King, R. M. (2013, February). The Enteric Nervous System: The Brain in the Gut. *King's Psychology Network*. Retrieved November 18, 2015, from http://www.psyking.net/id36.htm

[1014] Carabotti, M., Scirocco, A., Maselli, M. A., & Severi, C. (2015). The gut-brain axis: interactions between enteric microbiota, central and enteric nervous systems. *Annals of Gastroenterology : Quarterly Publication of the Hellenic Society of Gastroenterology*, 28(2), 203–209.

[1015] Biology Online. (2004, August 4). Enteric Nervous System. *Biology Online*. Retrieved November 19, 2015, from http://www.biology-online.org/articles/enteric_nervous_system.html

[1016] Ibid

[1017] Carabotti, M., Scirocco, A., Maselli, M. A., & Severi, C. (2015). The gut-brain axis: interactions between enteric microbiota, central and enteric nervous systems. *Annals of Gastroenterology : Quarterly Publication of the Hellenic Society of Gastroenterology*, 28(2), 203–209.

[1018] King, R. M. (2013, February). The Enteric Nervous System: The Brain in the Gut. *King's Psychology Network*. Retrieved November 19, 2015, from http://www.psyking.net/id36.htm

[1019] Camilleri, M. (2009). Serotonin in the Gastrointestinal Tract. *Current Opinion in Endocrinology, Diabetes, and Obesity*, 16(1), 53–59.

[1020] Dfarmud, D., Malmir, M., & Khanahmadi, M. (2014). *Happiness & Health: The Biological Factors- Systematic Review Article*. Iranian Journal of Public Health, 43(11), 1468–1477.

[1021] Bouchez, C. (2011, October 12). Reviewed by Brunilda Nazario, MD. Serotonin and Depression: 9 Questions and Answers. *WebMD*. Retrieved November 19, 2015, from http://www.webmd.com/depression/features/serotonin

[1022] Dfarmud, D., Malmir, M., & Khanahmadi, M. (2014). *Happiness & Health: The Biological Factors- Systematic Review Article*. Iranian Journal of Public Health, 43(11), 1468–1477.

[1023] Ibid

[1024] Weng, R., Shen, S., Burton, C., Yang, L., Nie, H., Tian, Y., . . . Liu, H. (2016). Lipidomic profiling of tryptophan hydroxylase 2 knockout mice reveals novel lipid biomarkers associated with serotonin deficiency. *Analytical and Bioanalytical Chemistry*, 408(11), 2963-2973. doi:10.1007/s00216-015-9256-3

[1025] Bouchez, C. (2011, October 12). Reviewed by Brunilda Nazario, MD. Serotonin and Depression: 9 Questions and Answers. *WebMD*. Retrieved November 19, 2015, from http://www.webmd.com/depression/features/serotonin?page=3

[1026] Integrative Psychiatry. (2007, November 7). ADHD Alternative Treatment. *Integrative Psychiatry*. Retrieved November 19, 2015, from http://www.integrativepsychiatry.net/adhd.html

[1027] Brown, H. (2005, August 22). The Other Brain Also Deals With Many Woes. *The New York Times*. Retrieved November 19, 2015, from http://www.nytimes.com/2005/08/23/health/23gut.html?pagewanted=all&_r=4&

[1028] Krajmalnik-Brown, R., Lozupone, C., Kang, D., & Adams, J. B. (2015). Gut bacteria in children with autism spectrum disorders: challenges and promise of studying how a complex community influences a complex disease. *Microbial Ecology in Health & Disease*, 26(0). doi:10.3402/mehd.v26.26914

[1029] Adams, J. B., Johansen, L. J., Powell, L. D., Quig, D., & Rubin, R. A. (2011). Gastrointestinal flora and gastrointestinal status in children with autism – comparisons to typical children and correlation with autism severity. BMC Gastroenterology, 11(1). doi:10.1186/1471-230x-11-22

[1030] Ibid

[1031] Jandhyala, S. M., Talukdar, R., Subramanyam, C., Vuyyuru, H., Sasikala, M., & Reddy, D. (2015). Role of the normal gut microbiota. *World Journal of Gastroenterology*, 21(29), 8787. doi:10.3748/wjg.v21.i29.8787

[1032] Probiotic.org. (2010, February 19). Intestinal Flora. *Probiotic.org*. Retrieved November 19, 2015, from http://www.probiotic.org/intestinal-flora.htm

[1033] Vieira, A. T., Teixeira, M. M., & Martins, F. S. (2013). The Role of Probiotics and Prebiotics in Inducing Gut Immunity. *Frontiers in Immunology*, 4. doi:10.3389/fimmu.2013.00445

[1034] FDA. (2013, September 1). Prevention is Key to Avoiding borne Illness Outbreaks | Food Service Employee Health and Hygiene Matters. *U.S. Food and Drug Administration*. Retrieved September 3, 2014, from http://www.fda.gov/Food/GuidanceRegulation/RetailFoodProtection/FoodborneIllnessRiskFactorReduction/ucm122832.htm

[1035] Taylor, M. (2012, September 11). Progress on FSMA, Changes within the FDA Foods Program, and on Partnerships. *U.S. Food and Drug Administration*. Retrieved November 19, 2015, from http://www.fda.gov/food/guidanceregulation/fsma/ucm319053.htm

[1036] Wilson, L, MD. (2013, March). YOUR INTESTINAL FLORA. *The Center For Development | by Lawrence Wilson*, MD. Retrieved November 19, 2015, from http://www.drlwilson.com/ARTICLES/FLORA.htm

[1037] Farhud, D. D. (2015). Impact of Lifestyle on Health. *Iranian Journal of Public Health*, 44(11), 1442–1444.

[1038] Ibid

[1039] Langdon, A., Crook, N., & Dantas, G. (2016). The effects of antibiotics on the microbiome throughout development and alternative approaches for therapeutic modulation. *Genome Medicine*, 8(1). doi:10.1186/s13073-016-0294-z

[1040] Ghabril, M., Chalasani, N., & Björnsson, E. (2010). Drug-induced liver injury: a clinical update. *Current Opinion in Gastroenterology, 26*(3), 222-226. doi:10.1097/mog.0b013e3283383c7c

[1041] MSU. (2009, December 26). CAUSES OF YEAST INFECTIONS. *Michigan State University*. Retrieved November 19, 2015, from https://www.msu.edu/~eisthen/yeast/causes.html

[1042] Ibid

[1043] Snedeker, S. M., & Hay, A. G. (2011). Do Interactions Between Gut Ecology and Environmental Chemicals Contribute to Obesity and Diabetes? *Environmental Health Perspectives*, 120(3), 332-339. doi:10.1289/ehp.1104204

[1044] Wilson, L, MD. (2013, March). YOUR INTESTINAL FLORA. *The Center For Development | by Lawrence Wilson*, MD. Retrieved November 19, 2015, from http://www.drlwilson.com/ARTICLES/FLORA.htm

[1045] Ibid

[1046] Abou-Donia, M. B., El-Masry, E. M., Abdel-Rahman, A. A., Mclendon, R. E., & Schiffman, S. S. (2008). Splenda Alters Gut Microflora and Increases Intestinal P-Glycoprotein and Cytochrome P-450 in Male Rats. *Journal of Toxicology and Environmental Health*, Part A, 71(21), 1415-1429. doi:10.1080/15287390802328630

[1047] Savcheniuk, O. A., Virchenko, O. V., Falalyeyeva, T. M., Beregova, T. V., Babenko, L. P., Lazarenko, L. M., . . . Spivak, M. (2014). The efficacy of probiotics for monosodium glutamate-induced obesity: dietology concerns and opportunities for prevention. *EPMA Journal*, 5(1), 2. doi:10.1186/1878-5085-5-2

[1048] Wilson, L, MD. (2013, March). YOUR INTESTINAL FLORA. *The Center For Development | by Lawrence Wilson*, MD. Retrieved November 19, 2015, from http://www.drlwilson.com/ARTICLES/FLORA.htm

[1049] Høst, A., & Samuelsson, E. (1988). Allergic reactions to raw, pasteurized, and homogenized/pasteurized cow milk: a comparison. *Allergy*, 43(2), 113-118. doi:10.1111/j.1398-9995.1988.tb00404.x

[1050] Phillips, M. L. (2009). Gut Reaction: Environmental Effects on the Human Microbiota. *Environmental Health Perspectives*, 117(5), A198–A205.

[1051] Baldwin, H. B. (1916). Some Observations On Homogenized Milk And Cream. *American Journal of Public Health*, 6(8), 862-864. doi:10.2105/ajph.6.8.862

[1052] Augustin (Marcus), S. A. (2015). *The hungry brain: the nutrition/cognition connection*. New York, NY: Skyhorse Publishing.

[1053] Oster, K. A., Ross, D. J., Dawkins, H. H., Sampsidis, N., & Morrison, M. D. (1983). *The XO factor: Homogenized Milk May Cause Your Heart Attack*. New York: Park City Press.

[1054] Ibid

[1055] Goldes, M. (1989, September 25). Studies Confirm Cholesterol-Heart Attack Link; The Fault in the Milk. *The New York Times*. Retrieved April 05, 2017, from http://www.nytimes.com/1989/09/26/opinion/l-studies-confirm-cholesterol-heart-attack-link-the-fault-in-the-milk-466689.html

[1056] Engen, P. A., Green, S. J., Voigt, R. M., Forsyth, C. B., & Keshavarzian, A. (2015). The Gastrointestinal Microbiome: Alcohol Effects on the Composition of Intestinal Microbiota. *Alcohol Research: current reviews*. 37(2):223-36

[1057] Purohit, V., Bode, J. C., Bode, C., Brenner, D. A., Choudhry, M. A., Hamilton, F., . . . Turner, J. R. (2008). Alcohol, intestinal bacterial growth, intestinal permeability to endotoxin, and medical consequences: Summary of a symposium. *Alcohol*, 42(5), 349-361. doi:10.1016/j.alcohol.2008.03.131

[1058] Walker, W. A. (1975, November). Antigen absorption from the small intestine and gastrointestinal disease. Pediatric Clinics of North America. 22(4):731-46. PMID: 1196680

[1059] Hazenberg, M. P., Klasenm, I. S., Kool, J., Embden, J. G., & Severijnen, A. J. (1992). Are Intestinal bacteria involved in the etiology of rheumatoid arthritis? *Apmis*, 100(1-6), 1-9. doi:10.1111/j.1699-0463.1992.tb00833.x

[1060] Peters, T. J., & Bjarnason, I. (1988). Uses and Abuses of Intestinal Permeability Measurements. *Canadian Journal of Gastroenterology, 2*(3), 127-132. doi:10.1155/1988/867416

[1061] Deitch, E.A.(1990, March). The role of intestinal barrier failure and bacterial translocation in the development of systemic infection and multiple organ failure. *Archives of Surgery.* 125(3):403-4. PMID: 2407230

[1062] Bischoff, S. C., Barbara, G., Buurman, W., Ockhuizen, T., Schulzke, J., Serino, M., . . . Wells, J. M. (2014). Intestinal permeability – a new target for disease prevention and therapy. *BMC Gastroenterology, 14*(1). doi:10.1186/s12876-014-0189-7

[1063] Rooney, P. J., Jenkins, R. T., & Buchanan, W. W. (1990, Jan-Feb). A short review of the relationship between intestinal permeability and inflammatory joint disease. *Clinical and experimental rheumatology.* 8(1):75-83. PMID: 2189626

[1064] Michielan, A., & D'Incà, R. (2015). Intestinal Permeability in Inflammatory Bowel Disease: Pathogenesis, Clinical Evaluation, and Therapy of Leaky Gut. *Mediators of Inflammation, 2015*, 1-10. doi:10.1155/2015/628157

[1065] Fasano, A. (2011). Leaky Gut and Autoimmune Diseases. *Clinical Reviews in Allergy & Immunology,42*(1), 71-78. doi:10.1007/s12016-011-8291-x

[1066] Visser, J., Rozing, J., Sapone, A., Lammers, K., & Fasano, A. (2009). Tight Junctions, Intestinal Permeability, and Autoimmunity. *Annals of the New York Academy of Sciences, 1165*(1), 195-205. doi:10.1111/j.1749-6632.2009.04037.x

[1067] Berkeley Wellness. (2015, April 17). Are Antibiotics Making Us Fat?. *University of California, Berkeley Wellness.* Retrieved July 06, 2017, from http://www.berkeleywellness.com/healthy-eating/food/food-safety/article/are-antibiotics-food-making-people-fat

[1068] CBS News. (2010, February 11). Chemicals in Food Can Make You Fat. *CBS News.* Retrieved July 06, 2017, from http://www.cbsnews.com/news/chemicals-in-food-can-make-you-fat/

[1069] Zuckerbrot, T. (2017, February 7). 6 foods that can damage your metabolism the moment you eat them. *Fox News Health.* Retrieved July 06, 2017, from http://www.foxnews.com/health/2017/02/07/6-foods-that-can-damage-your-metabolism-moment-eat-them.html

[1070] The Dr. Oz Show. (2014, April 07). The Fat Drug: How Antibiotics Can Make You Gain Weight, Pt 1. *The Dr. Oz Show Televised Episode.* Retrieved July 07, 2017, from http://www.doctoroz.com/episode/fat-drug-how-antibiotics-make-you-gain-weight

[1071] Berkeley Wellness. (2015, April 17). Are Antibiotics Making Us Fat?. *University of California, Berkeley Wellness.* Retrieved July 06, 2017, from http://www.berkeleywellness.com/healthy-eating/food/food-safety/article/are-antibiotics-food-making-people-fat

[1072] Riley, L. W., Raphael, E., & Faerstein, E. (2013). Obesity in the United States – Dysbiosis from Exposure to Low-Dose Antibiotics? *Frontiers in Public Health*, 1. doi:10.3389/fpubh.2013.00069

[1073] Ibid

[1074] Berkeley Wellness. (2015, April 17). Are Antibiotics Making Us Fat?. *University of California, Berkeley Wellness.* Retrieved July 06, 2017, from http://www.berkeleywellness.com/healthy-eating/food/food-safety/article/are-antibiotics-food-making-people-fat

[1075] Jeong, S., Kang, D., Lim, M., Kang, C., & Sung, H. (2010). Risk Assessment of Growth Hormones and Antimicrobial Residues in Meat. *Toxicological Research, 26*(4), 301-313. doi:10.5487/tr.2010.26.4.301

[1076] Holtcamp, W. (2011). Poultry Relief? Organic Farming May Reduce Drug Resistance. *Environmental Health Perspectives, 119*(11). doi:10.1289/ehp.119-a489b

[1077] Hackert, J. (2013, April 19). Understanding Probiotics . *University of Missouri Extension.* Retrieved November 19, 2015, from http://extension.missouri.edu/harrison/documents/understandingprobiotics.pdf

[1078] The Dr. Oz Show. (2012, September 6). Fact Sheet: Probiotics. *The Dr. Oz Show.* Retrieved November 19, 2015, from http://www.doctoroz.com/videos/fact-sheet-probiotics?page=2

[1079] Raak, C., Ostermann, T., Boehm, K., & Molsberger, F. (2014). Regular Consumption of Sauerkraut and Its Effect on Human Health: A Bibliometric Analysis. *Global Advances in Health and Medicine*, 3(6), 12–18. doi: 10.7453/gahmj.2014.038

[1080] Plengvidhya, V., Breidt, F., Lu, Z., & Fleming, H. P. (2007). DNA Fingerprinting of Lactic Acid Bacteria in Sauerkraut Fermentations. *Applied and Environmental Microbiology*, 73(23), 7697-7702. doi:10.1128/aem.01342-07

[1081] Kwak, C. S., Lee, M. S., Oh, S. I., & Park, S. C. (2010). Discovery of Novel Sources of Vitamin B12 in Traditional Korean Foods from Nutritional Surveys of Centenarians. *Current Gerontology and Geriatrics Research*, 2010, 374897. doi: 10.1155/2010/374897

[1082] Patra, J. K., Das, G., Paramithiotis, S., & Shin, H.-S. (2016). Kimchi and Other Widely Consumed Traditional Fermented Foods of Korea: A Review. *Frontiers in Microbiology.* 7, 1493. doi: 10.3389/fmicb.2016.01493

[1083] Ibid

[1084] Raymond, J. (2008, February 1). World's Healthiest Foods: Kimchi (Korea). *Health Magazine - Digestive Health.* Retrieved November 19, 2015, from http://www.health.com/health/article/0,,20410300,00.html

[1085] Hackert, J. (2013, April 19). Understanding Probiotics . *University of Missouri Extension.* Retrieved November 19, 2015, from http://extension.missouri.edu/harrison/documents/understandingprobiotics.pdf

[1086] WebMD. (2014, December 21). Foods With Probiotics That Help Digestion. *WebMD.* Retrieved November 19, 2015, from http://www.webmd.com/digestive-disorders/probiotics-10/slideshow-probiotics

[1087] Ibid

[1088] Liem, I. T., Steinkraus, K. H., & Cronk, T. C. (1977). Production of vitamin B-12 in tempeh, a fermented soybean food. *Applied and Environmental Microbiology*, 34(6), 773–776

[1089] GHC. (2013, November 14). Probiotic Foods. *Global Healing Center.* Retrieved November 19, 2015, from http://www.globalhealingcenter.com/natural-health/probiotic-foods/

[1090] WebMD. (2014, December 21). Foods With Probiotics That Help Digestion. *WebMD*. Retrieved November 19, 2015, from http://www.webmd.com/digestive-disorders/probiotics-10/slideshow-probiotics

[1091] Ehrlich, S. D. (2011, June 11). Spirulina. *University of Maryland Medical Center*. Retrieved November 19, 2015, from http://umm.edu/health/medical/altmed/supplement/spirulina

[1092] Ibid

[1093] Ibid

[1094] WebMD. (2009). CHLORELLA: Uses, Side Effects, Interactions and Warnings. *WebMD*. Retrieved November 19, 2015, from http://www.webmd.com/Vitamins-supplements/ingredientmono-907-CHLORELLA.aspx?activeIngredientId=907&activeIngredientName=CHLORELLA

[1095] The Dr. Oz Show. (2012, September 6). Fact Sheet: Probiotics. *The Dr. Oz Show*. Retrieved April 04, 2015, from http://www.doctoroz.com/article/fact-sheet-probiotics

[1096] Plengvidhya, V., Breidt, F., Lu, Z., & Fleming, H. P. (2007). DNA Fingerprinting of Lactic Acid Bacteria in Sauerkraut Fermentations. *Applied and Environmental Microbiology*, 73(23), 7697-7702. doi:10.1128/aem.01342-07

[1097] Bloomfield, S. F., Rook, G. A., Scott, E. A., Shanahan, F., Stanwell-Smith, R., & Turner, P. (2016). Time to abandon the hygiene hypothesis: new perspectives on allergic disease, the human microbiome, infectious disease prevention and the role of targeted hygiene. *Perspectives in Public Health*, 136(4), 213-224. doi:10.1177/1757913916650225

[1098] Savilahti, E. (2011). Probiotics in the Treatment and Prevention of Allergies in Children. *Bioscience and Microflora*, 30(4), 119-128. doi:10.12938/bifidus.30.119

[1099] Franco, R., Oñatibia-Astibia, A., & Martínez-Pinilla, E. (2013). Health Benefits of Methylxanthines in Cacao and Chocolate. *Nutrients*, 5(10), 4159-4173. doi:10.3390/nu5104159

[1100] Chairperson Reid, G.,Dr., & Rapporteur Stanton, C.,Dr. (2001, October 1-4). Health and Nutritional Properties of Probiotics in Food including Powder Milk with Live Lactic Acid Bacteria | Report of a Joint FAO/WHO Expert Consultation. Food *and Agriculture Organization of the United Nations*. Retrieved September 5, 2014, from http://www.who.int/foodsafety/publications/fs_management/en/probiotics.pdf

[1101] Patel, S., & Goyal, A. (2012). The current trends and future perspectives of prebiotics research: a review. *3 Biotech*, 2(2), 115-125. doi:10.1007/s13205-012-0044-x

[1102] Raposo, M. D., Morais, A. D., & Morais, R. D. (2016). Emergent Sources of Prebiotics: Seaweeds and Microalgae. *Marine Drugs*, 14(2), 27. doi:10.3390/md14020027

[1103] Dahl, W. J., & Mai, V. (2011, January 10). Go With Your Gut: Understanding Microbiota and Prebiotics1. *University of Florida EDIS Publications RSS*. Retrieved from http://edis.ifas.ufl.edu/fs171

[1104] Migliozzi, M., Thavarajah, D., Thavarajah, P., & Smith, P. (2015). Lentil and Kale: Complementary Nutrient-Rich Whole Food Sources to Combat Micronutrient and Calorie Malnutrition. *Nutrients*, 7(11), 9285-9298. doi:10.3390/nu7115471

[1105] WomenHealth.gov. (2011, August 4). Why breastfeeding is important. *Office on Women's Health, U.S. Department of Health and Human Services*. Retrieved September 7, 2014, from http://www.womenshealth.gov/breastfeeding/why-breastfeeding-is-important/ http://womenshealth.gov/breastfeeding/breastfeeding-benefits.html

[1106] Ibid

[1107] Dahl, W. J., & Mai, V. (2011, July 10). Go With Your Gut: Understanding Microbiota and Prebiotics1. *University of Florida EDIS Publications RSS Publication #FSHN11-10*. Retrieved November 19, 2015, from http://edis.ifas.ufl.edu/fs171

[1108] McKeith, G. (2005). *You are what you eat: the plan that will change your life*. New York: Dutton.

[1109] Ibid

[1110] Ibid

[1111] Ibid

[1112] Ibid

[1113] Cheung, T. (2008). Lose weight for Christmas with the Lemon Juice Diet. *Associated Newspapers - Mail Online*. Retrieved November 19, 2015, from http://www.dailymail.co.uk/health/article-501148/Lose-weight-Christmas-Lemon-Juice-Diet.html

[1114] McKeith, G. (2005). *You are what you eat: the plan that will change your life*. New York: Dutton.

[1115] The Dr. Oz Show. (2012, September 6). Dr. Oz's Complete Body Restart Guide. The Dr. Oz Show. Retrieved November 19, 2015, from http://www.doctoroz.com/videos/dr-oz-complete-body-restart-guide?page=3

[1116] Ibid

[1117] Spivey, A. (2010). Lose Sleep, Gain Weight: Another Piece of the Obesity Puzzle. *Environmental Health Perspectives*, 118(1). doi:10.1289/ehp.118-a28

[1118] Spivey, A. (2010). Lose Sleep, Gain Weight: Another Piece of the Obesity Puzzle. *Environmental Health Perspectives*, 118(1). doi:10.1289/ehp.118-a28

[1119] Taheri, S., Lin, L., Austin, D., Young, T., & Mignot, E. (2004). Short Sleep Duration Is Associated with Reduced Leptin, Elevated Ghrelin, and Increased Body Mass Index. *PLoS Medicine*, 1(3). doi:10.1371/journal.pmed.0010062

[1120] Wu, J. T., & Kral, J. G. (2004). Ghrelin Integrative Neuroendocrine Peptide in Health and Disease. *Annals of Surgery*, 239(4), 464-474. doi:10.1097/01.sla.0000118561.54919.61

[1121] Egecioglu, E., Skibicka, K. P., Hansson, C., Alvarez-Crespo, M., Friberg, P. A., Jerlhag, E., . . . Dickson, S. L. (2011). Hedonic and incentive signals for body weight control. *Reviews in Endocrine and Metabolic Disorders, 12*(3), 141-151. doi:10.1007/s11154-011-9166-4

[1122] Klok, M. D., Jakobsdottir, S., & Drent, M. L. (2007). The role of Leptin and ghrelin in the regulation of food intake and body weight in humans: a review. *Obesity Reviews, 8*(1), 21-34. doi:10.1111/j.1467-789x.2006.00270.x

[1123] Montmayeur, J., & Coutre, J. L. (2010). *Fat Detection Taste, Texture, and Post Ingestive Effects | Chapter 14 Fat-Rich Food Palatability and Appetite Regulation*. Hoboken: Taylor and Francis.

[1124] Pradhan, G., Samson, S. L., & Sun, Y. (2013). Ghrelin. *Current Opinion in Clinical Nutrition and Metabolic Care, 16*(6), 619-624. doi:10.1097/mco.0b013e328365b9be

[1125] Taheri, S., Lin, L., Austin, D., Young, T., & Mignot, E. (2004). Short Sleep Duration Is Associated with Reduced Leptin, Elevated Ghrelin, and Increased Body Mass Index. *PLoS Medicine, 1*(3). doi:10.1371/journal.pmed.0010062

[1126] Shaw, G. (2012, April 14). The Healing Power of Sleep; Reviewed by Louise Chang, MD. *WebMD Sleep Disorders Health Center*. Retrieved from http://www.webmd.com/sleep-disorders/features/healing-power-sleep

[1127] Knutson, K. L. (2007). Impact of Sleep and Sleep Loss on Glucose Homeostasis and Appetite Regulation. *Sleep Medicine Clinics, 2*(2), 187-197. doi:10.1016/j.jsmc.2007.03.004

[1128] NHLBI-NIH. (2012, February 22). How Much Sleep Is Enough?. *NHLBI, National Institutes of Health*. Retrieved November 20, 2015, from http://www.nhlbi.nih.gov/health/health-topics/topics/sdd/howmuch.html

[1129] Sehgal, A., & Mignot, E. (2011). Genetics of Sleep and Sleep Disorders. *Cell, 146*(2), 194-207. doi:10.1016/j.cell.2011.07.004

[1130] Weise, E. (2009, August 13). 6 hours of sleep? It's not enough. *USA TODAY*. Retrieved November 20, 2015, from http://usatoday30.usatoday.com/tech/science/2009-08-13-sleep-gene_N.htm

[1131] Ibid

[1132] Kripke, D. F., Langer, R. D., & Kline, L. E. (2012). Hypnotics' association with mortality or cancer: a matched cohort study. *BMJ Open, 2*(1). doi:10.1136/bmjopen-2012-000850

[1133] LoGiudice, P., & Bongiorno, P. (2012, March 9). What to Eat for Deep Sleep. *The Dr. Oz Show*. Retrieved November 20, 2015, from http://www.doctoroz.com/videos/what-eat-deep-sleep

[1134] Ibid

[1135] Searing, L. (2012, March 5). Study finds sleeping pills associated with higher risk of cancer and death. *Washington Post*. Retrieved November 20, 2015, from http://www.washingtonpost.com/national/health-science/study-finds-sleeping-pills-associated-with-higher-risk-of-cancer-and-death/2012/02/29/gIQAufQ4sR_story.html

[1136] DeNoon, D. (2012, February 27). Sleeping Pills Called "as Risky as Cigarettes". *WebMD*. Retrieved November 20, 2015, from http://www.webmd.com/sleep-disorders/news/20120227/sleeping-pills-called-as-risky-as-cigarettes

[1137] Kripke, D. F., Langer, R. D., & Kline, L. E. (2012). Hypnotics' association with mortality or cancer: a matched cohort study. *BMJ Open, 2*(1). doi:10.1136/bmjopen-2012-000850

[1138] Salahi, L. (2012, February 27). Sleeping Pills Linked to Almost Fourfold Increase in Death Risk. *ABC News*. Retrieved November 20, 2015, from http://abcnews.go.com/Health/Sleep/sleeping-pills-linked-times-increased-death-risk/story?id=15803687

[1139] Psychology Today. (2015, November 19). Circadian Rhythm - body clock, sleep cycle, jet lag | What is the Circadian Rhythm?. *Psychology Today*. Retrieved November 20, 2015, from http://www.psychologytoday.com/basics/circadian-rhythm

[1140] Ibid

[1141] NIH. (n.d.). Brain Basics: Understanding Sleep. *National Institute of Neurological Disorders and Stroke (NINDS)*. Retrieved November 20, 2015, from http://www.ninds.nih.gov/disorders/brain_basics/understanding_sleep.htm

[1142] Butler, C. (2010, June 29). Circadian rhythms are powerful, but people can change their sleep-wake cycles. *The Washington Post*. Retrieved November 20, 2015, from http://www.washingtonpost.com/wp-dyn/content/article/2010/06/28/AR2010062803820.html

[1143] Duffy, J. F., & Czeisler, C. A. (2009). Effect of Light on Human Circadian Physiology. *Sleep Medicine Clinics, 4*(2), 165-177. doi:10.1016/j.jsmc.2009.01.004

[1144] RPI News. (2012, August 27). Light From Self-Luminous Tablet Computers Can Affect Evening Melatonin, Delaying Sleep. *Rensselaer Polytechnic Institute*. Retrieved April 06, 2017, from https://news.rpi.edu/luwakkey/3074

[1145] Ibid

[1146] Burkhart, K., & Phelps, J. (2009). Amber Lenses To Block Blue Light And Improve Sleep: A Randomized Trial. *Chronobiology International, 26*(8), 1602-1612. doi:10.3109/07420520903523719

[1147] Alberts, B., Johnson, A., Lewis, J., Raff, M., Roberts, K., & Walter, P. (2002). *Molecular biology of the cell*. New York: Garland Science.

[1148] Picco, M. F., M.D.(2012, October 30). Digestion: How long does it take?. *Mayo Clinic*. Retrieved November 20, 2015, from http://www.mayoclinic.org/digestive-system/expert-answers/FAQ-20058340

[1149] Murphy, P., & Campbell, S. (1997). Nighttime Drop in Body Temperature: A Physiological Trigger for Sleep Onset? *Sleep*. doi:10.1093/sleep/20.7.505

[1150] Columbia University. (2011, February 26). HLC Pilot Program Tips. *Columbia University Work-Life*. Retrieved November 20, 2015, from http://worklife.columbia.edu/healthy-lifestyles-challenge-weekly-tips

[1151] Ibid

[1152] Silver, J. K., MD. (2008, February 25). Don't eat before you go to sleep—good advice or medical myth?. *Health Gather*. Retrieved February 25, 2014, from http://health.gather.com/viewArticle.action?articleId=281474977268011

[1153] Andrén-Sandberg (2002). René G. Holzheimer & J. A. Mannick(Eds):Surgical treatment. Evidence-based and problem-oriented., P Gorecki, M.D. Gastro-esophageal reflux disease (GERD). W. Zuckschwerdt Verlag, München, Bern, Wien, New York, 2001.(843 pages). ISBN 3-88603-714-2. *European Journal of Surgery, 168*(5), 310-310. doi:10.1002/ejs.52

[1154] MNSU. (2006, October 23). Tips for Getting a Good Night's Sleep – The Counseling Center. *Minnesota State University, Mankato*. Retrieved November 20, 2015, from http://www.mnsu.edu/counseling/students/sleep.html

[1155] University of Maryland Medical Center. (2006, May 22). Tryptophan. *University of Maryland Medical Center*. Retrieved from http://umm.edu/health/medical/ency/articles/tryptophan

[1156] Ibid

[1157] Ibid

[1158] MNSU. (2006, October 23). Tips for Getting a Good Night's Sleep – The Counseling Center. *Minnesota State University, Mankato*. Retrieved November 20, 2015, from http://www.mnsu.edu/counseling/students/sleep.html

[1159] Murray, M. (2006, April 28). Insomnia & Sleep-wake Cycle Disorder. Dr. Michael Murray. Retrieved November 20, 2015, from http://doctormurray.com/health-conditions/insomnia-sleep-wake-cycle-disorder/

[1160] Niccals, M. (2009, July 16). Hypoglycemia Insomnia Sleep Problems Due to Hypoglycemia. *Ezine Articles*. Retrieved November 20, 2015, from http://ezinearticles.com/?Hypoglycemia-Insomnia---Sleep-Problems-Due-to-Hypoglycemia&id=2618159

[1161] Golokhov, D. (2012, April 15). 10 foods to avoid before bed. *Fox News*. Retrieved November 20, 2015, from http://www.foxnews.com/health/2012/04/13/10-foods-to-avoid-before-bed/

[1162] Baratloo, A., Rouhipour, A., Forouzanfar, M. M., Safari, S., Amiri, M., & Negida, A. (2016). The Role of Caffeine in Pain Management: A Brief Literature Review. *Anesthesiology and Pain Medicine, 6*(3). doi:10.5812/aapm.33193

[1163] Diamond, S. (2000). Ibuprofen plus caffeine in the treatment of tension-type headache. *Clinical Pharmacology & Therapeutics, 68*(3), 312-319. doi:10.1067/mcp.2000.109353

[1164] Antonaci, F., Ghiotto, N., Wu, S., Pucci, E., & Costa, A. (2016). Recent advances in migraine therapy. *SpringerPlus, 5*(1). doi:10.1186/s40064-016-2211-8

[1165] Cleveland Clinic. (2014, December 29). Caffeine & Headaches: Treatment & Sources | Caffeine can be a double-edged sword for those with headache. *Cleveland Clinic*. Retrieved April 13, 2017, from https://my.clevelandclinic.org/health/articles/caffeine-and-headache

[1166] Drake, C., Roehrs, T., Shambroom, J., & Roth, T. (2013). Caffeine Effects on Sleep Taken 0, 3, or 6 Hours before Going to Bed. *Journal of Clinical Sleep Medicine*. doi:10.5664/jcsm.3170

[1167] CBC News. (2013, November 14). Caffeine may harm sleep 6 hours before bedtime. *CBCnews | CBC/Radio Canada*. Retrieved November 20, 2015, from http://www.cbc.ca/news/health/caffeine-may-harm-sleep-6-hours-before-bedtime-1.2426901

[1168] Ibid

[1169] CBC News. (2013, November 14). Caffeine may harm sleep 6 hours before bedtime. *CBCnews | CBC/Radio Canada*. Retrieved November 20, 2015, from http://www.cbc.ca/news/health/caffeine-may-harm-sleep-6-hours-before-bedtime-1.2426901

[1170] MNSU. (2006, October 23). Tips for Getting a Good Night's Sleep – The Counseling Center. *Minnesota State University, Mankato*. Retrieved November 20, 2015, from http://www.mnsu.edu/counseling/students/sleep.html

[1171] Perricone, N. (2008). *Ageless Face, Ageless Mind: Erase Wrinkles and Rejuvenate the Brain*. New York: Ballantine Books.

[1172] Stenson, J. (2005, August 23). Is exercising at night really so bad?. *MSNBC News*. Retrieved November 20, 2015, from http://www.nbcnews.com/id/8986839/ns/health-fitness/#.UxOOz-NdWdI

[1173] Myllymäki, T., Kyröläinen, H., Savolainen, K., Hokka, L., Jakonen, R., Juuti, T., . . . Rusko, H. (2011). Effects of vigorous late-night exercise on sleep quality and cardiac autonomic activity. *Journal of Sleep Research, 20*(1pt2), 146-153. doi:10.1111/j.1365-2869.2010.00874.x

[1174] Uchida, S., Shioda, K., Morita, Y., Kubota, C., Ganeko, M., & Takeda, N. (2012). Exercise Effects on Sleep Physiology. *Frontiers in Neurology, 3*. doi:10.3389/fneur.2012.00048

[1175] UMM. (2013, July 31). Sleep Hygiene. *University of Maryland Medical Center*. Retrieved November 20, 2015, from http://umm.edu/programs/sleep/patients/sleep-hygiene http://umm.edu/health/medical/reports/articles/insomnia

[1176] Valham, F., Sahlin, C., Stenlund, H., & Franklin, K. A. (2012). Ambient Temperature and Obstructive Sleep Apnea: Effects on Sleep, Sleep Apnea, and Morning Alertness. *Sleep*. doi:10.5665/sleep.1736

[1177] Doheny, K. (2010, March 29). Best Temperature For Sleep, Effects of Temperature on Sleep. *WebMD*. Retrieved November 20, 2015, from http://www.webmd.com/sleep-disorders/features/cant-sleep-adjust-the-temperature

[1178] Okamoto-Mizuno, K., & Mizuno, K. (2012). Effects of thermal environment on sleep and circadian rhythm. *Journal of Physiological Anthropology, 31*(1), 14. doi:10.1186/1880-6805-31-14

[1179] National Sleep Foundation. (2014, November 21). Best Temperature for Sleep. *National Sleep Foundation*. Retrieved April 13, 2017, from https://sleep.org/articles/temperature-for-sleep/

[1180] Harvard Health Letter. (2009, November). Snoozing without guilt — a daytime nap can be good for health, reports the Harvard Health Letter. *Harvard Health Publications | Harvard Medical School*. Retrieved November 20, 2015, from
http://www.health.harvard.edu/press_releases/snoozing-without-guilt--a-daytime-nap-can-be-good-for-health

[1181] Ibid

[1182] Ibid

[1183] JAD. (2009, July 1). Researchers find possible environmental causes for Alzheimer's, diabetes. *JAD - Press Releases | Journal of Alzheimer's Disease*. Retrieved October 26, 2015, from http://www.j-alz.com/press/2009/20090706.html

[1184] DeLaMonte, S. M., Neusner, A., Chu, J., & Lawton, M. (2009). Epidemiological Trends Strongly Suggest Exposures as Etiologic Agents in the Pathogenesis of Sporadic Alzheimers Disease, Diabetes Mellitus, and Non-Alcoholic Steatohepatitis. *Journal of Alzheimers Disease, 17*(3), 519-529. doi:10.3233/jad-2009-1070

[1185] Rosedale, R. (2008, December). Insulin Resistance: The Real Culprit by Ron Rosedale, M.D.. *Nourished Magazine : Wisdom to thrive by*. Retrieved November 23, 2015, from http://nourishedmagazine.com.au/blog/articles/Insulin-resistance-the-real-culprit
also Retrieved September 27, 2017, https://www.sott.net/article/236090-Insulin-Resistance-The-Real-Culprit

[1186] Ibid

[1187] Ibid

[1188] Rosedale, R., Westman, E. C., & Konhilas, J. P. (2009). Clinical Experience of a Diet Designed to Reduce Aging. *The Journal of Applied Research*, 9(4), 159–165.

[1189] Guyton, A. C., & Hall, J. E. (2000). *Textbook of medical physiology*. Philadelphia: Saunders.

[1190] Rosedale, R. (2008, December). Insulin Resistance: The Real Culprit by Ron Rosedale, M.D.. *Nourished Magazine : Wisdom to thrive by*. Retrieved November 23, 2015, from http://nourishedmagazine.com.au/blog/articles/Insulin-resistance-the-real-culprit
also Retrieved September 27, 2017, https://www.sott.net/article/236090-Insulin-Resistance-The-Real-Culprit

[1191] Siegel, L. J. (2004, April 4). Are Telomeres the Key to Aging and Cancer?. *N.C. State University*. Retrieved November 23, 2015, from http://www.ncsu.edu/project/bio183de/Black/genelinkage_disorders/genelinkage_disorders_reading/telomeres.html

[1192] Ibid

[1193] Ibid

[1194] SpectraCell Laboratories. (2014). Telomere Testing. *SpectraCell Laboratories*. Retrieved November 23, 2015, from http://www.spectracell.com/clinicians/products/telomere-testing/

[1195] Telomeretesting.net. (2013, February 5). Telomere Testing. *Telomere Testing*. Retrieved November 23, 2015, from http://www.telomeretesting.net/

[1196] Kahn, B. B., & Flier, J. S. (2000). Obesity and insulin resistance. *Journal of Clinical Investigation, 106*(4), 473-481. doi:10.1172/jci10842

[1197] Berg, J. M., Tymoczko, J. L., Stryer, L., & Stryer, L. (2002). *Biochemistry | Chapter 21 Glycogen Metabolism*. New York: W.H. Freeman.

[1198] Orthomolecular. (2001, February 1). Glycogen. *Orthomolecular.org*. Retrieved November 23, 2015, from http://www.orthomolecular.org/nutrients/glycogen.html

[1199] NIH. (2016, June 22). What Is Metabolic Syndrome? .*U.S National Library of Medicine, NIH*. Retrieved October 13, 2016, from http://www.nhlbi.nih.gov/health/health-topics/topics/ms

[1200] Rundek, T., Gardener, H., Xu, Q., Goldberg, R. B., Wright, C. B., Boden-Albala, B., . . . Sacco, R. L. (2010). Insulin Resistance and Risk of Ischemic Stroke Among Nondiabetic Individuals From the Northern Manhattan Study. *Archives of Neurology, 67*(10). doi:10.1001/archneurol.2010.235

[1201] Bingham, E. M., Hopkins, D., Smith, D., Pernet, A., Hallett, W., Reed, L., . . . Amiel, S. A. (2002). The Role of Insulin in Human Brain Glucose Metabolism: An 18Fluoro-Deoxyglucose Positron Emission Tomography Study. *Diabetes, 51*(12), 3384-3390. doi:10.2337/diabetes.51.12.3384

[1202] Woolley, E. (2012, February 29). How Insulin Works In the Body. *About Health*. Retrieved November 23, 2015, from http://diabetes.about.com/od/whatisdiabetes/a/How-Insulin-Works-In-The-Body.htm

[1203] NIH. (2016, June 22). What Is Metabolic Syndrome? .*U.S National Library of Medicine, NIH*. Retrieved October 13, 2016, from http://www.nhlbi.nih.gov/health/health-topics/topics/ms

[1204] Rosedale, R. (2008, December). Insulin Resistance: The Real Culprit by Ron Rosedale, M.D.. *Nourished Magazine : Wisdom to thrive by*. Retrieved November 23, 2015, from http://nourishedmagazine.com.au/blog/articles/Insulin-resistance-the-real-culprit
also Retrieved September 27, 2017, https://www.sott.net/article/236090-Insulin-Resistance-The-Real-Culprit

[1205] Mercola, J. (2006, July 18). More Evidence Sugar Feeds Cancer. *Latest and Current Health News and Information by Dr. Mercola*. Retrieved November 23, 2015, from http://articles.mercola.com/sites/articles/archive/2006/07/18/more-evidence-sugar-feeds-cancer.aspx

[1206] Ibid

[1207] Ibid

[1208] Hamdy, O., Porramatikul, S., & Al-Ozairi, E. (2006, November). Metabolic Obesity: The Paradox Between Visceral and Subcutaneous Fat. *Bentham Science Publisher Bentham Science Publisher Current Diabetes Reviews, 2*(4), 367-373. doi:10.2174/1573399810602040367

[1209] Ibid

[1210] Klein, S. (2004). The case of visceral fat: argument for the defense. *Journal of Clinical Investigation*, 113(11), 1530-1532. doi:10.1172/jci200422028

1211 Lee, J. S., Kim, S. H., Jun, D. W., Han, J. H., Jang, E. C., Park, J. Y., et al. (2009). Clinical Implications Of Fatty Pancreas: Correlations Between Fatty Pancreas And Metabolic Syndrome. *World Journal of Gastroenterology*. 15(15), 1869.

1212 Tsushima, Y., & Endo, K. (2000, January). Spleen enlargement in patients with nonalcoholic fatty liver: correlation between degree of fatty infiltration in liver and size of spleen. *Digestive diseases and sciences, Japan*. 45(1):196-200 PMID: 10695635

1213 Foster, M. C., Hwang, S., Porter, S. A., Massaro, J. M., Hoffmann, U., & Fox, C. S. (2011). Fatty Kidney, Hypertension, And Chronic Kidney Disease: The Framingham Heart Study. *Hypertension*, 58(5), 784-790.

1214 Chang, M. The Associated Press. (2007, May 10). DIET: Thin People May Be Fat Inside. *The Washington Post*. Retrieved October 14, 2016, from http://www.washingtonpost.com/wp-dyn/content/article/2007/05/10/AR2007051001171.html

1215 Sifferlin, A. (2012, September 5). Can You Be Fat and Fit — or Thin and Unhealthy?. *Time*. Retrieved November 23, 2015, from http://healthland.time.com/2012/09/05/can-you-be-fat-and-fit-or-thin-and-unhealthy/

1216 Hartley, M. (2009, September 24). About Visceral Fat. Calorie Count. Retrieved November 23, 2015, from http://caloriecount.about.com/visceral-fat-b337280

1217 Donohoe, C. L., Doyle, S. L., & Reynolds, J. V. (2011). Visceral adiposity, insulin resistance and cancer risk. *Diabetology & Metabolic Syndrome*, 3(1), 12. doi:10.1186/1758-5996-3-12

1218 Ishikawa, T., Glidewell-Kenney, C., & Jameson, J. L. (2006). Aromatase-independent Testosterone conversion into Estrogenic steroids is inhibited by a 5α-reductase inhibitor. *The Journal of Steroid Biochemistry and Molecular Biology*, 98(2-3), 133-138. doi:10.1016/j.jsbmb.2005.09.004

1219 Lee, H., Lee, J. K., & Cho, B. (2013). The Role of Androgen in the Adipose Tissue of Males. *The World Journal of Mens Health*, 31(2), 136. doi:10.5534/wjmh.2013.31.2.136

1220 BodyMeasure. (2013, November 26). Visceral Fat turning Men into Women!. *Body Measure Body Composition Scan Sydney Australia*. Retrieved November 23, 2015, from http://bodymeasure.com.au/2013/11/26/the-impact-of-visceral-fat-and-aromatase-on-the-body/

1221 Johnson, R. E., & Murad, M. H. (2009). Gynecomastia: Pathophysiology, Evaluation, and Management. *Mayo Clinic Proceedings*, 84(11), 1010-1015. doi:10.1016/s0025-6196(11)60671-x

1222 American Society of Plastic Surgeons. (2016, February 25). New Statistics Reflect the Changing Face of Plastic Surgery. Retrieved April 14, 2017, from https://www.plasticsurgery.org/news/press-releases/new-statistics-reflect-the-changing-face-of-plastic-surgery

1223 Steriti, R. S., PhD & Wright, J. V., MD. (2010, November 23). Natural Aromatase Inhibitors for Men With Metabolic Syndrome. *NDNR*. Retrieved November 23, 2015, from http://ndnr.com/mens-health/natural-aromatase-inhibitors-for-men-with-metabolic-syndrome/

1224 Rajfer, J. (2003). Decreased Testosterone in the Aging Male. *Reviews in Urology*, 5(Suppl 1), S1–S2.

1225 Ibid

1226 Harvard Medical School. (2005, September 1). Abdominal fat and what to do about it. *The Harvard Medical School*. Retrieved November 23, 2015, from http://www.health.harvard.edu/fhg/updates/Abdominal-fat-and-what-to-do-about-it.shtml

1227 Mayo Clinic Staff. (2013, June 8). Belly fat in women: Taking — and keeping — it off. *Mayo Clinic - Women's Health*. Retrieved November 23, 2015, from http://www.mayoclinic.com/health/belly-fat/WO00128

1228 Paoletti, R., Bolego, C., Poli, A., & Cignarella, A. (2006). Metabolic Syndrome, Inflammation and Atherosclerosis. *Vascular Health and Risk Management*, 2(2), 145–152.

1229 Lee, J., Lee, H., Lee, D., Chu, S., Jeon, J. Y., Kim, N., & Lee, J. (2014). Visceral Fat Accumulation Is Associated with Colorectal Cancer in Postmenopausal Women. *PLoS ONE*, 9(11). doi:10.1371/journal.pone.0110587

1230 Mayo Clinic Staff. (2013, June 8). Belly fat in women: Taking — and keeping — it off. *Mayo Clinic - Women's Health*. Retrieved November 23, 2015, from http://www.mayoclinic.com/health/belly-fat/WO00128

1231 Carr, MD, M., & Tannock, PhD, L. (2009, April 9). Body-Fat Distribution and Mortality Risk: Thinking Small. *American Heart Association*. Retrieved November 24, 2015, from http://my.americanheart.org/professional/General/Body-Fat-Distribution-and-Mortality-Risk-Thinking-Small_UCM_433097_Article.jsp#.VlPVBLNdE_w

1232 Mcneely, M. J., Shofer, J. B., Leonetti, D. L., Fujimoto, W. Y., & Boyko, E. J. (2011). Associations Among Visceral Fat, All-Cause Mortality, and Obesity-Related Mortality in Japanese Americans. *Diabetes Care*, 35(2), 296-298. doi:10.2337/dc11-1193

1233 Lim, E. L., Hollingsworth, K. G., Aribisala, B. S., Chen, M. J., Mathers, J. C., & Taylor, R. (2011). Reversal of type 2 diabetes: normalization of beta cell function in association with decreased pancreas and liver triacylglycerol. *Diabetologia*, 54(10), 2506-2514. doi:10.1007/s00125-011-2204-7

1234 Ha, J., Satin, L. S., & Sherman, A. S. (2016). A Mathematical Model of the Pathogenesis, Prevention, and Reversal of Type 2 Diabetes. *Endocrinology*, 157(2), 624-635. doi:10.1210/en.2015-1564

1235 Taylor, R. (2013). Type 2 Diabetes: Etiology and reversibility. *Diabetes Care Institute of Cellular Medicine, Newcastle University, Newcastle upon Tyne, U.K.*, 36(4), 1047-1055. doi:10.2337/dc12-1805

1236 Ornish, D., Brown, S. E., Scherwitz, L. W., Billings, J. H., Armstrong, W. T., Ports, T. A., et al. (1990). Can Lifestyle Changes Reverse Coronary Heart Disease? The Lifestyle Heart Trial. *The Lancet*, 336(8708), 129-133

1237 Aronson, D., MS, RD. (2009). Cortisol — Its Role in Stress, Inflammation, and Indications for Diet Therapy. *Today's Dietitian - The Magazine for Nutrition Professionals*. Vol. 11 No. 11 P. 38

1238 Khani, S., & Tayek, J. A. (2001). Cortisol increases gluconeogenesis in humans: its role in the metabolic syndrome. *Clinical Science*, 101(6), 739. doi:10.1042/cs20010180

[1239] Randall, M. (2011, February 03). The Physiology of Stress: Cortisol and the Hypothalamic-Pituitary-Adrenal Axis. *Dartmouth Undergraduate Journal of Science*. Retrieved June 26, 2016, from http://dujs.dartmouth.edu/2011/02/the-physiology-of-stress-cortisol-and-the-hypothalamic-pituitary-adrenal-axis/#.V3AVULgrKHs

[1240] Aronson, D., MS, RD. (2009). Cortisol — Its Role in Stress, Inflammation, and Indications for Diet Therapy. *Today's Dietitian - The Magazine for Nutrition Professionals*. Vol. 11 No. 11 P. 38

[1241] Ibid

[1242] Moyer, A. E., Rodin, J., Grilo, C. M., Cummings, N., Larson, L. M., & Rebuffé-Scrive, M. (1994). Stress-Induced Cortisol Response and Fat Distribution in Women. *Obesity Research*, 2(3), 255-262. doi:10.1002/j.1550-8528.1994.tb00055.x

[1243] Whitworth, J. A., Williamson, P. M., Mangos, G., & Kelly, J. J. (2005). Cardiovascular Consequences of Cortisol Excess. *Vascular Health and Risk Management*, 1(4), 291–299.

[1244] Dedovic, K., & Ngiam, J. (2015). The cortisol awakening response and major depression: examining the evidence. *Neuropsychiatric Disease and Treatment*, 1181. doi:10.2147/ndt.s62289

[1245] Burke, H. M., Davis, M. C., Otte, C., & Mohr, D. C. (2005). Depression and cortisol responses to psychological stress: A meta-analysis. *Psychoneuroendocrinology*, 30(9), 846-856. doi:10.1016/j.psyneuen.2005.02.010

[1246] Basta, M., Chrousos, G. P., Vela-Bueno, A., & Vgontzas, A. N. (2007). Chronic Insomnia and the Stress System. *Sleep Medicine Clinics*, 2(2), 279-291. doi:10.1016/j.jsmc.2007.04.002

[1247] Ehlert, U., Nater, U. M., & Böhmelt, A. (2005). High and low unstimulated salivary cortisol levels correspond to different symptoms of functional gastrointestinal disorders. *Journal of Psychosomatic Research*, 59(1), 7-10. doi:10.1016/j.jpsychores.2005.03.005

[1248] Kelly, J. R., Kennedy, P. J., Cryan, J. F., Dinan, T. G., Clarke, G., & Hyland, N. P. (2015). Breaking down the barriers: the gut microbiome, intestinal permeability and stress-related psychiatric disorders. *Frontiers in Cellular Neuroscience*, 9. doi:10.3389/fncel.2015.00392

[1249] Basta, M., Chrousos, G. P., Vela-Bueno, A., & Vgontzas, A. N. (2007). Chronic Insomnia and the Stress System. *Sleep Medicine Clinics*, 2(2), 279-291. doi:10.1016/j.jsmc.2007.04.002

[1250] Sasson, R. (2002, October 1). Positive Thinking Quotes to Inspire and Motivate - Remez Sasson Quotes. *SuccessConsciousness: Self Improvement and Spiritual Growth*. Retrieved November 24, 2015, from http://www.successconsciousness.com/index_000033.htm

[1251] Stevenson, S. (2012, June 25). There's Magic In Your Smile. *Psychology Today: Health, Help, Happiness*. Retrieved November 23, 2015, from http://www.psychologytoday.com/blog/cutting-edge-leadership/201206/there-s-magic-in-your-smile

[1252] Ibid

[1253] Guyton, A. C., & Hall, J. E. (2000). *Textbook of medical physiology*. Philadelphia: Saunders.

[1254] Ibid

[1255] Guyton, A. C., & Hall, J. E. (2000). *Textbook of medical physiology*. Philadelphia: Saunders.

[1256] Mercola, J. (2013, September 19). What Happens in Your Body When You Exercise?. *Peak Fitness | Mercola.com*. Retrieved November 23, 2015, from http://fitness.mercola.com/sites/fitness/archive/2013/09/20/exercise-health-benefits.aspx

[1257] Goodyear, L. J., Hirshman, M. F., Horton, E. D., Knutson, S. M., Wardzala, L. J., & Horton, E. S. (1991). Exercise training normalizes glucose metabolism in a rat model of impaired glucose tolerance. *Metabolism*, 40(5), 455-464.doi:10.1016/0026-0495(91)90224-k

[1258] Kellow, J. (2004, September 20). Dieting and Metabolism. *Weight Loss Resources*. Retrieved November 23, 2015, from http://www.weightlossresources.co.uk/calories/burning_calories/starvation.htm

[1259] Miller, M. B., Pearcey, G. E., Cahill, F., Mccarthy, H., Stratton, S. B., Noftall, J. C., . . . Button, D. C. (2014). The Effect of a Short-Term High-Intensity Circuit Training Program on Work Capacity, Body Composition, and Blood Profiles in Sedentary Obese Men: A Pilot Study. *BioMed Research International*, 2014, 1-10. doi:10.1155/2014/191797

[1260] Paoli, A., Pacelli, Q. F., Moro, T., Marcolin, G., Neri, M., Battaglia, G., . . . Bianco, A. (2013). Effects of high-intensity circuit training, low-intensity circuit training and endurance training on blood pressure and lipoproteins in middle-aged overweight men. *Lipids in Health and Disease*, 12(1), 131. doi:10.1186/1476-511x-12-131

[1261] Hill, E. E., Zack, E., Battaglini, C., Viru, M., Viru, A., & Hackney, A. C. (2008). Exercise and circulating Cortisol levels: The intensity threshold effect. *Journal of Endocrinological Investigation*, 31(7), 587-591. doi:10.1007/bf03345606

[1262] Randall, M. (2011, February 03). The Physiology of Stress: Cortisol and the Hypothalamic-Pituitary-Adrenal Axis. *Dartmouth Undergraduate Journal of Science*. Retrieved June 26, 2016, from http://dujs.dartmouth.edu/2011/02/the-physiology-of-stress-cortisol-and-the-hypothalamic-pituitary-adrenal-axis/#.V3AVULgrKHs

[1263] Aronson, D., MS, RD. (2009). Cortisol — Its Role in Stress, Inflammation, and Indications for Diet Therapy. *Today's Dietitian - The Magazine for Nutrition Professionals*. Vol. 11 No. 11 P. 38

[1264] Ominchanski, L. (1992). Hunger Scale | Adapted from You Count, Calories: Don't. *MIT Medical*. Retrieved November 25, 2015, from https://medical.mit.edu/gsearch/Hunger+Scale+-+MIT+Medical Also https://medical.mit.edu/sites/default/files/hunger_scale.pdf

[1265] Wood, M. (2011, December 27). The Hunger Level Scale for Weight Loss. *Melissa Wood ND*. Retrieved November 24, 2015, from http://stayhealthyandwell.com/the-hunger-level-scale-for-weight-loss/

[1266] Killoran, E. (2014, January 7). The Hunger Scale: Mindful Eating for Weight Loss. *Pritikin Longevity Center*. Retrieved January 25, 2016, from https://www.pritikin.com/your-health/healthy-living/eating-right/1838-hunger-scale-mindful-eating-weight-loss.html

[1267] http://media-cache-ak0.pinimg.com/736x/f3/fe/6e/f3fe6ee4241ea24fa9e6276c7a276c48.jpg

[1268] Ziauddeen, H., Subramaniam, N., Gaillard, R., Burke, L. K., Farooqi, I. S., & Fletcher, P. C. (2011). Food images engage subliminal motivation to seek food. *International Journal of Obesity, 36*(9), 1245-1247. doi:10.1038/ijo.2011.239

[1269] National Museum of Natural History. (2001, February, 1). Introduction to Human Evolution. *Human Evolution by The Smithsonian Institution's Human Origins Program.* Retrieved November 23, 2015, from http://humanorigins.si.edu/resources/intro-human-evolution

[1270] Ibid

[1271] IQWiG. (2016, August 22). How does the liver work?. *Institute for Quality and Efficiency in Health Care | U.S. National Library of Medicine.* Retrieved April 15, 2017, from https://www.ncbi.nlm.nih.gov/pubmedhealth/PMH0072577/

[1272] Ibid

[1273] Liver Doctor. (2012, December 7). Are toxins accumulating in your liver?. *Liver Doctor - Love Your Liver and Live Longer.* Retrieved November 23, 2015, from http://www.liverdoctor.com/are-toxins-accumulating-in-your-liver/

[1274] Doheny, K. (2009, May 29). Environmental Toxins & Liver Disease: A Link?. *WebMD - Better information. Better health..* Retrieved November 23, 2015, from http://www.webmd.com/digestive-disorders/news/20090529/environmental-toxins-and-liver-disease

[1275] Ibid

[1276] Colorado State University. (2001, Novermber 23). Secretion of Bile and the Role of Bile Acids In Digestion. *Colorado State University .* Retrieved November 23, 2015, from http://www.vivo.colostate.edu/hbooks/pathphys/digestion/liver/bile.html

[1277] NIH. (2013, March 22). Bile duct obstruction: MedlinePlus Medical Encyclopedia. *National Library of Medicine - National Institutes of Health.* Retrieved November 23, 2015, from http://www.nlm.nih.gov/medlineplus/ency/article/000263.htm

[1278] Ibid

[1279] Spittle, B. (2008). *Fluoride fatigue: An abridged version of, Fluoride poisoning: Is fluoride in your drinking water, and from other sources, making you sick?* (p. 4). Dunedin, N.Z.: Paua.

[1280] Ibid

[1281] Ibid

[1282] CDC. (2013, April 22). Facts About Hydrogen Fluoride (Hydrofluoric Acid*). Centers for Disease Control and Prevention.* Retrieved November 29, 2015, from http://www.bt.cdc.gov/agent/hydrofluoricacid/basics/facts.asp

[1283] Mercola, J. (2013, April 30). 10 Fluoride Facts You Should Know. *Mercola.com.* Retrieved November 25, 2015, from http://articles.mercola.com/sites/articles/archive/2013/04/30/water-fluoridation-facts.aspx#_edn2

[1284] Choi, A. L., Sun, G., Zhang, Y., & Grandjean, P. (2012). Developmental Fluoride Neurotoxicity: A Systematic Review and Meta-Analysis. *Environmental Health Perspectives, 120*(10), 1362-1368. doi:10.1289/ehp.1104912

[1285] Dwyer, M. (2012, July 25). Harvard School of Public Health. Impact of fluoride on neurological development in children. *Harvard School of Public Health.* Retrieved November 25, 2015, from http://www.hsph.harvard.edu/news/features/fluoride-childrens-health-grandjean-choi/

[1286] Ibid

[1287] Choi, A. L., Sun, G., Zhang, Y., & Grandjean, P. (2012). Developmental Fluoride Neurotoxicity: A Systematic Review and Meta-Analysis. *Environmental Health Perspectives, 120*(10), 1362-1368. doi:10.1289/ehp.1104912

[1288] Dwyer, M. (2012, July 25). Harvard School of Public Health. Impact of fluoride on neurological development in children. *Harvard School of Public Health.* Retrieved November 25, 2015, from http://www.hsph.harvard.edu/news/features/fluoride-childrens-health-grandjean-choi/

[1289] Ibid

[1290] Peckham, S., & Awofeso, N. (2014). Water Fluoridation: A Critical Review of the Physiological Effects of Ingested Fluoride as a Public Health Intervention. *The Scientific World Journal, 2014,* 1-10. doi:10.1155/2014/293019

[1291] Ibid

[1292] Muller, F., Zeitz, C., Mantz, H., Ehses, K., Soldera, F., Schmauch, J., . . . Jacobs, K. (2010). Elemental Depth Profiling of Fluoridated Hydroxyapatite: Saving Your Dentition by the Skin of Your Teeth?. *American Chemical Society Publication. Langmuir, 26*(24), 18750-18759. doi:10.1021/la102325e

[1293] Ibid

[1294] AAAS. (2011, March 11). Does fluoride really fight cavities by 'the skin of the teeth'?. *EurekAlert!.* Retrieved November 25, 2015, from http://www.eurekalert.org/pub_releases/2011-03/acs-dfr030211.php

[1295] Ibid

[1296] Ibid

[1297] Fluoride Action Network. (2012, August 28). FAN's Grocery Store Guide: 7 Ways to Avoid Fluoride in Beverages and Food. *Fluoride Action Network.* Retrieved November 25, 2015, from http://fluoridealert.org/content/grocery_guide/

[1298] Vermont Department of Health. (2013). Office Air Quality. *Vermont Department of Health.* Retrieved November 25, 2015, from http://www.healthvermont.gov/enviro/indoor_air/air_office.aspx

[1299] Śmiełowska, M., Marć, M., & Zabiegała, B. (2017). Indoor air quality in public utility environments—a review. *Environmental Science and Pollution Research, 24*(12), 11166-11176. doi:10.1007/s11356-017-8567-7

[1300] Oz, M., & Roizen, M. F. (2007). *You, staying young: the owners manual to extending your warranty.* New York: Simon & Schuster.

[1301] Francis, R., & Cotton, K. (2002). Never be sick again: health is a choice, learn how to choose it: one disease, two causes, six pathways. Deerfield Beach, Fla.: Health Communications.

[1302] Ibid

1303 Ibid

1304 Le, H. H., Carlson, E. M., Chua, J. P., & Belcher, S. M. (2008). Bisphenol A is released from polycarbonate drinking bottles and mimics the neurotoxic actions of estrogen in developing cerebellar neurons. *Toxicology Letters*, 176(2), 149-156. doi:10.1016/j.toxlet.2007.11.001

1305 Ibid

1306 Yang, C. Z., Yaniger, S. I., Jordan, V. C., Klein, D. J., & Bittner, G. D. (2011). Most Plastic Products Release Estrogenic Chemicals: A Potential Health Problem That Can Be Solved. *Environmental Health Perspectives*, 119(7), 989-996. doi:10.1289/ehp.1003220

1307 Douglas, B. H. (1990). *AgeLess: living younger longer*. Brandon, Miss.: QRP Books.

1308 Douglas, B. H. (1990). *AgeLess: living younger longer*. Brandon, Miss.: QRP Books.

1309 Vatansever, F., & Hamblin, M. R. (2012). Far infrared radiation (FIR): Its biological effects and medical applications. *Photonics & Lasers in Medicine*, 1(4). doi:10.1515/plm-2012-0034

1310 Shape Magazine. (2013, September 13). Glycation, GlyTerra, and Aging: Does Sugar Cause Wrinkles?. *Shape Magazine*. Retrieved October 15, 2015, from http://www.shape.com/lifestyle/beauty-style/sugar-giving-you-wrinkles

1311 Kowatzki, D., Macholdt, C., Krull, K., Schmidt, D., Deufel, T., Elsner, P., & Fluhr, J. (2008). Effect of Regular Sauna on Epidermal Barrier Function and Stratum Corneum Water-Holding Capacity in vivo in Humans: A Controlled Study. *Dermatology*, 217(2), 173-180. doi:10.1159/000137283

1312 Prystupa, T., Wołyńska, A., & Ślężyński, J. (2009). The Effects Of Finish Sauna On Hemodynamics Of The Circulatory System In Men And Women. *Journal of Human Kinetics*, 22(-1), 61-68.

1313 Ibid

1314 Ibid

1315 Ibid

1316 Ibid

1317 Ibid

1318 Ernst, E., Pecho, E., Wirz, P., & Saradeth, T. (1990). Regular Sauna Bathing and the Incidence of Common Colds. *Annals of Medicine*, 22(4), 225-227. doi:10.3109/07853899009148930

1319 Chiu, C. (n.d.). THAT WARM, FUZZY FEELING – THE HEALING POWER OF HEAT. Retrieved November 30, 2015, from http://www.eastyorkanimalclinic.com/.../The Healing Power of Heat.pdf

1320 The Free Online Library. (n.d.). The Benefits of Sauna for Raising Body Heat. *News, Magazines, Newspapers, Journals, Reference Articles and Classic Books - Free Online Library*. Retrieved August 22, 2013, from http://www.thefreelibrary.com/ /search/Search.aspx?SearchBy=0&q=The+Benefits+of+Sauna+for+Raising+Body+Heat&Search=Search&By=0

1321 International Steam Therapy Association. (2001, February 1). Steam Sauna Healing Benefits. *Oxygen Healing Therapies*. Retrieved November 29, 2015, from http://www.oxygenhealingtherapies.com/steam_sauna_rejuvenation_benefits.html

1322 Leppäluoto, J., Tuominen, M., Väänänen, A., Karpakka, J., & Vuor, J. (1986). Some cardiovascular and metabolic effects of repeated sauna bathing. *Acta Physiologica Scandinavica*, 128(1), 77-81. doi:10.1111/j.1748-1716.1986.tb07952.x

1323 Podstawski, R., Boraczyński, T., Boraczyński, M., Choszcz, D., Mańkowski, S., & Markowski, P. (2014). Sauna-Induced Body Mass Loss in Young Sedentary Women and Men. *The Scientific World Journal*, 2014, 1-7. doi:10.1155/2014/307421

1324 Stellner, A. (2011, March 10). Sauna Benefits: Calories Burned. *Livestrong.com - Lose Weight & Get Fit with Diet, Nutrition & Fitness Tools*. Retrieved November 29, 2015, from http://www.livestrong.com/article/242883-sauna-benefits-calories-burned/

1325 Bauer, B. (2011, June 3). Do infrared saunas have any health benefits?. *Mayo Clinic*. Retrieved November 29, 2015, from http://www.mayoclinic.com/health/infrared-sauna/AN02154

1326 Mercola, J. (2014, September 9). Saunas - Mercola.com. *Natural Health Products by Dr. Joseph Mercola - Mercola.com*. Retrieved November 29, 2015, from http://products.mercola.com/saunas/

1327 Kukkonen-Harjula, K., & Kauppinen, K. (1988). How the sauna affects the endocrine system. *Annals of Clinical Research*. 20(4):262-6 PMID: 3218898

1328 Ibid

1329 MedicineNet.com. (2011, February 14). MedicineNet.com.Medical Dictionary. *Definition of Endorphin*. Retrieved f November 29, 2015, from www.medterms.com/script/main/art.asp?articlekey=10812

1330 Blum, N., & Blum, A. (2007). Beneficial effects of sauna bathing for heart failure patients. *Experimental & Clinical Cardiology*, 12(1), 29–32

1331 Ibid

1332 Ibid

1333 Oz, M. (2009, March 24). Dr. Oz Explains an Infrared Sauna's Benefits - Oprah.com. *Oprah Winfrey's Official Website - Live Your Best Life - Oprah.com*. Retrieved Retrieved November 29, 2015, from http://www.oprah.com/health/Life-Extension-Technology-and-Tissue-Regeneration/6

1334 Ibid

1335 Richards, B. J. (2012, April 16). B. J. Richards, Board Certified Clinical Nutritionist, Why Toxins and Waste Products Impede Weight Loss - The Leptin Diet Weight Loss Challenge #3. *Wellness Resources*. Retrieved Retrieved August 22, 2013, from http://www.wellnessresources.com/weight/articles/why_toxins_and_waste_products_impede_weight_loss_-_the_Leptin_diet_weight_l

[1336] Lieberman, A., M.D., F.A.A.E.M.. (n.d.). Chemical Toxicity & Sensitivity | The Role of Biodetoxification in Overcoming Illness. *Center for Occupational & Environmental Medicine*. Retrieved April 17, 2017, from http://www.coem.com/demo/site/programstreatment_ChemicalToxicity_wearepolluted.shtml

[1337] Ibid

[1338] Merrill, M. L., Emond, C., Kim, M. J., Antignac, J., Bizec, B. L., Clément, K., . . . Barouki, R. (2013, February). Toxicological Function of Adipose Tissue: Focus on Persistent Organic Pollutants. *Environmental Health Perspectives*, 121(2), 162-169. doi:10.1289/ehp.1205485

[1339] Ibid

[1340] Richards, B. J. (2012, April 16). B. J. Richards, Board Certified Clinical Nutritionist, Why Toxins and Waste Products Impede Weight Loss - The Leptin Diet Weight Loss Challenge #3. *Wellness Resources*. Retrieved Retrieved August 22, 2013, from http://www.wellnessresources.com/weight/articles/why_toxins_and_waste_products_impede_weight_loss_-_the_Leptin_diet_weight_l

[1341] Ibid

[1342] Merrill, M. L., Emond, C., Kim, M. J., Antignac, J., Bizec, B. L., Clément, K., . . . Barouki, R. (2013, February). Toxicological Function of Adipose Tissue: Focus on Persistent Organic Pollutants. *Environmental Health Perspectives*, 121(2), 162-169. doi:10.1289/ehp.1205485

[1343] bid

[1344] bid

[1345] Sears, M. E. (2013). Chelation: Harnessing and Enhancing Heavy Metal Detoxification—A Review. *The Scientific World Journal*, 2013, 1-13. doi:10.1155/2013/219840

[1346] Subramoniam, A., Asha, V. V., Nair, S. A., Sasidharan, S. P., Sureshkumar, P. K., Rajendran, K. N., . . . Ramalingam, K. (2011). Chlorophyll Revisited: Anti-inflammatory Activities of Chlorophyll a and Inhibition of Expression of TNF-α Gene by the Same. *Inflammation*, 35(3), 959-966. doi:10.1007/s10753-011-9399-0

[1347] Simonich, M. T., Mcquistan, T., Jubert, C., Pereira, C., Hendricks, J. D., Schimerlik, M., . . . Bailey, G. S. (2008). Low-dose dietary chlorophyll inhibits multi-organ carcinogenesis in the rainbow trout. *Food and Chemical Toxicology*, 46(3), 1014-1024. doi:10.1016/j.fct.2007.10.034

[1348] Jubert, C., Mata, J., Bench, G., Dashwood, R., Pereira, C., Tracewell, W., . . . Bailey, G. (2009). Effects of Chlorophyll and Chlorophyllin on Low-Dose Aflatoxin B1 Pharmacokinetics in Human Volunteers. *Cancer Prevention Research*, 2(12), 1015-1022. doi:10.1158/1940-6207.capr-09-0099

[1349] Charles, A. L., Chang, C., Wu, M., & Huang, T. (2007). Studies on the expression of liver detoxifying enzymes in rats fed seaweed (Monostroma nitidum*). Food and Chemical Toxicology*, 45(12), 2390-2396. doi:10.1016/j.fct.2007.06.014

[1350] Rector-Page, L. G., Ph.D. (2004). *Healthy healing: a guide to self-healing for everyone*. Del Rey Oaks, CA: Healthy Healing, Inc.

[1351] Bhat, G., Dodwad, V., & Kudva, P. (2011). Aloe vera: Nature's soothing healer to periodontal disease. *Journal of Indian Society of Periodontology*, 15(3), 205. doi:10.4103/0972-124x.85661

[1352] Freiburg, A. (2012, July 2). Natural intestinal flora strengthen immune system. ScienceDaily. Retrieved Retrieved November 29, 2015, from http://www.sciencedaily.com/releases/2012/07/120702152940.htm

[1353] Pagnini, C., Saeed, R., Bamias, G., Arseneau, K. O., Pizarro, T. T., & Cominelli, F. (2009). Probiotics promote gut health through stimulation of epithelial innate immunity. *Proceedings of the National Academy of Sciences*, 107(1), 454-459. doi:10.1073/pnas.0910307107

[1354] Gagnon, T. (2014, June). From Harm to Able. *Men's Fitness Magazine, Men's Fitness*, 54.

[1355] Harvard Heart Letter. (2010, October). Beating high blood pressure with food. *Harvard Health Publication*. Retrieved April 17, 2017, from http://www.health.harvard.edu/newsletter_article/beating-high-blood-pressure-with-food

[1356] Reviewed by Harvey Simon, MD, Associate Professor of Medicine, Harvard Medical School; Physician, Massachusetts General Hospital. Also reviewed by David Zieve, MD, MHA, Medical Director, A.D.A.M., Inc . (2012, May 22). High blood pressure. *University of Maryland Medical Center*. Retrieved April 17, 2017, from http://www.umm.edu/health/medical/reports/articles/high-blood-pressure

[1357] Oki, T., Kano, M., Watanabe, O., Goto, K., Boelsma, E., Ishikawa, F., & Suda, I. (2016). Effect of consuming a purple-fleshed sweet potato beverage on health-related biomarkers and safety parameters in Caucasian subjects with elevated levels of blood pressure and liver function biomarkers: a 4-week, open-label, non-comparative trial. *Bioscience of Microbiota, Food and Health*, 35(3), 129-136. doi:10.12938/bmfh.2015-026

[1358] Koufman, J., Stern, J., & Bauer, M. M. (2010). *Dropping acid: the reflux diet cookbook & cure*. New York, N.Y.: Reflux Cookbooks, L.L.C..

[1359] Prasad, S., & Tyagi, A. K. (2015). Ginger and Its Constituents: Role in Prevention and Treatment of Gastrointestinal Cancer. *Gastroenterology Research and Practice*, 2015, 1-11. doi:10.1155/2015/142979

[1360] Zelman, K. M. (2005, March 29). 5 Heart-Healthy Foods. WebMD. Retrieved November 29, 2015, from http://www.webmd.com/heart-disease/features/5-heart-healthy-foods

[1361] Eisenstein, D. (2004, October). 10 Superfoods for Heart Disease. *Better Homes & Gardens*. Retrieved November 29, 2015, from http://www.bhg.com/health-family/conditions/heart-disease/superfoods-for-heart-disease/

[1362] Bowen, K. J., Harris, W. S., & Kris-Etherton, P. M. (2016). Omega-3 Fatty Acids and Cardiovascular Disease: Are There Benefits? *Current Treatment Options in Cardiovascular Medicine*, 18(11). doi:10.1007/s11936-016-0487-1

[1363] Gröber, U., Schmidt, J., & Kisters, K. (2015). Magnesium in Prevention and Therapy. *Nutrients*, 7(9), 8199-8226. doi:10.3390/nu7095388

[1364] Weaver, C. M. (2013). Potassium and Health. *Advances in Nutrition: An International Review Journal*,4(3). doi:10.3945/an.112.003533

[1365] UCLA:LONI. (2008). Brain Trivia, UCLA. *LONI: Laboratory of Neuro Imaging*. Retrieved August 29, 2013, from http://loni.usc.edu/about_loni/education/brain_trivia.php

[1366] Tugend, A. (2012, March 23). Praise Is Fleeting, but Brickbats We Recall, The *New York Times*. Retrieved November 29, 2015, from http://www.nytimes.com/2012/03/24/your-money/why-people-remember-negative-events-more-than-positive-ones.html?_r=0

[1367] izquotes. (2012, July 13). Shirley MacLaine Quote. *Quotes and Sayings - iz quotes*. Retrieved November 29, 2015, from http://izquotes.com/quote/284578

[1368] Friedman, M. (1991). Nutritional and Toxicological Consequences of Food Processing. *Advances in Experimental Medicine and Biology*. doi:10.1007/978-1-4899-2626-5

[1369] WebMD. (2013, December 2). Reviewed by Maryann Tomovich Jacobsen, MS, RD. Raw Food Diet Review: Benefits, What You Eat, & More. *WebMD*. Retrieved November 29, 2015, from http://www.webmd.com/diet/raw-foods-diet

[1370] Stephens, B. (2013, January 23). Raw or Cooked: Which Vegetables Are Healthier? *Health magazine | Health.com*. Retrieved December 1, 2015, from http://www.health.com/health/gallery/0,,20667296,00.html

[1371] MSN. (n.d.). Raw or cooked: Which vegetables are healthier?. *MSN Healthy Living*. Retrieved August 29, 2013, from http://healthyliving.msn.com/nutrition/raw-or-cooked-which-vegetables-are-healthier#1

[1372] UC Health. (2010, April 14). The raw vs. the cooked | UC Health. *University of California Health*. Retrieved November 30, 2015, from http://health.universityofcalifornia.edu/2010/04/14/the-raw-vs-the-cooked/

[1373] Stephens, B. (2013, January 23). Raw or Cooked: Which Vegetables Are Healthier? *Health magazine | Health.com*. Retrieved December 1, 2015, from http://www.health.com/health/gallery/0,,20667296,00.html

[1374] MSN. (n.d.). Raw or cooked: Which vegetables are healthier?. *MSN Healthy Living*. Retrieved August 29, 2013, from http://healthyliving.msn.com/nutrition/raw-or-cooked-which-vegetables-are-healthier#1

[1375] World Health Organization, Regional Office for South-East Asia. (2013). Self-Care for Health. *World Health Organizations*. ISBN 978-92-9022-443-3. pg. 9. Retrieved December 1, 2015, from http://apps.searo.who.int/PDS_DOCS/B5084.pdf

[1376] Franklin Institute. (2015, June 17). White Blood Cells. *The Franklin Institute*. Retrieved November 30, 2015, from https://www.fi.edu/heart/white-blood-cells

[1377] Kouchakoff, P., MD. (1930). The Influence of Food Cooking on the Blood Formula of Man. *Proceedings: First International Congress of Microbiology, Paris*. pp. 1-8.

[1378] Medical Dictionary. (2010, April 18). Digestive Leukocytosis. *TheFreeDictionary.com*. Retrieved from http://medical-dictionary.thefreedictionary.com/digestive+leukocytosis

[1379] McKeith, G. (2005). *Dr. Gillian McKeith's living food for health: 12 natural superfoods to transform your health*. North Bergen, NJ: Basic Health Publications.

[1380] Ibid

[1381] Mihalik, R. (2012, May). KOUCHAKOFF 2.0. *Whole Foods Magazine NEC Health News*. Retrieved November 30, 2015, from http://www.wholefoodsmagazine.com/sites/default/files/nechealth_0.pdf

[1382] Rogers, K. (2011). *Blood: physiology and circulation*. New York, NY: Britannica Educational Pub., in association with Rosen Educational Services.

[1383] Colquhoun, J. (Director). (2008). *Food Matters* [Documentary]. United States: Distributed by Permacology Productions.

[1384] Ibid

[1385] Kouchakoff, P., MD. (1930). The Influence of Food Cooking on the Blood Formula of Man. *Proceedings: First International Congress of Microbiology, Paris*. pp. 1-8.

[1386] Ibid

[1387] Colquhoun, J. (Director). (2008). *Food Matters* [Documentary]. United States: Distributed by Permacology Productions.

[1388] Kouchakoff, P., MD. (1930). The Influence of Food Cooking on the Blood Formula of Man. *Proceedings: First International Congress of Microbiology, Paris*. pp. 1-8.

[1389] Ibid

[1390] Mihalik, R. (2012, May). KOUCHAKOFF 2.0. *Whole Foods Magazine NEC Health News*. Retrieved November 30, 2015, from http://www.wholefoodsmagazine.com/sites/default/files/nechealth_0.pdf

[1391] Colquhoun, J. (Director). (2008). *Food Matters* [Documentary]. United States: Distributed by Permacology Productions.

[1392] Ibid

[1393] Patisaul, H., & Adewale, H. (2009). Long-term effects of environmental endocrine disruptors on reproductive physiology and behavior. *Frontiers in Behavioral Neuroscience*, 3. doi:10.3389/neuro.08.010.2009

[1394] CDC.gov. (2011, September 13). Eat More, Weigh Less? How to manage your weight without being hungry. *Centers for Disease Control and Prevention*. Retrieved November 30, 2015, from http://www.cdc.gov/healthyweight/healthy_eating/energy_density.html

[1395] Janick, J., & Paull, R. E. (2008). *The encyclopedia of fruit & nuts*. Wallingford, UK: CABI North American Office.

[1396] Sharma, K. D., Karki, S., Thakur, N. S., & Attri, S. (2011). Chemical composition, functional properties and processing of carrot—a review. *Journal of Food Science and Technology*, 49(1), 22-32. doi:10.1007/s13197-011-0310-7

[1397] El-Mageed, N. A. (2011). Hepatoprotective effect of feeding celery leaves mixed with chicory leaves and barley grains to hypercholesterolemic rats. *Pharmacognosy Magazine*, 7(26), 151. doi:10.4103/0973-1296.80675

[1398] Janick, J., & Paull, R. E. (2008). *The encyclopedia of fruit & nuts*. Wallingford, UK: CABI North American Office.

[1399] Boyer, J., & Liu, R. H. (2004). Apple phytochemicals and their health benefits. *Nutrition Journal, 3*(1). doi:10.1186/1475-2891-3-5

[1400] Deng, R., & Chow, T. (2010). Hypolipidemic, Antioxidant, and Antiinflammatory Activities of Microalgae Spirulina. *Cardiovascular Therapeutics, 28*(4). doi:10.1111/j.1755-5922.2010.00200.x

[1401] Tremblay, L. (2013, October 30). Vitamins in Spirulina. *LIVESTRONG.COM*. Retrieved November 30, 2015, from http://www.livestrong.com/article/261312-Vitamins-in-spirulina/

[1402] Huang, W., Zhang, H., Liu, W., & Li, C. (2012). Survey of antioxidant capacity and phenolic composition of blueberry, blackberry, and strawberry in Nanjing. *Journal of Zhejiang University SCIENCE B, 13*(2), 94-102. doi:10.1631/jzus.b1100137

[1403] Benzie, I. F., & Wachtel-Galor, S. (2011). *Herbal medicine biomolecular and clinical aspects*. Boca Raton: CRC Press.

[1404] Ibid

[1405] Cervo, M. M., Llido, L. O., Barrios, E. B., & Panlasigui, L. N. (2014). Effects of Canned Pineapple Consumption on Nutritional Status, Immunomodulation, and Physical Health of Selected School Children. *Journal of Nutrition and Metabolism, 2014*, 1-9. doi:10.1155/2014/861659

[1406] Hunter, III, J. P. (2014). *Health Benefits: From Foods and Spices*. Washington , DC: Copyrights: Library of Congress.

[1407] Janick, J., & Paull, R. E. (2008). *The encyclopedia of fruit & nuts*. Wallingford, UK: CABI North American Office.

[1408] Guyton, A. C., & Hall, J. E. (2000). *Textbook of medical physiology*. Philadelphia: Saunders.

[1409] Pray, L. A. (2015). *Relationships among the brain, the digestive system, and eating behavior: workshop summary*. Washington, D.C.: The National Academies Press.

[1410] Fulkerson, L. (Director). (2011). *Forks over knives* [Documentary]. Doug Lisle, Ph.D. United States: Monica Beach Media.

[1411] Wilde, P. J., Ph.D. (2009). Eating for Life: Designing Foods for Appetite Control. *Journal of Diabetes Science and Technology, 3*(2), 366-370. doi:10.1177/193229680900300219

[1412] Institute of Medicine. (2015). Relationships Among the Brain, the Digestive System, and Eating Behavior. *Food Forum; Food and Nutrition Board; Institute of Medicine. Washington (DC): National Academies Press (US); 2015 Feb 27*. doi:10.17226/21654

[1413] Ibid

[1414] Fulkerson, L. (Director). (2011). *Forks over knives* [Documentary]. Doug Lisle, Ph.D. United States: Monica Beach Media.

[1415] Ibid

[1416] Schuna, C. (2014, January 8). Is Eating Fruit After a Meal Bad for You?. *LIVESTRONG.COM*. Retrieved November 30, 2015 from http://www.livestrong.com/article/457270-is-eating-fruit-after-a-meal-bad-for-you/

[1417] Theophilus, P. A., Victoria, M. J., Socarras, K. M., Filush, K. R., Gupta, K., Luecke, D. F., & Sapi, E. (2015). Effectiveness of Stevia rebaudiana whole leaf extract against the various morphological forms of Borrelia burgdorferi in vitro. *European Journal of Microbiology and Immunology, 5*(4), 268-280. doi:10.1556/1886.2015.00031

[1418] WebMD. (2014, October 13). STEVIA: Uses, Side Effects, Interactions and Warnings. *WebMD*. Retrieved November 30, 2015, from http://www.webmd.com/Vitamins-supplements/ingredientmono-682-STEVIA.aspx?activeIngredientId=682&activeIngredientName=STEVIA

[1419] Odonnell, S., Baudier, K., Fiocca, K., & Marenda, D. R. (2017). Erythritol ingestion impairs adult reproduction and causes larval mortality in Drosophila melanogaster fruit flies (Diptera: Drosophilidae). *Journal of Applied Entomology*. doi:10.1111/jen.12409

[1420] Mäkinen, K. K. (2016). Gastrointestinal Disturbances Associated with the Consumption of Sugar Alcohols with Special Consideration of Xylitol: Scientific Review and Instructions for Dentists and Other Health-Care Professionals. *International Journal of Dentistry, 2016*, 1-16. doi:10.1155/2016/5967907

[1421] Duncan, L., ND, CN. (2011, October 14). Chia: Ancient Super-Seed Secret. *The Dr. Oz Show*. Retrieved November 30, 2015, from http://www.doctoroz.com/blog/lindsey-duncan-nd-cn/chia-ancient-super-secret

[1422] Segura-Campos, M. R., Ciau-Solís, N., Rosado-Rubio, G., Chel-Guerrero, L., & Betancur-Ancona, D. (2014). Chemical and Functional Properties of Chia Seed (Salvia hispanicaL.) Gum. *International Journal of Food Science, 2014*, 1-5. doi:10.1155/2014/241053

[1423] Ibid

[1424] Jampolis, M. (2009, August 28). Can eating too much fruit keep me from losing weight?. *CNN*. Retrieved November 30, 2015, from http://www.cnn.com/2009/HEALTH/expert.q.a/08/28/fruit.weightloss.jampolis/

[1425] Ibid

[1426] Ibid

[1427] Grioni, S., Agnoli, C., Sieri, S., Pala, V., Ricceri, F., Masala, G., . . . Krogh, V. (2015). Espresso Coffee Consumption and Risk of Coronary Heart Disease in a Large Italian Cohort. *Plos One, 10*(5). doi:10.1371/journal.pone.0126550

[1428] Roberts, C. (2016, November 23). Is There More Caffeine in Espresso Than in Coffee?. *Consumer Reports*. Retrieved September 14, 2017, from https://www.consumerreports.org/coffee/is-there-more-caffeine-in-espresso-than-in-coffee/

[1429] Lovallo, W. R., Farag, N. H., Vincent, A. S., Thomas, T. L., & Wilson, M. F. (2006). Cortisol responses to mental stress, exercise, and meals following caffeine intake in men and women. *Pharmacology Biochemistry and Behavior, 83*(3), 441-447. doi:10.1016/j.pbb.2006.03.005

[1430] Randall, M. (2011, February 03). The Physiology of Stress: Cortisol and the Hypothalamic-Pituitary-Adrenal Axis. *Dartmouth Undergraduate Journal of Science*. Retrieved June 26, 2016, from http://dujs.dartmouth.edu/2011/02/the-physiology-of-stress-cortisol-and-the-hypothalamic-pituitary-adrenal-axis/#.V3AVULgrKHs

[1431] Aronson, D., MS, RD. (2009). Cortisol — Its Role in Stress, Inflammation, and Indications for Diet Therapy. *Today's Dietitian - The Magazine for Nutrition Professionals*. Vol. 11 No. 11 P. 38

[1432] Ibid

[1433] Lovallo, W. R., Farag, N. H., Vincent, A. S., Thomas, T. L., & Wilson, M. F. (2006). Cortisol responses to mental stress, exercise, and meals following caffeine intake in men and women. *Pharmacology Biochemistry and Behavior*, 83(3), 441-447. doi:10.1016/j.pbb.2006.03.005

[1434] Petrie H.J., Chown S.E., Belfie L.M., Duncan A.M., McLaren D.H., Conquer J.A., Graham, T.E .(2004, July). Caffeine ingestion increases the insulin response to an oral-glucose-tolerance test in obese men before and after weight loss. *American Journal of Clinical Nutrition*. 80(1):22-8. PMID: 15213023

[1435] Benvenga, S., Bartolone, L., Pappalardo, M. A., Russo, A., Lapa, D., Giorgianni, G., . . . Trimarchi, F. (2008). Altered Intestinal Absorption of L-Thyroxine Caused by Coffee. *Thyroid: Journal of American Thyroid Association*, 18(3), 293-301. doi:10.1089/thy.2007.0222

[1436] Morck T.A., Lynch S.R., Cook J.D. (1983, March). Inhibition of food iron absorption by coffee. *American Journal of Clinical Nutrition*. 37(3):416-20. PMID: 6402915

[1437] Ibid

[1438] Ulvik, A., Vollset, S. E., Hoff, G., & Ueland, P. M. (2008). Coffee Consumption and Circulating B-Vitamins in Healthy Middle-Aged Men and Women. *Clinical Chemistry*, 54(9), 1489-1496. doi:10.1373/clinchem.2008.103465

[1439] Lohsiriwat, S., Hirunsai, M., & Chaiyaprasithi, B. (2011). Effect of caffeine on bladder function in patients with overactive bladder symptoms. *Urology Annals*, 3(1), 14. doi:10.4103/0974-7796.75862

[1440] Massey, L. K., & Sutton, R. A. (2004). Acute Caffeine Effects On Urine Composition And Calcium Kidney Stone Risk In Calcium Stone Formers. *The Journal of Urology*, 172(2), 555-558. doi:10.1097/01.ju.0000129413.87024.5c

[1441] Seal, A. D., Bardis, C. N., Gavrieli, A., Grigorakis, P., Adams, J. D., Arnaoutis, G., . . . Kavouras, S. A. (2017). Coffee with High but Not Low Caffeine Content Augments Fluid and Electrolyte Excretion at Rest. *Frontiers in Nutrition*, 4. doi:10.3389/fnut.2017.00040

[1442] Boekema, P. J., Samsom, M., Van Be, G. P. (1999). Coffee and Gastrointestinal Function: Facts and Fiction: A Review. *Scandinavian Journal of Gastroenterology*, 34(230), 35-39. doi:10.1080/003655299750025525

[1443] Wendl, B., Pfeiffer, A., Pehl, C., Schmidt, T., & Kaess, H. (2007). Effect of decaffeination of coffee or tea on gastro-oesophageal reflux. *Alimentary Pharmacology & Therapeutics*, 8(3), 283-287. doi:10.1111/j.1365-2036.1994.tb00289.x

[1444] Meredith, S. E., Juliano, L. M., Hughes, J. R., & Griffiths, R. R. (2013). Caffeine Use Disorder: A Comprehensive Review and Research Agenda. *Journal of Caffeine Research*, 3(3), 114-130. doi:10.1089/jcr.2013.0016

[1445] Juliano, L. M., & Griffiths, R. R. (2004). A critical review of caffeine withdrawal: empirical validation of symptoms and signs, incidence, severity, and associated features. *Psychopharmacology*, 176(1), 1-29. doi:10.1007/s00213-004-2000-x

[1446] Ibid

[1447] Addicott, M. A., Ph.D. (2014). Caffeine Use Disorder: A Review of the Evidence and Future Implications. *Current Addiction Reports*, 1(3), 186–192. doi: 10.1007/s40429-014-0024-9. PMCID: PMC4115451

[1448] Juliano, L. M., & Griffiths, R. R. (2004). A critical review of caffeine withdrawal: empirical validation of symptoms and signs, incidence, severity, and associated features. *Psychopharmacology*, 176(1), 1-29. doi:10.1007/s00213-004-2000-x

[1449] Ibid

[1450] Greger, M., MD. (2012, November 8). Does "organic" chicken contain less arsenic?. *NutritionFacts.org*. Retrieved from http://nutritionfacts.org/questions/does-organic-chicken-contain-less-arsenic/

[1451] Kennedy, D. (2016). B Vitamins and the Brain: Mechanisms, Dose and Efficacy—A Review. *Nutrients*,8(2), 68. doi:10.3390/nu8020068

[1452] NIH. (2017, April 17). B Vitamins. *MedlinePlus U.S. Department of Health and Human Services National Library of Medicine*. Retrieved May 26, 2017, from https://medlineplus.gov/bVitamins.html

[1453] Joshi, G., Rawat, M., Bisht, V., Negi, J., & Singh, P. (2010). Chemical constituents of Asparagus. *Pharmacognosy Reviews*, 4(8), 215. doi:10.4103/0973-7847.70921

[1454] Dreher, M. L., & Davenport, A. J. (2013). Hass Avocado Composition and Potential Health Effects. *Critical Reviews in Food Science and Nutrition*, 53(7), 738-750. doi:10.1080/10408398.2011.556759

[1455] Clifford, T., Howatson, G., West, D., & Stevenson, E. (2015). The Potential Benefits of Red Beetroot Supplementation in Health and Disease. *Nutrients*,7(4), 2801-2822. doi:10.3390/nu7042801

[1456] University of Wisconsin. (1997, November 12). Scientists Get the Facts on Folic Acid in Red Beets. *University of Wisconsin News*. Retrieved May 25, 2017, from http://news.wisc.edu/scientists-get-the-facts-on-folic-acid-in-red-beets/

[1457] Vasanthi, H., Mukherjee, S., & Das, D. (2009). Potential Health Benefits of Broccoli- A Chemico-Biological Overview. *Mini-Reviews in Medicinal Chemistry*, 9(6), 749-759. doi:10.2174/138955709788452685

[1458] George Mateljan Foundation (2013, June 9). WHFoods Site Search. *The George Mateljan Foundation for The World's Healthiest Foods*. Retrieved November 30, 2015, from http://www.whfoods.com/sitesearch.php

[1459] Sharma, K. D., Karki, S., Thakur, N. S., & Attri, S. (2011). Chemical composition, functional properties and processing of carrot—a review. *Journal of Food Science and Technology*, 49(1), 22-32. doi:10.1007/s13197-011-0310-7

[1460] Ahmed, F. A., & Ali, R. F. (2013). Bioactive Compounds and Antioxidant Activity of Fresh and Processed White Cauliflower. *BioMed Research International*, 2013, 1-9. doi:10.1155/2013/367819

[1461] USDA. (2016, May). Basic Report:11297, Parsley, fresh. *Agricultural Research Service National Nutrient Database*. Retrieved May 26, 2017, from https://ndb.nal.usda.gov/ndb/foods/show/3045?manu=&fgcd=&ds=Standard%20Reference

[1462] USDA. (2016, May). Basic Report | Nutrient values and weights for edible portion. *United States Department of Agriculture, Agricultural Research Service, National Nutrient Database for Standard Reference*. Retrieved May 26, 2017, from https://ndb.nal.usda.gov/ndb/search/list

[1463] George Mateljan Foundation (2013, June 9). Cucumbers. *The George Mateljan Foundation for The World's Healthiest Foods*. Retrieved November 30, 2015, from http://www.whfoods.com/genpage.php?tname=foodspice&dbid=42

[1464] Nachman, K. E., Baron, P. A., Raber, G., Francesconi, K. A., Navas-Acien, A., & Love, D. C. (2013). Roxarsone, Inorganic Arsenic, and Other Arsenic Species in Chicken: A U.S.-Based Market Basket Sample. *Environmental Health Perspectives, 121*(7), 818-824. doi:10.1289/ehp.1206245

[1465] Greger, M., MD. (2012, November 8). Does "organic" chicken contain less arsenic? . *NutritionFacts.org*. Retrieved November 30, 2015, from http://nutritionfacts.org/questions/does-organic-chicken-contain-less-arsenic/

[1466] Ibid

[1467] USDA. (2001, February 1). Meat and Poultry Labeling Terms. *USDA Food Safety Information*. Retrieved November 30, 2015, from http://www.fsis.usda.gov/wps/wcm/connect/e2853601-3edb-45d3-90dc-1bef17b7f277/Meat_and_Poultry_Labeling_Terms.pdf?MOD=AJPERES

[1468] USDA. (2004, June 24). Organic Certification - How does USDA define the term organic?. *U.S. Department of Agriculture - USDA*. Retrieved November 30, 2015, from http://usda.gov/wps/portal/usda/usdahome?parentnav=FAQS_BYTOPIC&FAQ_NAVIGATION_ID=ORGANIC_FQ&FAQ_NAVIGATION_TYPE=FAQS_BYTOPIC&contentid=faqdetail-3.xml&edeployment_action=retrievecontent

[1469] MayoClinic. (2002, November 3). Hypoglycemia: Causes. *Mayo Clinic*. Retrieved October 16, 2015, from http://www.mayoclinic.org/diseases-conditions/hypoglycemia/basics/causes/con-20021103

[1470] MedlinePlus. (2013, February 18). Vitamins: MedlinePlus Medical Encyclopedia. *U.S National Library of Medicine | National Institutes of Health*. Retrieved November 30, 2015, from http://www.nlm.nih.gov/medlineplus/ency/article/002399.htm

[1471] FDA. (varies by document). ACE inhibitors by name. *U.S. Food and Drug Administration*. Retrieved November 10, 2016, from
http://www.accessdata.fda.gov/drugsatfda_docs/label/2014/019888s056lbl.pdf
http://www.accessdata.fda.gov/drugsatfda_docs/label/2013/019901s060lbl.pdf
http://www.accessdata.fda.gov/drugsatfda_docs/label/2014/019221s044lbl.pdf
http://www.accessdata.fda.gov/drugsatfda_docs/label/2015/020364s061lbl.pdf
http://www.accessdata.fda.gov/drugsatfda_docs/label/2012/018343s084lbl.pdf
http://www.accessdata.fda.gov/drugsatfda_docs/label/2016/020528s024lbl.pdf
http://www.accessdata.fda.gov/drugsatfda_docs/label/2010/020729s021lbl.pdf
http://www.accessdata.fda.gov/drugsatfda_docs/label/2013/020125s015lbl.pdf
http://www.accessdata.fda.gov/drugsatfda_docs/label/2014/019221s044lbl.pdf
http://www.accessdata.fda.gov/drugsatfda_docs/label/2003/19915se5-037_monopril_lbl.pdf
http://www.accessdata.fda.gov/drugsatfda_docs/label/2005/020184s011lbl.pdf

[1472] FDA. (varies by document). Beta blockers by name. *U.S. Food and Drug Administration*. Retrieved November 10, 2016, from
http://www.accessdata.fda.gov/drugsatfda_docs/label/2011/018760s028lbl.pdf
http://www.accessdata.fda.gov/drugsatfda_docs/label/2008/017963s062,018704s021lbl.pdf
http://www.accessdata.fda.gov/drugsatfda_docs/label/2010/018031s036lbl.pdf
http://www.accessdata.fda.gov/drugsatfda_docs/label/2011/018063s062lbl.pdf
http://www.accessdata.fda.gov/drugsatfda_docs/label/2007/019386s039lbl.pdf
http://www.accessdata.fda.gov/drugsatfda_docs/label/2014/075541Orig1s010lbl.pdf
http://www.accessdata.fda.gov/drugsatfda_docs/label/2006/020297s018lbl.pdf
http://www.accessdata.fda.gov/drugsatfda_docs/label/2011/021742s013lbl.pdf
http://www.accessdata.fda.gov/drugsatfda_docs/label/2011/018976s012lbl.pdf
http://www.accessdata.fda.gov/drugsatfda_docs/label/2011/021151s010lbl.pdf
http://www.accessdata.fda.gov/drugsatfda_docs/label/2011/018917s025lbl.pdf
http://www.accessdata.fda.gov/drugsatfda_docs/label/2014/075541Orig1s010lbl.pdf
http://www.accessdata.fda.gov/drugsatfda_docs/label/2007/020186s023lbl.pdf

[1473] FDA. (2014, March 1). CFR - Code of Federal Regulations Sec. 101.22 Foods; labeling of spices, flavorings, colorings and chemical preservatives. *U.S. Food and Drug Administration*. Retrieved November 30, 2015, from http://www.accessdata.fda.gov/scripts/cdrh/cfdocs/cfcfr/cfrsearch.cfm?fr=101.22

[1474] FDA. (2013, April 1). CFR - Code of Federal Regulations Title 21 | 21CFR172.510 . *U.S. Food and Drug Administration*. Retrieved November 30, 2015, from http://www.accessdata.fda.gov/scripts/cdrh/cfdocs/cfcfr/CFRSearch.cfm?fr=172.510

[1475] FDA. (2013, April 1). CFR - Code of Federal Regulations Title 21 | 21CFR182.10. *U.S. Food and Drug Administration*. Retrieved November 30, 2015, from http://www.accessdata.fda.gov/scripts/cdrh/cfdocs/cfcfr/CFRSearch.cfm?fr=182.10

[1476] FDA. (2013, April 1). CFR - Code of Federal Regulations Title 21 | 21CFR182.20. *U.S. Food and Drug Adminstration*. Retrieved November 30, 2015, from http://www.accessdata.fda.gov/scripts/cdrh/cfdocs/cfcfr/CFRSearch.cfm?fr=182.20

[1477] FDA. (2013, April 1). CFR - Code of Federal Regulations Title 21 | 21CFR182.40. *U.S. Food and Drug Administration*. Retrieved November 30, 2015, from http://www.accessdata.fda.gov/scripts/cdrh/cfdocs/cfcfr/CFRSearch.cfm?fr=182.40

[1478] FDA. (2013, April 1). CFR - Code of Federal Regulations Title 21 | 21CFR182.50. *U.S. Food and Drug Administration*. Retrieved November 30, 2015, from http://www.accessdata.fda.gov/scripts/cdrh/cfdocs/cfcfr/CFRSearch.cfm?fr=182.50

[1479] FDA. (2013, June 1). CFR - Code of Federal Regulations Title 21 | PART 184 DIRECT FOOD SUBSTANCES AFFIRMED AS GENERALLY RECOGNIZED AS SAFE. *U.S. Food and Drug Administration*. Retrieved November 30, 2015, from http://www.accessdata.fda.gov/scripts/cdrh/cfdocs/cfcfr/CFRSearch.cfm?CFRPart=184

Made in the USA
Middletown, DE
04 April 2018